Issues in Correctional Health

Issues in Correctional Health

edited by

Rick Ruddell
Eastern Kentucky University

Mark Tomita
California State University, Chico

Newgate Press
Richmond, Kentucky

Issues in Correctional Health
edited by Rick Ruddell and Mark Tomita

Published by Newgate Press
Richmond, Kentucky
http:www.newgatepress.com

Newgate Press publishes works in criminology and criminal justice, with an emphasis on corrections, including correctional policy, reference works, and historical studies of jails and prisons.

ISBN 978-0-9796455-0-1

LLCN: 2007903663

Printed in the United States of America on acid-free paper.

Contents

FOREWORD

Personal Observations from an Ex-Con Academician

Having spent in excess of five years confined in the Federal Bureau of Prisons (FBOP)—and a majority of that time in Federal Medical Centers—I am especially well suited to comment on the state of health care in American prisons. Post-incarceration I earned a Master of Arts and Ph.D. degrees in Sociology and am presently an Assistant Professor of Criminal Justice at Appalachian State University. I have published extensively on the topics of medical health care in prison, and the psychological impact of imprisonment upon ex-prisoners.

The present book, edited by Drs. Rick Ruddell and Mark Tomita, addresses issues heretofore under-studied within the field of corrections: *Issues in Correctional Health*. Ruddell provides an insightful overview of health care issues in his chapter addressing "Correctional Health." Parker and Fearn discuss the challenges faced by "Mothers Behind Bars." Women are the fastest growing sector of the prison population, and a key issue is that many are pregnant or parents, and this fact has forced correctional administrators to develop health care responses that accommodate those conditions, and best prepare these women to assume their role as parents. Thomas gives insight into the medical and psychological problems of incarcerated adolescents in his discussion of "Juvenile Correctional Health." Franklin, Fearn and Franklin describe one of the largest challenges facing correctional health in their analysis of "Communicable Diseases in Corrections."

One issue that has seldom been addressed in the corrections literature is the issue of dental health—a significant problem considering the effects of methamphetamine on long-term users who develop a disfiguring condition that some dentists have labeled "meth mouth." Dias and Vaughn shed light on the legal remedies available to prisoners denied health care in their discussion of "Section 1983 Civil Liability." Of all the factors that have driven changes in correctional health care, the most significant has been prisoner litigation.

It is not the intent of the sentencing judge to impose a death penalty and this issue is discussed by Franklin and Franklin in their chapter on "Violence Reduction" in corrections. One of the challenges confronting many prisoners who survive incarceration is that the effects of their victimization in prison follow them into the streets after they are released. While issues of psychological health are not always at the forefront of our attention, the mental health status of prisoners poses a significant challenge. Many prisoners bring with them drug addiction problems as outlined by Dirks-Linhorst, and she describes the challenges of providing effective programs for this group. Additionally, many prisoners enter jail or prison suffering mental illness as outlined by Dirks-Linhorst in her chapter on "Correctional Mental Health." Moreover, Tartaro and Lester address the issue of "Saving Lives Through Suicide Prevention."

Given the extreme lengths of sentences currently imposed on some offenders, elderly prisoners pose a challenge the corrections system must address as described by Kuhlmann. The fact that states are building living units specifically for prisoners with dementia, and hiring prison gerontologists speaks volumes about the state of American corrections. Linder, by contrast, examines how some correctional and jail systems are developing palliative care and hospice to help prisoners die with dignity. This is a significant problem as some 3,000 inmates die in state prisons each year, and the total is much higher when one adds local jails and the FBOP.

Yet, the reality is that prisoners are not the only persons confined. Humphrey discusses a much neglected area in the prison literature in her chapter "Doing Time Together: Correctional Officer Health" and she outlines that when officers are mentally and physically healthier, they are apt to treat prisoners in a more humanitarian manner. Ruddell and Tomita conclude the volume with a discussion of "Opportunities for Change," an area I shall expand upon.

Prison health care has been described as the nation's largest health maintenance organization (HMO). Funding for prison health care is budgeted by the Federal Congress and State legislatures. Funding is determined upon projected need and is allocated on an annual basis. In light of the prison population explosion (and the more serious cases confronting correctional health care providers today), funding consistently fails to keep pace. In essence, as the correctional population grows, the amount of health care available for any inmate decreases.

The 1976 U.S. Supreme Court case, *Estelle v. Gamble,* and cases that followed, decreed that deliberate indifference to a prisoner's serious medical needs was prohibited. In a civilized society it is realized that if health care is not provided, prisoners would die from neglect. This stated, and governed by law, corrections faces the reality of not being able to fiscally maintain the standards delineated by the Supreme Court.

To address the crisis in correctional health care, the courts, Congress, state legislatures and local officials are seeking alternatives to alleviate the burgeoning problem posed by health care expenditures. In November 2006 I testified in Federal Court as to the inadequacies of health care provided in the FBOP. I testified on behalf of a first-time non-violent offender who suffers Chrohn's Disease, which I suffer also. I explained to the sentencing judge the "reality" of health care which is symbolically "provided" behind the razor wire of prison. Testifying on behalf of the FBOP was the Regional Director of Health Care Services. In describing the challenges the prison system faces in efforts to provide health care, it became clear to the judge that the prison system was unable to provide appropriate health care. As a result, the judge ruled that sentencing the defendant to the FBOP would be tantamount to a death sentence. As an alternative to prison, the judge imposed home confinement and in this instance the defendant was in a position to provide for his own heath care.

Attorney Margaret Colgate Love, representing the American Bar Association, testified before the United States Sentencing Commission in Washington, D.C. on March 15, 2006 (Proposed Guidelines Amendment on Reduction of Term of Imprisonment Based on Bureau of Prisons Motion under 18 U.S.C. Section 3582§(1)(A)(i)). Her comments spoke to subsection (i) which outline the possibility of sentence reduction for "extraordinary and compelling reasons." Her testimony was in response to recommendations of the American Bar Association's Justice Kennedy Commission which urged jurisdictions to establish standards for sentence reduction based upon "medical and non-medical circumstances." Of importance to the present work is the fact that "extraordinary and compelling reasons" is written to *include poor health.*

Prior to this new interpretation of medical circumstances, compassionate release was based upon two doctors stating the prisoner had six or less months to live. The expansion of sentencing guidelines to include "poor health" underscores the magnitude of the challenge(s) faced by corrections in providing health care. This clearly illuminates the scope of the problem as understood by the Courts, Congress, and State Legislatures as relates to providing health care for those confined. Please allow me to be clear: this is not a "get out of prison pass." To the contrary, this is a rational realization that the health care crisis in prison is beyond the ability of correctional facilities to provide adequate health care.

This stated, should those who break the law have a loophole based upon their physical condition? The answer to this is clearly NO. However, a balance need be made between societal safety, the medical needs of those confined, and the mandates of a civilized society. The contributors to this book have outlined a number of deficiencies in the medical and psychological care of inmates and providing a safe environment for them. I hope that future scholars, students, correctional practitioners and advocates use this insight to understand and study the problem of correctional health care more thoroughly, urge politicians to support the expansion of evidence-based practices that reduce suffering, and correctional practitioners to provide safer and more humane conditions of confinement.

Daniel S. Murphy
Assistant Professor of Criminal Justice
Appalachian State University

Introduction

There is increased interest in correctional health care, in part because of the 2.3 million Americans who are living in jails or prisons, but also in recognition of the relationships between correctional and community health. Prisoners and jail inmates have high rates of communicable diseases, injuries (both unintentional and due to violence), chronic health problems, and poor histories of community health care. This population is also likely to be involved in risky behaviors (including crime and substance abuse) and suffer from some type of psychological disorder. Inmates cycle in and out of correctional facilities: there are some 14 million arrests annually and most of these persons will spend some time in a juvenile detention center or county jail. Moreover, 650,000 Americans are released from prison each year, and most will return within a year or two. This constantly changing population suggests that if left untreated, the health problems of jail or prison inmates will quickly find their way back to the community. Many practitioners, scholars, and policy analysts believe that medical, public health, and health promotion interventions in juvenile halls, jails, or prisons will have a long-term positive impact upon community health.

To respond to this interest in correctional health, a number of scholarly journals and professional publications have emerged in the past few years, including *CorrectCare*, the *Infectious Diseases in Corrections Report*, the *International Journal of Prison Health*, and the *Journal of Correctional Health Care*. In addition, other journals have published themed issues that have addressed correctional health, including the *Prison Journal* (March, 2002), the *Californian Journal of Health Promotion* (June, 2005), and the *American Journal of Public Health* (October, 2005).

Despite the growing number of scholarly publications, one gap in the correctional health literature was the lack of a comprehensive work that could introduce readers to the main challenges or issues in the field. We thought that the time was right to gather a number of experts in community and correctional health and put their work together in a single book that would serve as a reference for students, scholars, and policy analysts. The contributors to this book address issues in correctional health from inmate nurseries to hospice care. The authors come from a wide variety of backgrounds—practitioners, health promotion specialists, as well as academics and public policy analysts—and they have highlighted specific problems, described some promising interventions, and mapped out a research agenda for future scholars.

Our contributors explain the difficulties that medical and health care providers, correctional administrators, and policy makers face in delivering care to incarcerated juveniles and adults. Some times the demands on these practitioners can be overwhelming: each year in the United States thousands of infants are born behind bars, and at least 3,000 inmates die, with approximately 90 percent from natural causes. Practitioners also confront an array of serious health care problems, from providing emergency care, preventing the spread of communicable diseases, managing chronic illnesses, and preparing for pandemics. Correctional institutions were seldom designed to deliver these types of services, and many under-funded and overcrowded facilities do not have the medical or health care staff to provide appropriate care.

The correctional health practitioner is further burdened by the fact that inmate populations have higher levels of psychological and medical problems than their community counterparts. Subsequently, they are likely to be difficult-to-manage, prone to malingering, and noncompliant with treatment. Moreover, medical staff members employed within correctional facilities are working with antiquated equipment, in professional isolation, and receive uncompetitive salaries. Sometimes their best efforts are undermined by the correctional officers. Last, despite the fact that they can be implemented and delivered with little cost there is little public or political support for health promotion and prevention programs. Altogether the challenges are daunting, but investments in correctional health payoff in the long-term with healthier communities, something even the most "tough on crime" politicians can support.

Acknowledgments

Preparing any book involves a cast of dozens, yet only the editor's names appear on the cover. In this case, we first have to acknowledge its thirteen contributors. We thank you for your insights into correctional health, your patience with the lengthy peer review and publication process, and your tolerance when we edited the products of your hard work. It is our hope that our colleagues will continue to research and publish about issues in correctional health care, as these studies will inform the policy debate, especially in terms of evidence-based practice and health promotion, issues that many of our contributors discuss.

We would also like to extend our appreciation to the reviewers, including Marilyn McShane (University of Houston—Downtown) who critiqued an early version of this work, our reviewers from the Federal Bureau of Prisons, and the health care providers who critiqued the first versions of the manuscript. All combined, their excellent suggestions greatly aided our efforts to bring the chapters together and address issues that we had overlooked. Reviewing is sometimes a thankless task, and we do appreciate all of the comments that we received. We are also very grateful for the hard work and insight of Jeff Hopkins who provided valuable editorial comments. We would like to credit Bob Morris for the cover photograph of the elderly inmates (taken at Bostick State Prison, GA., in 2000).

Rick Ruddell would like to thank his colleagues for their encouragement and support while editing this manuscript. The College of Behavioral and Social Sciences at the California State University, Chico also provided course release time that enabled him to work on this book, and he is thankful for that support. Rick is also blessed with unwavering support and frequent care packages from Renu James (his favorite Canadian!), Alister and Lucie Sutherland, and Eric Owen. Writing is often a solitary task, and knowing that one has friends and family in his corner is a constant source of inspiration. Last, Rick would like to thank Mark Tomita for the opportunity to work together on this project—and for the great job on the cover artwork!

Mark Tomita would like to thank Rick Ruddell and all of the authors for the countless number of hours spent working on this book. This book will be an excellent resource to correctional health professionals, academics, and students.

Contact Information

We encourage readers to provide feedback about this book on correctional health care, and we can be reached at:

rick.ruddell@eku.edu
Department of Correctional and Juvenile Justice Studies
Eastern Kentucky University

mtomita@csuchico.edu
Health and Community Services Department
California State University, Chico

Contributors

Clarissa F. Dias is a Doctoral Student in the Department of Political Science at Georgia State University. Clarissa Dias current research interest is gender and politics, particularly feminist political theories and policy implications.

P. Ann Dirks-Linhorst is an Assistant Professor at Southern Illinois University Edwardsville. She received her Ph.D. in Criminology from the University of Missouri St. Louis in 2003, and her Juris Doctorate from the University of Missouri Kansas City in 1984. She spent five years as an Assistant Attorney General for Missouri representing the Department of Mental Health, and then joined that Department in a variety of roles (Forensic Director, Policy Deputy, Assistant General Counsel, and HIPAA Privacy Officer) for fourteen years. Her research interests include the intersection of the criminal justice and mental health systems, and has been published in *Law and Human Behavior, Social Service Review, International Journal of Forenisc Mental Health,* and the *Journal of Criminal Justice Education.*

Noelle E. Fearn received her Ph.D. in Criminology and Criminal Justice from the University of Missouri, St. Louis in 2003 and is an Assistant Professor in the Department of Sociology and Criminal Justice at Saint Louis University. Her work has appeared in *Justice Quarterly, Criminal Justice Studies: A Critical Journal of Crime, Law, and Society,* the *International Journal of Comparative Criminology,* the *International Journal of Offender Therapy and Comparative Criminology,* and the *Californian Journal of Health Promotion.* Her current research focuses on multilevel influences on criminal justice decision making and evaluations of community and custodial programming for female offenders.

Cortney A. Franklin, M.A. is a Doctoral Candidate in the Criminal Justice Program at Washington State University. Her recent work has appeared in *Women and Criminal Justice*, *Journal of Criminal Justice*, *Journal of Offender Rehabilitation*, and the *Californian Journal of Health Promotion*. Her current research focuses on violence against women and gender and justice issues—more specifically on the role of gendered peer groups in influencing behavioral outcomes. She also conducts research on institutional and community corrections, custodial health care and communicable diseases, and female inmate and offender populations.

Travis W. Franklin received his M.A. from Washington State University where he is currently finishing his Ph.D. in Criminal Justice. His research focuses on correctional policy and practices, criminal sentencing and theories of judicial decision making, structural theories of prosecutorial decision making, and fear of crime. His recent work has appeared in the *Californian Journal of Health Promotion* and the *Journal of Criminal Justice*.

Amanda Mathias Humphrey is an Assistant Professor in the Criminal Justice Department at Mount Mercy College in Cedar Rapids, Iowa. Amanda obtained her Bachelor and Master of Criminal Justice degrees from New Mexico State University. Dr. Mathias Humphrey obtained her Doctor of Philosophy degree with a major in criminal justice from the University of Nebraska-Omaha in 2004. Amanda's primary areas of research and teaching interest are corrections, women and crime, victims of crime, and drug use.

Robynn Kuhlmann received her Bachelor's degree from the University of San Francisco in 2000. She has also served in Burkina Faso, West Africa as a Peace Corps volunteer. She recently received her Master's degree in Political Science at the California State University, Chico and is currently a Ph.D. student and Crescent City Doctoral Scholarship recipient in Political Science at the University of New Orleans. Her research areas of interest include political participation, democratic theory, social capital, and minority politics.

David Lester has Ph.D. degrees in Psychology (Brandeis University, USA) and in Social and Political Science (Cambridge University, UK). He has written extensively on suicide and homicide and other aspects of death and dying. He has served as President of the International Association for the Prevention of Suicide and is presently Professor of

Psychology at the Richard Stockton College of New Jersey.

John F. Linder is a Licensed Clinical Social Worker and principal therapist at the Cancer Counseling and Support Clinic at the U.C. Davis Cancer Center. John has worked in medical social work for 17 years. In addition to clinical work, John teaches and participates in ongoing research in psycho-oncology and palliative care. John was awarded a Project on Death in America Social Work Leadership Development award in 2000. John is currently a Doctoral Fellow at the Smith College School for Social Work, Northampton, MA. and recipient of a doctoral training grant in oncology social work from the American Cancer Society.

Kelly Parker received her J.D. from the University of Idaho in 2005. She served as a law clerk in the Fourth Judicial District of Idaho in 2005–2006. Her work has appeared in the *Idaho Law Review, Journal of Law and Health,* and the *Californian Journal of Health Promotion*. She was also a participant in the 2005 University of Idaho International Law Symposium.

Rick Ruddell is the Graduate Program Director in the Department of Correctional and Juvenile Justice Studies at Eastern Kentucky University. Dr. Ruddell was a supervisor and manager within the Department of Corrections and Public Safety in Saskatchewan, Canada, and served as Associate Professor of Political Science at the California State University, Chico. His research has been published in 35 scholarly articles, and focuses upon corrections and criminal justice policy. Rick Ruddell is the co-author of *Making Sense of Criminal Justice* (Oxford University Press), and author of *America Behind Bars: Trends in Imprisonment, 1950 to 2000* (LFB Scholarly Press).

Christine Tartaro is an Associate Professor of Criminal Justice at the Richard Stockton College of New Jersey. She received her Masters' and Ph.D. in Criminal Justice from Rutgers University. Prior to entering the teaching field, she worked as a researcher for the New Jersey Department of Corrections and Police Foundation and as a research consultant with the New Jersey Juvenile Justice Commission. Her research interests include prison and jail violence, suicide, sentencing, the history of punishment, and crime prevention.

Matthew O. Thomas is an Associate Professor at California State University, Chico. His research interests include police administration, community policing, juvenile justice, and urban politics and policy.

He previously served as a research consultant for the Urban Institute, where he participated in an analysis of reform and reorganization in the Metropolitan Police Department, Washington, D.C. He authored several reports for the National Institute of Justice and has published work in criminal justice and political science journals.

Mark Tomita, Ph.D., R.N., C.H.E.S, is an Associate Professor in the Department of Health and Community Services, California State University, Chico. He is also the Editor of the *Californian Journal of Health Promotion,* a peer-reviewed, scholarly journal that is fully electronic, and publishes on the web and on CD-ROM. Dr. Tomita specializes in the integration of technology in public health and public health professional development.

Michael S. Vaughn is a Professor in the College of Criminal Justice at Sam Houston State University. He is the Co-Director for the Institute of Legal Studies in Criminal Justice at Sam Houston. Professor Vaughn's research interests are primarily related to legal issues, specializing in the area of legal liabilities of criminal justice personnel.

CHAPTER ONE

Correctional Health

Rick Ruddell

Since the 1970s the jail and prison population within the United States has grown fivefold. As a result, America now has higher rates of incarceration than any other nation (Walmsley 2007). On any given day, some 2.3 million Americans are incarcerated in juvenile detention facilities, adult jails, or prisons operated by state or federal governments (Harrison and Beck 2006). Another 4.9 million offenders are supervised in the community by probation or parole officers (Glaze and Bonczar 2006). Imprisonment cost U.S. taxpayers approximately $60.8 billion in 2003 (Hughes 2006), but the indirect costs of incarceration may even be higher if one considers the impact of imprisonment on individuals, families, and communities. Two of the issues that are seldom considered in the public debates over the use of incarceration is the delivery of correctional health care, and the relationships between correctional and community health. This chapter provides a brief orientation to correctional health care, the types of facilities that hold inmates, and the characteristics of inmate populations.

While correctional populations expanded, providing appropriate health care for the persons that we incarcerate has became a significant challenge for many local jails, juvenile facilities, and state or federal prison systems. Among these challenges, rates of illness in correctional facilities are much greater than in the community population and many of the inmates of juvenile or adult correctional facilities have serious health problems, including communicable diseases such as HIV/AIDS, tuberculosis, sexually transmitted infections, methicillin-resistant staphylococcus aureus (MRSA), and hepatitis. Other inmates suffer from the long-term effects of living on the street, addictions, risky lifestyles, poor community health-care, homelessness, poverty, and undiagnosed or untreated chronic diseases.

Incarcerated populations with untreated health problems pose a significant challenge to community health. Over 14 million arrestees cycle through juvenile facilities or county jails (Federal Bureau of Investigation 2006), and some 650,000 persons are released from prison each year (Office of Justice Programs 2007). As a result, there has been increased attention to the connections between correctional and community health (Potter and Krane-Rapposelli 2002). The Centers for Disease Control and Prevention observes that:

> Many ties connect the community with prisons and jails. For one, inmates are constantly moving back and forth between corrections and the community. Problems or risky behaviors begun in prison or jail return with inmates to the community after release (2001:2).

It is important to understand that modest investments in medical services, health education, health promotion, or public health interventions in correctional settings may have a significant effect on long-term community health. There are, however, a number of economic and political barriers to implementing these programs.

Attitudes Towards Correctional Health Care

One of the obstacles to delivering appropriate levels of correctional health care is the expense. For instance, a survey undertaken by the American Correctional Association (2004) found that up to one-quarter of all expenditures in one state prison system was used for health care, and the health care budget in large prison systems can exceed a billion dollars a year. A number of critics, however, have argued that the growth in the use of imprisonment has resulted in rationed health care spending, where the funds used to care for inmates remained constant as correctional populations rose (see Murphy 2005). Persuading the administrators of jails, juvenile correctional facilities, or prisons to increase spending on health care to levels consistent with community care is a challenge for prisoners, advocates for prisoner's rights, academics, and community advocates. An admission to a correctional facility shouldn't end in death, but cases of poor medical care or deliberate indifference may result in more inmate deaths than prison violence and capital punishment combined.

While jail or prison inmates are not populations that draw much public sympathy, it is important to understand that after the government incarcerates someone they also assume responsibility for that person's care, including treatment of his or her physical or psychological problems. Historically, jails and prisons provided poor health care to prisoners. In response, reformers such as Benjamin Rush and Elizabeth Fry advocated for better inmate care 200 years ago. Two centuries later, many of the same problems still exist: a lack of funding for correctional health care, jail and prison overcrowding, high percentages of persons with mental illness in jails or prison, and a lack of dedicated health care professionals who want to work in these settings.

The type of correctional system that a nation develops is often a function of that country's history and perceptions about justice. Cullen and Gendreau (2000) found that respondents to national polls in the United States generally supported rehabilitation for prison inmates. Yet, not everybody believes that offenders deserve assistance or support, and many citizens are downright hostile to the plight of jail or prison inmates. In other nations, by contrast, prisoners are seen as citizens who have made mistakes and are in need of encouragement and rehabilitation, and part of that support is providing high levels of correctional health care. When ex-prisoners re-enter society with a greater set of skills and fewer health problems, it has been speculated that they will commit fewer crimes, and less likely to be returned to prison (see MacDonald 2005).

Prisoner Litigation and Correctional Health Care

A number of problems emerge when we attempt to save money by reducing access to correctional health care. When medical services are rationed, or inmates don't have access to appropriate care, prisoners may be able to sue for damages, or more frequently, lawyers will sue on their behalf to improve the conditions of confinement for all inmates. In many of these cases, a judge will attempt to get the parties to enter into a consent decree, where the lawsuit is dropped in favor of a court-supervised agreement between the parties to remedy the situation. In the 1980s and 1990s, many jails or state correctional systems entered into these agreements to provide better conditions for inmates, including the delivery of more comprehensive health care.

While litigation is not a health promotion strategy *per se,* lawsuits have had a profound influence on the types of correctional health services provided to inmates. A recent study of litigation within jails and prisons revealed that inmate health care was the foremost cause of lawsuits (Schlanger 2003). The impact of this litigation, however, was generally perceived to be positive amongst the jail and prison administrators who responded to Schlanger's survey. There is an intuitive appeal to this finding: when conditions of confinement improve (including health care), inmate morale and institutional behavior are apt to be more positive. Accordingly, this creates better working conditions for the correctional officers who supervise these prisoners.

Correctional systems are required to abide by the Americans with Disabilities Act (ADA). Inmates have initiated lawsuits after state correctional officials and local jail administrators failed to provide reasonable accommodations for inmates with disabilities. Many jails and prisons were not designed for prisoners with physical disabilities, and correctional administrators were ordered to build ramps for wheelchairs, and provide railings or handholds in showers for elderly inmates. But the problem of accommodating inmates with special needs extends beyond the modification of the physical structure of a jail or prison. Inmates who are hard of hearing, for instance, occasionally require translators with sign language skills, as well as telecommunication devices for the deaf (TDD phones) that communicate using text. Despite these requirements, deaf inmates have attended administrative, disciplinary or parole eligibility hearings without the aide of an interpreter, placing them at considerable disadvantage.

One significant change to accommodate inmates with disabilities is the acknowledgement that many prisoners have some type of learning or cognitive disability (e.g., problems with the psychological processing of information), and others suffer from organic brain damage (James and Glaze 2006). Today, correctional officers have to understand and be sensitive to these special needs in order to provide effective supervision. Juvenile inmates with cognitive disabilities also require some accommodation for education or vocational training to comply with the Individuals with Disabilities Education Improvement Act (IDEIA) of 2004.

In response to inmate litigation, federal requirements such as the ADA, and state-level standards in a number of jurisdictions, some facilities also comply with standards of health care established by four national organizations, and the American Correctional Association (ACA) and the National Commission on Correctional Health Care (NCCHC) are the leading bodies. Of these organizations, the NCCHC was first to establish voluntary standards for correctional health care. Delivering an accredited correctional health care program increases staff awareness about the delivery of health care and the ultimate goal of these standards is to increase the quality of care.[1]

Although federal and state standards exist, along with the constant threat of prisoner litigation, it is important to acknowledge the dire consequences for some inmates whose health care needs were ignored, rationed, or denied. For example, in September 2004, a 27 year-old first-time offender in Washington DC who was also a quadriplegic sentenced to ten days incarceration for marijuana possession, died after being refused access to his ventilator (Cauvin 2004). The following year an Arizona jail inmate awaiting a court date died after being denied access to her insulin for two days by jail deputies, despite the fact that it was a prescribed medication (Whiting 2005). These are not isolated cases, and inmates die every year because their health care needs are ignored. As a result, a short period of jail incarceration for non-violent offenders can become a death sentence. Mumola (2007) reports that of the 3,138 inmates who died in state prisons in 2004, over 90 percent were of natural causes; although we do not know if any of these prisoners would have lived longer if they had been receiving care in the community.

Balancing Medical Care and Correctional Security

There is a delicate balance between ensuring the safety of a correctional facility and meeting the health care needs of the inmates. Some inmates with disabilities, for instance, require assistive devices such as prosthetic limbs, crutches, or wheelchairs. Others may require unrestricted possession of inhalers or testing and monitoring equipment (e.g., for diabetes or high blood pressure). Some of these devices, medications, or instruments are seen as threatening to the safety of the staff and other inmates. Correctional officers may be very reluctant to allow inmates to possess these items, even if they are considered necessary by the medical staff. Such issues create tension between the medical and security staff, and this sometimes results in the security staff undermining an inmate's treatment plan. The following paragraphs outline some of the security-related issues that may conflict with the ability of health care staff to deliver treatment to inmates.

One safety-related concern in corrections is the distribution of prescription medications. Most inmates are monitored when taking their medications, as some will either exchange their drugs with other prisoners, or hoard their tablets and then take them all at once in order to "get high" or to end their lives. Stanley (2006) outlines how inmates sometimes experience delays in getting their medications, and that inmates don't always receive the type of medication that they require. These factors can increase inmate stress, which in turn, compromises security. Furthermore, correctional officers are reluctant to dispense medications and nurses are often responsible for this task in correctional facilities. Unfortunately, health care professionals aren't always available when an inmate requires such care, especially in smaller facilities, and on occasion, this has resulted in tragedies.

Rates of communicable diseases in corrections are high (Maruschak 2006, 2006b). A few ways to reduce their transmission are by distributing condoms, exchanging dirty needles for clean syringes, and making bleach for cleaning needles available to prisoners. The rationale for offering these options is that preventing even one case of HIV/AIDS saves taxpayers $13,900 to $36,500 for HIV/AIDS medication per year (Infectious Diseases in Corrections Report 2006). In support of this, research from other nations suggests that these programs reduce the transmission of communicable diseases (MacDonald 2005). On the other hand, corrections officers have a legitimate fear that needles or bleach can be used as weapons and condoms can be used to hide contraband. Such issues raise an important question: Do we introduce these programs in order to reduce disease at the cost of alienating the security personnel?

In many small juvenile halls or jails inmates are transported to hospitals, health care facilities, or specialists for medical assessment and/or treatment. These transports create challenges for correctional officers, as most inmates require some type of mechanical restraints (such as handcuffs or leg irons) when leaving a facility. Additionally, when a physician is examining the inmate, these restraints are sometimes removed, increasing the hazards if the inmate is planning an escape, and placing both the physician and correctional officer at some risk. As a result, correctional officers often need to be skeptical when an inmate is requesting emergency health care during times when medical care staff members are not available.

Another issue that is seldom mentioned in the correctional literature is the problem of malingering. Malingering occurs when a prisoner feigns psychological or physical distress in order to receive some type of secondary gain. Some inmates may pretend to be ill to avoid an unpleasant work assignment, obtain psychotropic (mood altering) medications, avoid a potentially dangerous or unpleasant situation, or to receive some attention or sympathy from the medical staff. A more serious problem occurs when inmates either act as if they are hurt or deliberately injure themselves in order to participate in misconduct or facilitate an escape. Since correctional officers need to be mindful of these ploys, they sometimes ignore legitimate pleas for health care assistance, and this negligence has resulted in unnecessary suffering and fatalities.

Providing a safe and secure environment is a primary goal of the uniformed staff in a jail or prison. While the correctional officer's preoccupation with security is seen as counterproductive by some, it is one reason why the prison homicide rate dropped 93 percent in the past two decades (Mumola 2005). The provision of a safe environment has two important outcomes. First, it reduces tensions between inmates and second it lessens stress levels for correctional officers. Increasing safety and reducing chaos is also important for rehabilitation because it is difficult for a prisoner to focus on developing their vocational skills or work on their G.E.D. when they are fearful of being assaulted. Although there are a number of reasons for decreased violence, correctional experts attribute such changes to improvements in correctional leadership (Useem and Piehl 2006).

Correctional Health Care

Prisons with thousands of beds are much like self-contained cities. Unfortunately, correctional facilities often have trouble recruiting medical professionals since many would rather work in less depressing or stressful settings, with more sympathetic patients. Further, as a point of interest, Bick observed that medical staff spend much of their time on administrative duties such as approving amenities for inmates (e.g., extra blankets or special diets), rather than providing medical care, and "endure professional isolation while struggling in "clinics" that lack sinks, exam tables, common implements for examinations, computers, internet access, PDAs, electronic medical records, medical education, and timely access to diagnostic studies and specialists" (2006:3).

It has been suggested that prison medical care attracts some professionals who would otherwise have difficulty finding work due to prior incidents of malpractice or other legal troubles (Vaughn and Collins 2004). The austere environment of the prison, a lack of modern amenities, and unsympathetic clients make it difficult to recruit qualified health care specialists in competitive job markets. In addition, many prisons are located in rural areas where professionals are hesitant to reside. Further, few correctional facilities can compete with the higher wages offered by hospitals or other health care settings. Last, working in a correctional facility has little professional allure.

Physicians and other medical staff who are committed and hardworking are also discouraged by the bureaucracy of correctional system, and the high rates of inmate litigation. Before 1996, inmates could file an almost unlimited number of lawsuits without filing fees, and a large percentage of these lawsuits were frivolous. The enactment of the Prison Litigation Reform Act (PLRA) greatly reduced the amount of prisoner litigation. While correctional litigation has helped inmates improve the quality of life behind bars (including better access to correctional health care) it has also driven some dedicated practitioners to community careers.

A Short Orientation to Locked Institutions

There is an incredible diversity of services provided by facilities that hold inmates. The types of health care services that they deliver are shaped by the political, economic, historical, and cultural nature of these institutions, and the communities or states where they are located. Size matters: the care that an inmate might expect at a rural jail of less than ten beds may be significantly different than one who is admitted to a state prison system that delivers health care according to the NCCHC standards. The following pages outline some of the characteristics of juvenile facilities, as well as adult jails and prisons.

Juvenile Correctional Facilities

The upper age of juvenile court jurisdiction differs throughout the nation. In most states, juveniles become adults at either 17 or 18 years of age (although they can sometimes be held within juvenile correctional facilities until their 21st or 25th birthday in some states). Youths who are arrested are usually taken to detention facilities, which are often known as juvenile halls. In the majority of cases, juveniles are held for a few hours, until either their parents or a legal guardian takes responsibility for them. Youths who have committed more serious offenses or repeat offenders will be confined longer. Even though the average stay in juvenile halls is usually less than two weeks, some youth accused of committing serious offenses may wait months for their court dates.

Once arrested, juveniles are admitted directly from the streets into these detention facilities. Many of them are under the influence of drugs or alcohol. Most require careful assessment and monitoring because they are at some risk of alcohol or drug overdoses, and medical supervision is required. Others either are injured during the commission of their offense (such as involvement in an assault) or are hurt while resisting arrest. In such cases, police officers usually take these youths to an emergency room for initial assessment and treatment. Juvenile hall staff provides the follow-up care.

Many juvenile detention facilities are small. As a result, if a youth requires emergency or advanced care, they are often transported off-site to hospitals or specialists. Alternatively larger facilities often provide nursing care, on-site medical or dental facilities, and in some cases, physicians provide care at the detention facility. In most states, juvenile detention facilities are operated by local or county governments. This also influences the type of health care that inmates receive. Youths sentenced to a term of incarceration are generally placed in state juvenile correctional facilities (these are sometimes called training schools). In 2003, there were almost 100,000 youths held in these institutions (Harrison and Beck 2006). These state-operated facilities often provide better medical care than their local counterparts. This pattern is similar for adult facilities as well: state-operated agencies typically have larger budgets for health care as they can draw from a larger tax base.

A very small number of juveniles are held in adult jails or prisons. Some rural jurisdictions don't have detention facilities—so they are temporarily held in the jail. Other juveniles have been charged with a serious offense, and their cases are frequently transferred to adult courts. In some states, these adolescents are held with adults, and if convicted of serious crimes such as homicide, they may spend the rest of their life in an adult prison. In any case, placing juveniles in adult facilities puts them at a greater risk of suicide and victimization from the adult inmates (Elrod and Brooks 2003).

Jails and Detention Facilities

Jails were originally intended to be short-term facilities either to detain persons accused of crimes until their court dates, or to house defendants convicted of offenses until their sentencing. In fact, in most local jails today, over half the inmate population is awaiting their court dates. About one-third of jail inmates are actually serving sentences of incarceration of less than one year, while the remainder is awaiting transfer to prison. In some Southern states, however, inmates may serve their entire prison sentence in a county jail. Almost one half of Louisiana's prisoners, for example, reside in a parish jail (Harrison and Beck 2006).

Unlike prisons, most jails hold both males and females, and the typical stay is measured in days rather than years. In addition, the rich and famous and the poor and homeless are also admitted to jails, as well as people from every nationality, religion, and social or ethnic group. Jails also hold a diverse range of special needs inmates, including persons with mental illnesses, pregnant or nursing women, elderly inmates, and some detain juveniles. Jails are often described as the entry point to corrections, and every person serving a prison sentence or sitting on death row first spent time in a local jail. Yet, the person accused of being drunk in public or other minor offenses is also held in the same jail.

Almost every county in America has a jail, and some are very small. Ruddell and Mays (2007) reported that there were some 1,775 jails of less than 100 beds, and the types of health care that are delivered in small facilities tends to be much different than in larger institutions that may have special psychiatric, hospital, hospice units, and medical doctors on staff. The Los Angeles County jail, for example, holds some 3,500 persons with severe mental illness on any given day, and this facility has been described as the world's largest psychiatric hospital (Quanbeck,

Frye and Altshuler 2003). Jail populations are transient: the average stay in a California jail, for instance, is approximately 20 days (Corrections Standards Authority 2007), while the average term served in prison is 24.1 months (California Department of Corrections and Rehabilitation 2007). Thus, the health problems that develop (or go untreated) in a jail are likely to be transmitted to the community (Centers for Disease Control and Prevention 2001).

Prisons

Prisons differ from jails because they hold offenders who have either been convicted or have plead guilty to a felony. Thus, most are serving a period of incarceration in excess of one year. While the majority of jails are managed by local municipalities or counties, prisons are operated by state or federal governments. For instance, each state has a prison system to hold long-term offenders. The size of these state prison systems varies greatly and Harrison and Beck (2006) reported that while North Dakota imprisoned 1,385 inmates, other larger states, such as Texas, held approximately 170,000 inmates at year-end 2005. In addition, the federal government incarcerated about 196,000 prisoners at the end of March, 2007 (Federal Bureau of Prisons 2007).

At year-end 2005 over 100,000 persons were incarcerated in facilities operated by corporations (Harrison and Beck 2006). Some corporations confine low-security immigration detainees for the federal government, while other firms imprison inmates sentenced to terms of life imprisonment. There is an increasing presence of corporations in the delivery of correctional services: from food services to health care. Some scholars have questioned whether punishment should be delivered by corporations whose primary motivation is making a profit, and some companies have been accused of providing less than adequate correctional care to bolster profits (see Christie 2000).

Today prisons are also holding offenders for longer sentences. Accordingly, tens of thousands are now serving decades-long sentences due to tougher sentencing schemes that include "three-strikes," truth-in sentencing (which requires that the prisoner serves 85 percent of their sentence before being eligible for parole) and mandatory-minimum sentencing guidelines (where a judge imposes a minimum sentence regardless of mitigating factors). These practices have increased the numbers of aging prisoners, and the health care costs to hold these elderly inmates are contributing to an economic crisis in some states.

Prisoners sentenced to death are also held in prisons until their sentence is carried out. There are almost 3,300 death row prisoners, and approximately 60 are executed each year (Snell 2006). In most jurisdictions, inmates will remain on death row for over a decade before the death sentence is actually imposed, and this delay is caused by the lengthy appeals process. Many of these inmates die before their sentence is actually carried out, either by suicide or natural causes (Snell 2006). One ethical question that some prison physicians have had to confront is their role in the execution of the condemned: and the President of the American Association of Anesthesiologists has advised their members to steer clear of these acts (Guidry 2006)

When prison inmates are incarcerated for at least one year, there is an opportunity to undertake interventions that promote healthy lifestyles and improve the individual's health, both within the facility and after the prisoner returns to the community. Interventions that address the inmate's drug and alcohol addictions, for instance, are important as a large percentage of inmates have substance abuse problems. In a national survey conducted by the U.S. Bureau of Justice Statistics, for example, Karburg and James (2005) found that 68 percent of the persons admitted to jail were substance abusers. Despite the fact that alcohol and drug abuse counseling is an identified problem for many offenders, the percentage of persons receiving treatment in prison has actually decreased in recent years (Mumola 1999).

Many prisoners have lead difficult lives in the community. Often a combination of addictions, risky behaviors, and poor lifestyle choices contributes to premature aging, and a greater need for prison health care. In many cases, these prison inmates also have a history of chronic illnesses, and noncompliance with treatment. Sometimes these treatments are both expensive and controversial. Correctional officials in Arizona recently placed an inmate serving a term of life imprisonment on a waiting list for a kidney. The decision was not based on compassion, but economic benefits as the transplant would generate a cost-saving after three years (Arizona Phoenix 2005).

Regardless of the cause of their health problems, prisoners are unable to access community services so the lack of adequate medical care in both state and federal prisons adds to their problems. Murphy (2003, 2005) and Santos (2003) have outlined the limitations of health care within the Federal Bureau of Prisons, and they argue that there is a significant disconnect between the level of health care that is posited to be delivered and that which actually occurs.

Who Goes to Jail or Prison?

In order to understand the health care needs of offender populations, it is important to understand who actually resides in jails or prisons. Forty years ago, prison was reserved for the worst possible offenders. Today, however, a prison sentence is a routine milestone in some neighborhoods. For example, according to the U.S. Bureau of Justice Statistics, there is a 6.6 percent likelihood of going to prison for a child born in 2001 (Bonczar 2003). Racial make-up is another controversial factor in prison populations, and nearly a third of African-American men are expected to go to prison in their lifetime compared to one out of six Latinos, and one out of 17 white males (Bonczar 2003). Also accounting for gender, rates of imprisonment for women are much less than their male counterparts, but the pattern of African-American and Latina women closely follows the males, and white women are less likely to be incarcerated.

A large percentage of American jail or prison inmates have mental health problems (James and Glaze 2006). The challenges of living with mental illness are exacerbated by homelessness, addictions, and in some cases, jail or prison inmates may have all three problems prior to their incarceration (Hartwell 2004). Ruddell (2006) found that inmates with mental health problems were thought to be the most disruptive group in local jails, and they are at higher risk of being victimized both in the community and behind bars. Unfortunately, ignoring the needs of inmates with mental illness can result in significant long-term costs. We know that a large percentage of jail inmates with mental health problems are labeled "frequent fliers" by jail officers because they have been admitted dozens of times, and some have been arrested and admitted to jail over 100 times for being drunk in public, trespassing, and other "quality-of-life" offenses. Gladwell (2006) estimated that a single street person cost the Reno community upwards of a million dollars in health care and law enforcement costs, and this case prompted him to ask whether there is a better approach to working with these people.

Many incarcerated women are parents, some are pregnant, and a significant percentage of these women have given birth within the past year (Fearn and Parker 2004). These mothers face additional stress when their children are either placed in foster care or with relatives. In order to provide a more rehabilitative environment for these parents some jurisdictions are experimenting with prison-based programs that hold both the mother and child together in low-security settings.

Also while women represent approximately ten percent of the entire correctional population, they have a number of special needs that differ from their male counterparts. Correctional health services have been historically delivered on models developed from male correctional populations, who require less comprehensive physical or mental health care. Female inmates require higher levels of medical care for reproductive health, and sometimes these needs are ignored. In March 2004, for example, Kimberly Grey gave birth over a toilet after Tampa jail officers refused to transport her to a hospital (Crawley and Greenwood 2004). This case resulted in the death of Grey's infant, but the incident also underscores the treatment that some incarcerated women receive.

One emerging problem is providing care for the growing number of elderly prisoners. Imposing lengthy prison sentences has contributed to large numbers of inmates growing old behind bars (Aday 2003). In response to their specialized needs, state prisons have established separate units for these seniors. In addition to costing taxpayers three times as much as a younger prisoner, many of these elderly inmates also die in custody. Such cases have policy-makers questioning whether geriatric prisoners pose a risk to public safety, prompting the question of whether we should extend compassionate releases to this group (Legislative Analyst's Office 2003)? Moreover should we release elderly persons who were supposed to serve their entire life behind bars in order to reduce costs? A precedent has already been established for releasing prisoners who have terminal illnesses but who do not pose a risk to public safety. But with regard to elderly prisoners, the public may oppose such transfers, especially since it merely moves the health care costs from the correctional facility to the community.

Conclusions

A number of factors have converged to add to the burden of the delivery of correctional health programs. First, the political nature of punishment has contributed to an atmosphere where being "tough on crime" mandates that politicians are very unlikely to advocate for livable, rehabilitative, or safe jail or prison conditions. Second, the sheer number of Americans behind bars has led to administrators of under-funded facilities attempting to manage the problem as best as possible. Sadly, medical care in some places has not kept up with the increasing number of special needs populations who require a greater degree of medical and psychiatric services.

One goal of this book is to contribute to the debates about correctional health care. A key issue is whether or not to invest in prevention programs in jails or prisons in order to reduce long-term community health care costs. Incarceration represents a distinct opportunity for public health interventions with persons deemed high-risk. Yet, should jails and prisons become places of health interventions or health promotion?

We suggest that legislators and policy-makers become "smart on crime" and acknowledge the permeable relationships between correctional well-being and community health. Each year, some 650,000 inmates are discharged from prisons to our communities (Office of Justice Programs 2007). Providing basic health education, preventative health care and correctional facilities that are violence-free is an important long-term investment in community health. Sometimes the biggest challenges also represent the best opportunities to make a meaningful social change. The contributors to this book examine different dimensions of correctional health care, with the hope of defining the boundaries of this problem, highlighting successful programs, and acknowledging small victories whenever they occur. Community health is slowly shifting from a reactive to proactive orientation and so should correctional health care.

Endnote

1. According to the NCCHC (2006), their accreditation process monitors the following factors; facility governance and administration, maintaining a safe and healthy environment, personnel and training, health care services support, inmate care and treatment, health promotion and disease prevention, special inmate needs and services, health records, and medical-legal issues.

References

Aday, Ronald H. 2003. *Aging Prisoners: Crisis in American Corrections.* Westport, CT: Praeger.

American Correctional Association. 2004. *Inmate Health Care. Corrections Compendium* 29:10-29.

Arizona Republic. 2005. "Growing Old in Prison." Retrieved April 22, 2007 (http://www.azcentral.com/news/)

Bick, Joseph. 2006. "Letter from the Editor." *Infectious Diseases in Corrections Report* 9:3.

Bonczar, Thomas P. 2003. *Prevalence of Imprisonment in the U. S. Population, 1974-2001.* Washington DC: Bureau of Justice Statistics.

California Department of Corrections and Rehabilitation. 2007. *Second Quarter 2006 Facts and Figures.* Retrieved April 12, 2007 (http://www.cdc.state.ca.us/DivisionsBoards/AOAP/FactsFigures.html)

Cauvin, Henri E. 2004. D. C. Jail Stay ends in Death for Quadriplegic MD. Man. Washington Post, October 1, B01.

Centers for Disease Control and Prevention. 2001. *Drug Use, HIV, and the Criminal Justice System.* Atlanta, GA: Centers for Disease Control and Prevention.

Christie, Nils. 2000. *Crime Control as Industry: Towards Gulags Western Style.* London: Routledge.

Corrections Standards Authority. 2007. *Jail Profile Survey, 4th Quarter* 2006. Sacramento, CA: Corrections Standards Authority.

Crawley, Marcia and Jill King-Greenwood. 2004. "Mother Asks Why After Her Baby, Born in Jail, Dies." *Tampa Tribune.* Retrieved April 12, 2005 (http://www.tampatrib.com)

Cullen, Francis T. and Paul Gendreau. 2000. "Assessing Correctional Rehabilitation: Policy Practice, and Prospects." Pp. 109-176 in *Criminal Justice 2000: Policies, Process, and Decisions of the Criminal Justice System*, vol. 3. Washington, DC: U. S. Department of Justice.

Elrod, Preston and Michael T. Brooks. 2002. "Kids in Jail: I Mean You Ain't Really Learning Nothing [productive]." Pp. 325-346. in *Convict Criminology*, edited by J.I. Ross and S.C. Richards. Belmont, CA: Thompson/Wadsworth.

Federal Bureau of Investigation. 2006. *Crime in the United States.* Washington, DC: Author.

Federal Bureau of Prisons. 2007. *Quick Facts About the Bureau of Prisons.* Retrieved April 12, 2007 (http://www.bop.gov/about/facts.jsp#4)

Fearn, Noelle E. and Kelly Parker. 2004. "Washington State's Residential Parenting Program: An Integrated Public Health, Education, and Social Service Resource for Pregnant Inmates and Prison Mothers." *Californian Journal of Health Promotion* 2(4):34–48.

Gladwell, Malcolm. 2006. *Million-dollar Murray.* Retrieved April 21, 2007 (http://www.newyorker.com/fact/content/articles/060213fa_fact).

Glaze, Lauren and Thomas P. Bonczar. 2006. *Probation and Parole in the United States, 2005.* Washington, DC: Bureau of Justice Statistics.

Guidry, Orin F. 2006. Observations Regarding Lethal Injection. Retrieved April 12, 2007 (http://www.asahq.org/news/asanews063006.htm)

Harrison, Paige M. and Allen J. Beck. 2006. *Prisoners in 2005.* Washington, DC: Bureau of Justice Statistics.

Hartwell, Stephanie W. 2004. "Triple Stigma: Persons with Mental Illness and Substance Abuse Problems in the Criminal Justice System." *Criminal Justice Policy Review* 15:84-99.

Hughes, Kristen A. 2006. *Justice Expenditure and Employment in the United States,* 2003. Washington, DC: Bureau of Justice Statistics.

Infectious Diseases in Corrections Report. 2006. "News and Literature Reviews: HIV Costs Have Decreased." *Infectious Diseases in Corrections Report* 9:8.

James, Doris J. and Lauren E. Glaze. 2006. *Mental Health Problems of Prison and Jail Inmates.* Washington, DC: Bureau of Justice Statistics.

Karberg, Jennifer C. and Doris J. James. 2005. *Substance Dependence, Abuse, and Treatment of Jail Inmates, 2002.* Washington, DC: Bureau of Justice Statistics.

Legislative Analyst's Office. 2003. *Analysis of the 2003-04 Budget: Judiciary and Criminal Justice.* Sacramento, CA: Legislative Analyst's Office.

MacDonald, Morag. 2005. *A Study of the Health Care Provision, Existing Drug Services and Strategies Operating in Prisons in Ten Countries from Central and Eastern Europe.* Helsinki, Finland: European Institute for Crime Prevention and Control.

Maruschak, Laura M. 2006. *HIV in Prisons, 2004.* Washington, DC: Bureau of Justice Statistics.

Maruschak, Laura M. 2006b. *Medical Problems of Jail Inmates.* Washington, DC: Bureau of Justice Statistics.

Maruschak, Laura M. and Allen J. Beck. 2001. *Medical Problems of Inmates, 1997.* Washington, DC: Bureau of Justice Statistics.

Mumola, Christopher J. 1999. *Substance Abuse and Treatment – State and Federal Prisoners, 1997.* Washington, DC: Bureau of Justice Statistics.
------. 2005. *Suicide and Homicide in State Prisons and Local Jails.* Washington, DC: Bureau of Justice Statistics.
------. 2007. *Medical Causes of Death in State Prisons, 2001-2003.* Washington, DC: Bureau of Justice Statistics.
Murphy, Daniel S. 2003. "Aspirin Ain't Gonna Help the Kind of Pain I'm in." Pp. 247-266 in *Convict Criminology,* edited by J. I. Ross and S. C. Richards. Belmont, CA: Wadsworth.
------. 2005. "Health Care in the Federal Bureau of Prisons: Fact or Fiction." *Californian Journal of Health Promotion* 3(2):23-37.
National Commission on Correctional Health Care. 2006. Accreditation. Retrieved April 22, 2006 (http://www.ncchc.org/accred/index.html).
Office of Justice Programs. (2007). *Reentry.* Retrieved April 12, 2007 (http://www.ojp.usdoj.gov/reentry/learn.html).
Potter, Roberto H. and Karina Krane Rapposelli. 2002. "Why Public Health Must go to Jail." *Large Jail Network Exchange Annual Issue* 25-28.
Quanbeck, Cameron, Mark Frye, and Lori Altshuler. 2003. "Mania and the Law in California: Understanding the Criminalization of the Mentally Ill." *American Journal of Psychiatry* 160:1245-1250.
Ruddell, Rick. 2006. "Jail Interventions for Inmates with Mental Illnesses." *Journal of Correctional Health Care* 12: 118-131.
Ruddell, Rick and G. Larry Mays. 2007. "Rural Jails: Problematic Inmates, Overcrowded Cells, and Cash-Strapped Counties." *Journal of Criminal Justice*
Schlanger, Margo. 2003. "Inmate Litigation." *Harvard Law Review* 116:1555-1701.
Snell, Tracy L. 2006. *Capital Punishment, 2005.* Washington, DC: Bureau of Justice Statistics.
Stanley, Judith A. 2006. "Problematic Medication Practices: The Top 10." *CorrectCare* 20 (4): 19-20.
Useem, Burt and Anne M. Piehl. 2006. "Prison Buildup and Disorder." *Punishment & Society* 8:87-115.
Vaughn, Michael S. and Sue Carter Collins. 2004. "Medical Malpractice in Correctional Facilities: State Tort Remedies for Inappropriate and Inadequate Health Care Administered to Prisoners." *The Prison Journal* 84:505-534.
Walmsley, Roy. 2007. *World Prison Population List.* Retrieved April 12, 2007 (http://www.prisonstudies.org/).
Whiting, Brent. 2005. "20 Million Sought in Death of Diabetic Jail Inmate." *The Arizona Republic,* July 7, 2005.

CHAPTER TWO

Mothers Behind Bars: Challenges and Opportunities

Kelly Parker and Noelle E. Fearn

Most women in U.S. prisons are either mothers or mothers-to-be. Many of these women were the primary caretakers for their children at the time of their incarceration, hoping to resume that role upon release. However, incarceration can drastically disrupt the relationship between a woman and her infant/child. The consequences for both parties can be devastating. This chapter evaluates the circumstances of women behind bars, their infants, and young children, and highlights a range of correctional responses intended to help these women rebuild their families both during and after imprisonment (Morash, Bynum, and Koons 1998). The programs discussed throughout this chapter demonstrate a number of best practices for corrections and health officials seeking to develop strategies that may interrupt the cycle of intergenerational crime.

Women Inmates

As a result of anti-drug legislation and similar "get-tough" on crime policies, the number of women incarcerated has increased dramatically in recent years (Acoca and Raeder 1999; Belknap 2001; Richie 2000). Each year between 1995 and 2005, the annual increase in the number of women incarcerated grew at an average rate of 4.6 percent, outpacing the rate of men going to prison during the same period (Harrison and Beck 2006). Interestingly, women's patterns of criminal behavior are different than those of men (Chesney-Lind and Pasko 2004). Mumola (2000) found that the majority of incarcerated women's crimes were nonviolent property offenses (28 percent), drug offenses (35 percent), and public-order offenses (10 percent). By contrast, 45 percent of state prison inmate fathers are incarcerated for violent offenses (Mumola 2000). Drug use is often central to women's criminal activity. For example, one-third of the inmate mothers in state prisons, evaluated by Mumola (2000), had committed their crimes either to obtain drugs or to get money to buy drugs. Moreover, nearly three-quarters of the women in federal prisons had been convicted of drug-related offenses.

Despite steady increases in their rate of incarceration, women make up only a small fraction of the total number of people incarcerated in both state and federal prisons. At year-end 2005, women comprised seven percent of the nearly 1.4 million individuals incarcerated (Harrison and Beck 2006). The fact that women make up such a small proportion of prisoners has been used to justify "institutionalized sexism." This includes providing them with fewer treatment or programming opportunities, as well as incarceration in prisons located far from friends and loved ones (Belknap 2001:163). Often the programs and treatment these women receive was originally designed for male prisoners and labeled as "gender neutral." Treatment program offerings have historically been based on outdated stereotypes of women's capabilities (see Belknap 2001; Morash et al. 1998; Shearer 2003). These shortcomings are particularly glaring in the areas of health care (Belknap 1997; Ross and Lawrence 1998) and programming that is responsive to women's roles as mothers.

Women in prison and inmate mothers are likely to have been impoverished before their incarceration. Many either had no health insurance or lived in "medically underserved" locations (Marquart et al. 1996). Mothers in state prisons are also twice as likely as their male counterparts to have been homeless the year prior to their incarceration (Mumola 2000). In addition, these women are often further disadvantaged by prior drug use, mental illness, and histories of physical or sexual abuse (Fearn and Parker 2005) as well as sexually risky behaviors, particularly among drug users (Shearer 2003). Thus, women entering prison often lack many of the basic elements critical to functioning successfully in society, particularly as mothers. Knight and Plugge (2005:111) found that incarcerated women who were pregnant are "likely to smoke, drink alcohol to excess and take illegal drugs" and that "imprisoned women are clearly a high risk obstetric group."

It is estimated that American prisons hold 721,500 parents of minor children, and some 58 percent of these youngsters are less than ten years of age (Mumola 2000). Mumola (2000) found that female prisoners cannot easily be separated from their roles as mothers, as almost 60 percent of these women lived with their children prior to arrest, with approximately 31 percent of those heading single-parent households (comprised solely of the mother, now incarcerated, and her children). During the 1990s, the number of children with a mother in prison nearly doubled as the number of women inmates rose by 106 percent. The number of children with a father in prison, by contrast, rose only 58 percent during the same time (Mumola 2000). Estimates of the number of pregnant women entering prison range from five percent (Greenfeld and Snell 1999) to ten percent (Maeve 1999). Generally, it is posited that within the last year about 25 percent of women in correctional facilities either have been or still are pregnant (Barry, Ginchild and Lee 1995). Sadly, many of these pregnancies are deemed high risk since the mothers-to-be have histories of substance abuse or sexually transmitted diseases (Hufft, Fawkes and Lawson 1993).

While nearly 90 percent of inmate fathers sentenced to state prisons were able to entrust the care of a child to its mother, only 28 percent of inmate mothers were able to place at least one child in the care of the father (Mumola 2000). When looking to find a caregiver for their children, most inmate mothers must rely on either a grandparent (53 percent) or other relatives (26 percent) to provide care in their absence (Mumola 2000). Krisberg and Temin (2001) observed that women often place their children in the care of family members to reduce the likelihood they will lose them altogether (i.e., to the care of the state). However, in some cases, placing children with relatives may put them at risk of victimization. For example, Sharp (2005) found that some inmate mothers had reported knowingly placing their children with their own parents, persons who had sexually abused the inmate herself. Another potentially problematic issue surrounding familial placements is the financial burden it places on the "substitute" caregivers (Parke and Clarke-Stewart 2002). Children of inmate mothers, compared to those of inmate fathers, are five times more likely to be placed in foster care (Krisberg and Temin 2001). For many inmate mothers, foster care represents a "huge failure," (Kampfner 1995:91) since these placements pose difficulties for women who seek to maintain a bond with their children. For the children involved, it may result in confusion and less than optimal living conditions as well.

Separation from children for inmate mothers is often the most difficult consequence of incarceration (Hairston 2002). Although many inmate mothers in state prisons are able to maintain some sort of relationship with their children—by telephone, postal, or personal contact—this is often very stressful (Mumola 2000). Additionally, visiting mothers in prison may itself be a traumatic experience for the children, given the austere and frightening environment of these facilities (Krisberg and Temin

2001; Parke and Clarke-Stewart 2002). Phone calls and travel may also be an expense some families cannot bear (Hairston 2002). Christian (2005) found that travel to prison visits actually drew money away from already impoverished families and neighborhoods. A federal study found that 54 percent of inmate mothers had no personal contact with their children, 33 percent never spoke with their children on the telephone, and 12 percent had no contact with their children (Mumola 2000).

As corrections and health care officials became more aware of the harms that separation – due to incarceration – inflicts on the relationship between a mother and her child(ren), more humane methods have been developed to address this kind of familial disruption. These programs include community-based alternatives to incarceration (Morash et al. 1998), more flexible (and humane) visitation policies (Parke and Clarke-Stewart 2002), and correctional programs offering a broad range of services intended to address the multifaceted challenges of this population (Conly 1998).

In contrast to probation, which enables women to remain in the community under supervision, but receiving few rehabilitative opportunities, other alternatives to incarceration provide the sort of support that probation often lacks (Kubiak et al. 2004). Many of these programs recognize the importance of maintaining parent-child bonds in addition to providing inmates with the skills necessary to be successful parents and community members upon their release. Such programs include parenting classes, as well as vocational, educational, physical, psychological, and health-related services to facilitate successful re-entry to their communities and assist these women in establishing their independence (Morash et al. 1998). Additionally, as these parents near their release dates, it is important to provide them with bridges to outside agencies that can provide essential services to ensure their successful transitions back to society (Parke and Clarke-Stewart 2002).

Programs for Pregnant Inmates and Their Infants

Although the grim and sometimes primitive conditions women faced in prisons began to improve in the 1970s, a 1993 survey of state prisons found that medical care for pregnant inmates was not consistently delivered. For example, 48 percent of facilities provided prenatal care but appropriate diets were available only in 15 percent of state institutions (Wooldredge and Masters 1993). Some state correctional systems may adhere to accreditation standards established by the National Commission on Correctional Health Care (NCCHC) and the American Correctional Association (ACA). In some states, compliance with professional accreditation standards is mandatory. For example, women's prisons in Alabama were ordered to abide by guidelines established by the American College of Obstetricians and Gynecologists (*Laube v. Campbell* 2004). Other state prison systems have voluntarily taken steps to improve conditions for pregnant inmates, including designing programs that meet the health care needs of this special needs population.

Evaluations of the effects of incarceration on pregnancy outcomes are mixed. Some scholars and practitioners argue that the stresses of living in prison, which includes isolation from family and confusion over placement of infants following birth, are very harmful to women (Martin et al. 1997). Appropriate provision of care to pregnant women who are addicted to drugs is often lacking (Barry et al. 1995). Barry and colleagues (1995:163) contend that being incarcerated does not ensure pregnant women will remain either drug or alcohol free, because these substances are available in prisons and jails (either through distilling alcohol or contraband that is smuggled inside the prison by visitors or facility staff). Moreover, in the facilities that have tried to improve conditions for pregnant inmates, overcrowding—a persistent problem in many jails and prison systems — might dull the positive impact of these efforts. Rafter (1990:189) writing of prison improvements stated that "[t]he gains of today can be eradicated by overcrowding tomorrow."

Other scholars, however, have found that incarceration can benefit these pregnant women, insofar as it provides access to services not otherwise available to them. These typically include such amenities as shelter, meals (Martin et al. 1997), and health care (Marquart et al. 1996), especially for homeless and/or drug-addicted women who may lack these essentials "on the outside." Prison may also provide respite from physical and sexual abuse (Martin et al. 1997). Last, admission to a correctional facility might also reduce risky behaviors such as alcohol or drug use, smoking, or engaging in unprotected sex.

Once an inmate delivers her infant, the complications resulting from incarceration grow, especially after the woman has decided not to put her child(ren) up for adoption. According to the American Medical Association (AMA 1997), the first year of life is critical to a child's intellectual, emotional, and social development. During this time, an infant develops an attachment to its primary caregiver. Any disruption of this process can have negative effects on the child's development, including psychopathology or difficulty with intimacy resulting from the "'disorganized' attachment pattern" (AMA 1997). Separating children younger than two years of age, who have developed a sense of attachment to their parent(s) has been found to impair overall parent-child bonding as well (Johnston 1995).

One solution for addressing the possible ill-effects of separating women inmates from their infants is through nursery programs. This practice dates back to the nineteenth century. For instance, New York state correctional facilities have long been at the forefront of providing these kinds of services to pregnant inmates. According to Rafter (1990), the Mount Pleasant Reformatory in New York is suggested to have been the first state institution to open a nursery. Setting this precedent, it was not uncommon for women to keep their infants with them during their incarceration, although this was not the case in most American correctional facilities. The Bedford Hills prison, also in the New York corrections system, established a nursery in 1901 and such programs were common throughout the 1920s and 1930s, although they generally fell out of favor by the 1970s (Morton and Williams 1998).

Today, prison nurseries are still an alternative to the separation of the mother and her infant. Some nursery programs permit infants to stay with their mothers for a period of 12 to 18 months, while others permit babies to stay with their mothers for much shorter periods, ranging from two days to six weeks (Gabel and Girard 1995). Ironically, while they have many benefits, nursery programs are also controversial (Belknap 2001). Separating infants from their mothers may be traumatic, but some speculate that allowing infants to live in prisons may cause other problems. Catan (1992) found that, while overall development of nursery babies was not negatively affected (as compared to a control group), over time the nursery infants declined in their development of locomotor and cognitive skills. Catan (1992) attributed this decline to the deprivations of a prison environment. The AMA's evaluation (1997) speculated that infants in these kinds of institutional nurseries might develop behavioral problems as a result of the social and psychological challenges faced by their mothers. Others suggest that the placement of infants and young children in prisons with their mothers results in what may be perceived as an unfair punishment for the child(ren) (Parke and Clarke-Stewart 2002).

Practitioners and scholars, by contrast, have articulated the advantages in permitting these infants to remain with their mothers. Few empirical studies have evaluated the long-term impact of such nursery programs. However, preliminary results from an ongoing study of maternal and infant outcomes at Bedford Hills indicate that these infants achieved the proper developmental milestones during their first year (Byrne 2004; n.d.). At the same time, Byrne (2004) found that these women were able to identify themselves in parental roles and develop their parenting skills. Other anecdotal evidence suggests that prison nurseries are successful in providing these women with opportunities for stability and pre- and post-natal health care (AMA 1997). Nursery programs also enable mother and child to strengthen their attachment, which in turn may facilitate the underlying goals of such programs: to encourage family connections and develop stronger relationships with family members during incarceration that encourage rehabilitation and prevent recidivism (AMA 1997). While building their families, inmate mothers are provided with educational and vocational programming essential to their success after release (Parke and Clarke-Stewart 2002). The AMA (1997) cautions, however, that separation of an infant from its primary caregiver should be avoided after six months of age, a matter that has implications for women serving longer prison terms. The state of Washington has carefully weighed the potential harms associated with separating mothers from their infants and has implemented a comprehensive program that addresses the needs of pregnant (and parenting) inmates.

Washington State's Residential Parenting Program

The Residential Parenting Program (RPP) was started in 1999 at the Washington Corrections Center for Women (WCCW). Having housed approximately 100 inmates in the first five years of operation, this correctional program currently provides pregnant inmates with appropriate prenatal care as well as offering the mother and infant a long-term opportunity to bond (Fearn and Parker 2004). Today, the primary focus of the program is to provide inmates and their infants access to an enriched environment suitable for skill building and education. The RPP is a collaborative interagency initiative that partners with a number of local and state agencies, including the Puget Sound Educational Service District, the Woman, Infant, and Children (WIC) program, Tacoma Community College, the Department of Social and Health Services, and Child Protective Services.

The RPP enables pregnant, minimum-security inmates with relatively short sentences the opportunity to raise their infants in a correctional setting that has a residential appearance. The overall goals are to maximize the healthy growth and development of these babies, provide inmate mothers and their children with access to the Early Head Start (EHS) program, and, upon the inmate's release, assist these mothers and children to reintegrate successfully into their families and communities. RPP is a comprehensive program that uses its partnerships to respond to the broad range of health, educational, parenting, and life-skills challenges that many inmate mothers face.

Consistent with other prison nursery programs, there are strict eligibility criteria as well as application, screening, and operations processes. For instance, potential participants must have a minimum-security designation. They must expect to give birth during their term of incarceration; and they must possess the physical and mental capacities to care for their children. These women must also meet the EHS eligibility requirements. Subsequently, pregnant inmates admitted to the program are provided access to a variety of health-, education-, and parenting-related programs provided by RPP partners. These inmates also receive health services up to the time of birth and pediatric health care is provided to the infant afterwards. RPP participants (both mother and child) also receive special diets and nutritional counseling.

RPP participants work closely with community partners to develop and implement plans for community re-entry. EHS provides training and support in the areas of child development, parent training, community resources, childbirth, health and nutrition, and other needs specifically identified in the case plans that inmates develop in conjunction with correctional staff and community partners. Once ready to re-enter the community, EHS provides support to these families during their transition to parole.

Although the success of RPP has not been formally evaluated, it represents an innovative and promising strategy aimed at alleviating many of the potentially negative effects of family disruption when a mother (or mother-to-be) is incarcerated. The following section presents a general overview of the unique challenges and issues that inmate mothers and their young children face. Additionally, promising strategies and best practices programs aimed at strengthening mother-child bonds, family reunification, and preventing inter-generational cycles of crime and incarceration are also highlighted.

Programs for Inmate Mothers and Their Children

Children between the ages of two and six years may have very different challenges compared to infants born in a prison, particularly due to their exposure to dysfunctional family lifestyles and the traumatic incidents they may have witnessed. For example, some children may have been present at the time of a parent's arrest (Simmons 2000). As noted by Johnston (1995:72), "[Y]oung children are likely to be home at the time of a domestic crime, and the most likely of children of all ages to accompany their parent on [an] excursion for criminal activity." Also, toddlers separated from their parents may have experienced other deprivations —such as familial instability, abuse, poverty, or neglect—making it a challenge to attribute all subsequent problems to the parent's incarceration (Parke and Clarke-Stewart 2002). According to Johnston (1995), children between the ages of two and six years should show signs of development regarding perception, mobility, and the ability to remember. As a result, these children develop an ability to imagine and begin to develop a sense of autonomy and independence, although at this age they are not quite able to separate themselves from their parents.

Johnston (1995) found that children of prison inmates had higher rates of behavioral problems and difficulties in the classroom than other children. For example, these children often exhibit aggression, hostility, acting out, withdrawal, and poor conduct at school. Other studies that examined children of prison inmates, especially children with incarcerated mothers, support these results. Women incarcerated in Oklahoma prisons, for example, report that their children had experienced a variety of problems since their incarceration, ranging from trouble in school to depression and difficulties interacting with others (Sharp 2005). Older children of incarcerated women reportedly were more likely to struggle with substance abuse and as a result, become involved with the criminal justice system.

A wide range of developmental problems were also reported for two to six year-old children of incarcerated women. Being apart from a parent during this developmental period may result in separation anxiety and developmental regression. Furthermore, children who experience trauma at this age, such as witnessing a parent's arrest, may also develop stress reactions and survivor guilt. Youngsters are more likely to be influenced by traumatic events than are infants and are apt to experience long-term effects after a traumatic incident, particularly when no intervention follows, "because young children have the ability to perceive and remember traumatic events, but they cannot process or adjust to trauma without assistance" (Johnston 1995:74). Critical to a child's adjustment to a parent's incarceration is regular contact with that parent (Parke and Clarke-Stewart 2002). Given the likelihood that an inmate mother will be released and seek to resume parenting, programs that facilitate reunification are vital both to inmate mothers and their children. The following sections discuss several promising strategies and specific programs that focus on establishing and maintaining strong mother-child bonds in addition to reducing some of the challenges associated with incarcerated mothers who are or have been separated from their young child(ren).

California's Programs for Inmate Mothers

The California Department of Corrections and Rehabilitation (CDCR) has established two programs intended to help inmate mothers, the Community Prisoner Mother Program (CPMP) and the Family Foundations Program (FFP). According to the CDCR, the mission of both programs is "to provide a safe, stable, wholesome, and stimulating environment for both the mother and the child, using the least restrictive alternative to incarceration consistent with the needs for public safety" (CDCR, "Program Overview" n.d.). Programs and services are provided both to pregnant or parenting inmates as well as to their children, up to the age of six years.

Each program focuses on the best interests of the child, with the ultimate objective aimed at disrupting inter-generational involvement in crime and dependence on social service programs. Program goals consist of promoting or maintaining the bond between the inmate and her child, reuniting families, enhancing community reintegration, fostering successful independent living, and enhancing self-reliance and building self-esteem (CDCR, "Program Overview" n.d.). To accomplish these objectives, both CPMP and FFP provide services to develop educational, life skills, work preparation and social skills and each of these components emphasizes drug treatment, family reunification, and bonding (personal communication, Marc Stambuk). Services for CPMP and FFP are delivered by agencies that contract with the CDCR. For mothers who are expecting, prenatal education and parenting classes are available (CDCR, "Mother Infant Program" n.d.). Both programs provide a variety of activities for inmate mothers and their children, and a program coordinator arranges for childrens' pre-school and kindergarten placement. To accommodate these mothers and their children, these facilities offer children's furnishings and fixtures, nutritious diets, and children's books, as well as toys, play equipment, and games (CDCR, "Programs for Inmate Mothers" n.d.). The annual cost per bed for these programs is approximately $35,000 compared to the average inmate cost of $33,000 in other institutions during the 2004-2005 fiscal year (personal communication, Marc Stambuk).

For correctional officials, graduation from these programs and discharge to parole in the community are regarded as indicators of success. Consequently, while participants are not systematically tracked after leaving the program, the approximate recidivism rates—25 percent for CPMP and 15 percent for FFP—are notably lower than the overall CDCR recidivism rate of 47 percent (personal communication, Marc Stambuk). Perhaps contributing to this success, CDCR attempts to provide drug treatment, and women may also receive female-specific employment and treatment programs while on parole.

Despite the benefits of these programs it should be noted that the California corrections system has been severely criticized for providing substandard health care to women inmates generally (Hill 2002), and pregnant inmates at the Valley State Prison for Women specifically (Legal Services for Prisoners with Children n.d.). As a result, the California corrections system has been a frequent target for litigation by prisoners' rights groups (Barry 2001; 1989; Barry et al. 1995). In fact the entire California correctional system's medical care programs were placed under the supervision of a U.S. federal judge in 2005, and were operating under a consent decree at midyear 2007.

Community Prisoner Mother Program (CPMP)

Since 1985, some 840 inmate mothers have been housed in facilities located in Oakland, Pomona, and Bakersfield, California. The CPMP has the capacity to serve approximately 70 women at any given time (personal communication, Marc Stambuk) and the CPMP has been described as "another chance" for inmate mothers to "become good citizens and good mothers" (CDCR, "Where Do the Children Go" n.d.). The process works as follows; initially, women are housed in a state prison, where they may apply for admission to CPMP through a corrections counselor (CDCR, "Program Overview" n.d.). Similar to the RPP, candidates for these programs are carefully screened. The key criteria for eligibility include: having sentences of six years or less (accounting for good-time credit), no evidence of being an unfit parent, and no indications that the woman might pose an unreasonable risk to the public. The latter point is indicated by convictions for sexual, violent, and in some cases, drug offenses, as well as the woman's potential for escaping or engaging in institutional misconduct.

These criteria are important considering that CPMP facilities are low security and are based in the community. Women must also have been the primary caretaker of their child(ren) before being incarcerated. This requirement, however, does not exclude women who may have placed their child(ren) in the temporary care of relatives or other responsible adults if this placement was in the best interests of the child(ren). Pregnant inmates are also eligible for participation in this program. Finally, to be eligible for admission at CPMP, inmates must have at least 90 days remaining in their sentences (CDCR, "Program Overview" n.d.).

Once accepted into the CPMP, participants are then moved to a "home-like" residential facility. Here, inmates serve the remainder of their sentences while also living with and caring for their children (CDCR, "Where Do the Children Go" n.d.). Both the inmate and her child participate in individual treatment plans, which encourage development and growth (CDCR, "Community Prisoner Mother Program" n.d.). The staff members at CPMP focus on re-establishing the mother-child bond and enhancing social, life, and vocational skills in order to facilitate community re-entry. Since many of these women have a history of chemical dependency, drug education is typically an important part of their programming (CDCR, "Where Do the Children Go" n.d.). Other programs cover parenting skills, general health care and family planning, education, and vocational training.

Although the advocacy group Legal Services for Prisoners with Children (LSPC n.d.) reports high demand for admission to the CPMP, its research indicates that not all available spaces in the program are continuously occupied. This finding is attributed to the inability of some applicants to obtain either medical or security clearances before being granted their admissions. Some women, for example, were denied participation if they had been prescribed psychotropic medications, including Prozac and Welbutrin. Despite high demand for the program, efforts to open additional facilities have been opposed by community groups (Nieto 2003). Nevertheless, CPMP appears to be a very promising and cost-effective intervention.

Family Foundations Program (FFP)

FFP opened its first facility in 1999 in Santa Fe Springs, California and another in 2000 in San Diego (CDCR, "Program Overview" n.d.). Today this program has the capacity to serve 70 mothers. Since the opening of the first FFP facility the program has served 141 mothers (personal communication, Marc Stambuk). Different from the CPMP facilities, FFP participants do not spend time in prison (CDCR, "Programs for Inmate Mothers" n.d.). In fact, FFP is distinct from CPMP in that it is an alternative sentencing program for pregnant and/or parenting mothers with children under the age of six years (CDCR, "Family Foundations Program" n.d.). Some of its eligibility criteria—such as no convictions for certain violent crimes—are similar to those for the CPMP. It is distinct, however, in that it is open specifically to pregnant women or pregnant and parenting women with histories of substance abuse. Women eligible for program participation must have at least one child under the age of six years of age. Subsequently, at least one eligible child (under six years old) will live with his or her mother at the FFP facility. Additionally, the women must not have been sentenced for a period longer than 36 months.

To enter FPP, participants must complete a community substance abuse treatment program. The aims of the FFP are to help these women develop life skills, abstain from alcohol and drugs, and improve their parenting skills. In the longer term, FFP's goals also include preventing drug relapses and reducing recidivism rates. Courts, in collaboration with defense attorneys and probation officers, evaluate both a woman's interest in the program and her eligibility (CDCR, "Family Foundations Program" n.d.). Candidates must, however, be screened by correctional officials prior to the imposition of any prison term.

Following sentencing, women are housed in an FFP facility where they then participate in the 12-month program. Participants who fail to complete the program are returned to prison to complete their original sentences. Conversely inmates who graduate are released onto parole for at least 12 months of community supervision (CDCR, "Program Overview" n.d.).

One limitation of these programs is that they are relatively new. Accordingly, they have not been evaluated as of yet. However, the fact that these innovative programs are cost-effective and are a compassionate alternative to placing the infants into the care of relatives or with the state suggests that they be expanded. In June 2007, for instance, the West Virginia prison system will open their first prison nursery program (Porterfield 2007) and other state prison systems are also considering these programs.

However, even cost-effectiveness and positive outcomes are no guarantee when it comes to the survival of criminal justice programs. In some cases legislators have opposed correctional parenting programs as they are perceived to be soft on crime. Barkauskas, Low, and Pimlott (2002) report that one prominent residential program for pregnant women in the Midwest was discontinued after that state enacted "Truth in Sentencing" legislation (that mandated that inmates had to serve 85 percent of their sentence before being considered for parole) despite the fact that the program demonstrated positive health outcomes.

Conclusions

The programs described above illustrate constructive responses by state corrections officials to the difficulties presented by incarcerating pregnant and parenting women. When enacting criminal statutes, policymakers must realize the full ramifications of their decisions, especially those that go beyond building prisons (Fearn and Parker 2005). In this instance, it calls for an awareness of the role these women play as mothers. Because inmate mothers are likely to serve shorter sentences (see Mumola 2000) and are ultimately reunited with their children in many cases following incarceration, an awareness of these realities is essential to developing effective correctional strategies. Where incarceration for pregnant offenders (or parents) is appropriate, programs such as RPP, CPMP, and FFP are examples of how state corrections systems can respond proactively and sensitively to the challenges pregnant and parenting inmates present.

Addressing the health care needs of inmate mothers as well as their infants and children is a key issue confronting women's correctional health. Although the health care provided to these women is often limited by budget constraints, providing quality medical care creates long-term health benefits for both mothers and their children (Fearn and Parker 2005). Pregnancy screenings during admission, for example, allow inmates to begin receiving prenatal care and nutritional supplements quickly, and enable health care providers to test for complications (Parker 2005). Partnerships with local health care and community social service providers can help ensure the health and wellness of infants and children, even after mothers have been released. This is a vital option for ensuring the long-term health of these children and facilitating their physical and psychological development. Correctional health programs should also be attentive to children's mental health. Early Head Start (EHS) programs, for example, monitor mental health and help families who are juggling a variety of stressors, such as maternal depression, substance abuse, domestic violence, and behavioral problems (EHS n.d.).

While we focus primarily on interventions within state prisons, it is important to acknowledge that local jails also need to provide comprehensive medical services for pregnant women. The short-term nature of jail incarceration tends to reduce the need for medical care, but a recent Washington State study found that the median stay for pregnant women in jail was 14 days, and some were in jail for periods over six months (Bell et al. 2004). These longer jail terms necessitate better health care, and present an ideal place for public health practitioners to provide counseling regarding reproductive health, pregnancy, and prenatal care. Failure to provide such care can result in severe injuries or mortality. Morelli and Crawley (2004) describe the case of a woman who sued a Tampa jail after health officials failed to provide prenatal counseling, ultrasound testing, and vitamins or medication that ultimately led to a ruptured fallopian tube.

Jails and prisons should provide information about women's health and child development in order to benefit women inmates and their families. This is particularly critical in the area of prenatal education. Women often enter these facilities with inaccurate information about pregnancy, and ill-informed inmates may reinforce a pregnant inmate's existing misconceptions (Clark et al. 2006; Hufft et al. 1993). Providing education about health care issues, in general, and pregnancy-related issues, specifically, is one way corrections officials can begin to address this widespread problem and, by doing so, "dispel[ ] misinformation and the stress it causes for pregnant inmates" (Hufft et al. 1993:58). This education should continue after delivery. For women with young children, programs such as the EHS in Washington State can provide vital education about child development and children's health and development needs. Additionally, EHS provides tools and support for monitoring and evaluating children's progress. These programs work closely with parents to establish goals and participate in decision-making processes (EHS 2001).

It is unlikely that rates of incarceration will change in the near future, and the United States will continue to incarcerate many women. As a result, the innovative programs described in this chapter are essential in order to provide women and their infants and young children with a safe and structured environment in which to stabilize and start anew. By neglecting the medical care needs of women, we place their children at higher risk of health and social problems - including the greater risk of future imprisonment.

References

Acoca, Leslie and Myrna S. Raeder. 1999. "Severing Family Ties: The Plight of Nonviolent Female Offenders and Their Children." *Stanford Law and Policy Review* 11:133–143.

American Medical Association (AMA). 1997. *Report 3 of the Council on Scientific Affairs* (I-97). Washington, DC: Author.

Barkauskas, Violet H., Lisa Kane Low, and Sheryl Pimlott. 2002. "Health Outcomes of Incarcerated Pregnant Women and their Infants in a Community-Based Program." *Journal of Midwifery & Women's Health* 47:371-379.

Barry, Ellen. 2001. "Bad Medicine: Health Care Inadequacies in Women's Prisons." *Criminal Justice,* 16:39–43.

------. 1989. "Recent Developments: Pregnant Prisoners." *Harvard Women's Law Journal* 12:190-204.

Barry, Ellen, River Ginchild, and Doreen Lee. 1995. "Legal Issues for Prisoners with Children." Pp. 147–66 in *Children of Incarcerated Parents,* edited by K. Gabel and D. Johnston. New York: Lexington Books.

Belknap, Joanne. 2001. *The Invisible Woman: Gender, Crime, and Justice.* 2nd ed. Belmont, CA: Wadsworth.

------. 1997. "Access to Programs and Health Care for Incarcerated Women." *Federal Probation* 60:34–39.

Bell, Janice F., Frederick J. Zimmerman, Mary L. Cawthon, Colleen E. Huebner, Deborah H. Ward, and Carole A. Schroeder. 2004. "Jail Incarceration and Birth

Outcomes." *Journal of Urban Health* 81:630-644.

Byrne, Mary. 2004. "Ethnographic, Self-report Questionnaire, and Developmental Screening Data to Profile Maternal and Child Health Needs in a Prison Nursery." Presented at the National State of the Science Conference (poster session), October 6–9, Washington, DC.

------. n.d. "Maternal and Child Outcomes of a Prison Nursery Program." Report to the National Institutes of Health/National Institute for Nursing, RO1NR00778-01, 2003-2007.

California Department of Corrections and Rehabilitation (CDCR). n.d. "Community Prisoner Mother Program."

------. n.d. "Community Prisoner Mother Program & Family Foundations Program" [Program overview].

------. n.d. "Family Foundations Program."

------. n.d. "Mother Infant Program."

------. n.d. "Programs for Inmate Mothers."

------. n.d. "Where Do the Children Go When Moms Go to Prison?" [Where Do the Children Go].

Christian, Johnna. 2005. "Riding the Bus: Barriers to Prison Visitation and Family Management Strategies." *Journal of Contemporary Criminal Justice* 21:31-48.

Clarke, Jennifer G., Cynthia Rosengard, Jennifer Rose, Megan R. Hebert, Maureen G. Phipps, and Michael D. Stein. 2006. "Pregnancy Attitudes and Contraceptive Plans Among Women Entering Jail." Women & Health 43:111-130.

Conly, Catherine. 1998. *The Women's Prison Association: Supporting Women Offenders and Their Families.* Washington, DC: Department of Justice, National Institute of Justice.

Early Head Start (EHS). 2001. *Developmental Screening, Assessment, and Evaluation: Key Elements for Individualizing Curricula in Early Head Start Programs.* Technical Assistance Paper No. 4. Washington, DC: U.S. Department of Health and Human Services.

------. n.d. *Program Strategies: Responding to the Mental Health Needs of Infants, Toddlers and Families.* Washington, DC:U.S. Department of Health and Human Services.

Fearn, Noelle E. and Kelly Parker. 2005. "Health Care for Women Inmates: Issues, Perceptions and Policy Considerations." *Californian Journal of Health Promotion* 3(2):1-22.

------. 2004. "Washington State's Residential Parenting Program: An Integrated Public Health, Education, and Social Service Resource for Pregnant Inmates and Prison Mothers." *Californian Journal of Health Promotion* 2(4):34-48.

Gabel, Katherine and K. Girard. 1995. "Long-term Care Nurseries in Prisons: A Descriptive Study." Pp. 237-54 in *Children of Incarcerated Parents*, edited by K. Gabel and D. Johnston. New York: Lexington Books.

Greenfeld, Lawrence A. and Tracy L. Snell. 1999. *Women Offenders.* Washington, DC: Department of Justice, Bureau of Justice Statistics, NCJ 175688.

Hairston, Creasie Finney. 2002. "Prisoners and Families: Parenting Issues During Incarceration." Presented at the From Prison to Home Conference, Jan. 30-31. Washington, DC: Department of Health and Human Services.

Harrison, Paige M. and Allen J. Beck. 2006. *Prisoners in 2005.* Washington, DC: Department of Justice, Bureau of Justice Statistics.

Hill, Amy Petre. 2002 "Death Through Administrative Indifference: The PLRA Allows Women to Die in California's Substandard Prison Health Care System." *Hastings Women's Law Journal* 13:223-259.

Hufft, Anita G., Lena Sue Fawkes, and W. Travis Lawson. 1993. "Care of the Pregnant Offender." Pp. 54-59 in *Female Offenders: Meeting the Needs of a Neglected Population*, edited by J. A. Gondles, Jr. Baltimore, MD: United Book Press, Inc.

Johnston, Denise. 1995. "Effects of Parental Incarceration." Pp. 59-88 in *Children of Incarcerated Parents*, edited by K. Gabel and D. Johnston. New York: Lexington Books.

Kampfner, Cristina Jose. 1995. "Post-traumatic Stress Reactions in Children of Imprisoned Mothers." Pp. 89-100 in *Children of Incarcerated Parents,* edited by K. Gabel and D. Johnston. New York: Lexington Books.

Knight, Marian and Emma Plugge. 2005. "Risk Factors for Adverse Perinatal Outcomes in Imprisoned Pregnant Women: A Systematic Review." *BMC Public Health* 5:111-117.

Krisberg, Barry A. and Carolyn Engel Temin. 2001. *The Plight of Children Whose Parents are in Prison.* Oakland, CA: National Council on Crime and Delinquency.

Kubiak, Sheryl Pimlott, Amy Young, Kristine Siefert, and Abigail Stewart. 2004. "Pregnant, Substance-abusing, and Incarcerated: Exploratory Study of a Comprehensive Approach to Treatment." *Families in Society* 85:177-186.

Laube v. Campbell, 333 F.Supp.2d 1234, 1258 (M.D. Alabama, 2004). *Legal Services for Prisoners with Children (LSPC). n.d. Barriers to Care*. Retrieved January 27, 2006 (http://www.prisonerswithchildren/org/issues/overview.htm).

------. n.d. *Medical Clearance Approvals Plague Women Prisoners.* Retrieved January 17, 2006 (http://www.prisonerswithchildren.org/pf/medicalclearance.htm).

Maeve, M. Katherine. 1999. "Adjudicated Health: Incarcerated Women and the Social Construction of Health." *Crime, Law & Social Change* 31:49-71.

Marquart, James W., Dorothy E. Merianos, Steven J. Cuvelier, and Leo Carroll. 1996. "Thinking About the Relationship between Health Dynamics in the Free Community and the Prison." *Crime & Delinquency* 42:331-360.

Martin, Sandra L., Haesook Kim, Lawrence L. Kupper, Robert E. Meyer and Melissa Hays. 1997. "Is Incarceration During Pregnancy Associated With Infant Birthweight?" *American Journal of Public Health* 87:1526-1531.

Morelli, Keith and Marcia Crawley. 2004. "Ex-inmate Bemoans Medical Care in Jail." Tampa Tribune. March 24, Metro P.1.

Morton, J. B. and Deborah M. Williams. 1998. "Mother/child Bonding." *Corrections Today* 60:98-104.

Morash, Merry, Timothy S. Bynum, and Barbara A. Koons. 1998. *Women Offenders: Programming Needs and Promising Approaches.* Washington, DC: Department of Justice, National Institute of Justice, NCJ 171667.

Mumola, Christopher J. 2000. *Incarcerated Parents and Their Children.* Washington, DC: Department of Justice, Bureau of Justice Statistics, NCJ 182335.

Nieto, Marcus. 2003. *Adult Parole and Probation in California.* Sacramento, CA: California Research Bureau.

Parke, Ross and K. Allison Clarke-Stewart. 2002. "Effects of Parental Incarceration on Young Children." Presented at the From Prison to Home Conference, Jan. 30-31. Washington, DC: Department of Health and Human Services.

Parker, Kelly. 2005. "Pregnant Women Inmates: Evaluating Their Rights and Identifying Opportunities for Improvements in Their Treatment." *Journal of Law and Health* 19: 259-295.

Personal Communication. 2006. With Marc Stambuk, CCII, WCSU of the California Department of Corrections and Rehabilitation on January 24.

Porterfield, Mannix. 2007. "Governor Approves Prison Nursery For Pregnant Inmates." *The Register-Herald.* Retrieved April 12, 2007 (http://www.register-herald.com/)

Richie, Beth E. 2000. "Exploring the Link Between Violence Against Women and Women's Involvement in Illegal Activity." Pp. 1-15 in *Research on Women and Girls in the Justice System.* Washington, DC: Department of Justice, National Institute of Justice.

Ross, Phyllis Harrison and James E. Lawrence. 1998. "Health Care for Women Offenders." *Corrections Today* 60:122–129.

Sharp, Susan F. 2005. *Oklahoma Study of Incarcerated Mothers and Their Children, Phase II.* Oklahoma City, OK: Oklahoma Commission on Children and Youth.

Shearer, Robert A. 2003. "Identifying the Special Needs of Female Offenders." *Federal Probation* 67:46-51.

Simmons, Charlene Wear. 2000. *Children of Incarcerated Parents.* Sacramento, CA: California Research Bureau.

Wooldredge, John D. and Kimberly Masters. 1993. "Confronting Problems Faced by Pregnant Inmates in State Prisons." *Crime & Delinquency* 39:195–203.

CHAPTER THREE

Juvenile Correctional Health Care: Prevention and Education

Matthew O. Thomas

There are some 200,000 young persons held in juvenile correctional facilities within the United States. In addition to engaging in impulsive, risky and delinquent behaviors, this group is likely to have elevated rates of communicable diseases, high levels of mental disorders or learning difficulties, involvement in substance abuse, and poor histories of community health care. This population is also at high risk of violence and suicide, both within a correctional facility and in the community. These factors shape the type of medical and mental health care that these youths (also called wards, minors, residents or youthful offenders) require when they are incarcerated.

Various types of institutions and organizations provide residential services for delinquent youth, including detention facilities, group homes, boot camps, reception centers, state correctional facilities (also called training schools), and ranches. Considerable diversity exists in the types of programs that are offered, and a blend of public, private, and faith-based organizations offer residential programs. Significant differences in the style, security, and programming abound at these various facilities, but they are all expected to provide appropriate health care for their residents. Historically health care was an afterthought in many places, and some evidence suggests that training schools and ranches were less likely to conform to standards of care (Parent et al. 1994). There is, however, an increasing awareness between the relationships of physical and mental health care services and institutional behavior. Moreover, providing effective health care services for incarcerated youths may also contribute to success in the community once they are released.

For example, a study of Washington State juveniles found significant differences in the medical needs and care of juveniles in state versus county facilities. Those in county facilities had higher rates of emergency room visits, a greater number of acute health issues (such as pregnancy or sexually transmitted infections [STI]), and more suicide watches than those in state facilities. Conversely juveniles were more likely to have chronic health needs, such as dentistry, dermatology, or nutrition in state institutions (Anderson and Farrow 1998). There are several reasons for this difference in services. Juveniles in state facilities tend to stay longer and their health care needs are more likely to be identified. Moreover, because most state governments draw from a larger tax base, they may be able to provide a better standard of care.

A youth's admission to a correctional facility begins with establishing the legality of their detention or sentence, as well as an assessment of their current emotional and physical functioning. Information about the youth is also used to determine an appropriate classification. Classification enables officials to assign residents to units with levels of security based on several criteria: the youth's current and prior offenses (e.g., whether they are a violent offender), their age and gender, previous institutional behavior, and whether they have any significant physical or mental health concerns. This is not an option for all facilities though: smaller institutions may not have the capacity to segregate their residents due to their size. As a result, these facilities sometimes mix adolescent males and females, as well as youngsters and more mature adolescents on the same unit, thus creating further challenges to their supervision.

An initial medical assessment is critical for several reasons, including the need to identify communicable diseases, and also because juveniles who are taken into custody may be under the influence of drugs or alcohol. Intoxicated or impaired youth should be carefully evaluated and monitored by medically trained personnel as they are at some risk of overdose or poisoning (Roush 1996). In addition, newly admitted youth need to be checked for injuries or existing health problems. The American Correctional Association (ACA) sets a one hour standard timeframe for intake assessments, and staff conducting these evaluations should have appropriate training in suicide assessment and medical care (Parent et al. 1994) as the first few hours of incarceration are a time of high risk of self-harm or suicide.

In addition to the ACA, the National Commission on Correctional Health Care (NCCHC) also has comprehensive standards for juvenile health care. Correctional agencies are required to meet a set of health-related standards, such as health screening and assessment, availability of trained personnel, and the availability of emergency and recreational services. Few detention facilities, however, meet these standards. Gallagher and Dobrin reviewed data from over 700 juvenile halls and found facilities that provided better care tended to "have longer average lengths of stay, are larger, and are government owned" (2007: 991).

The quality of health screening often depends on the type of facility to which the juvenile is placed. Juvenile hall admissions often occur during hours when full-time medical staff members are unavailable, so a cursory screening is done and serious cases referred to a nurse or physician the next day. If immediate care is required, by contrast, the youth is taken to an emergency department in the community. Most youths stay for only a few days in juvenile detention, and this fact influences the types of health care that they receive. Health assessment in state correctional facilities, by contrast, tends to be more comprehensive because youths will be there much longer. Therefore, they are often screened for communicable diseases, chronic health conditions, and pregnancy.

One issue that juvenile correctional officers often encounter is the problem of malingering. Youths in confinement may exaggerate their health care conditions or needs. In some cases, the adolescent may have an ulterior motivation: such as missing educational classes, to get some sympathy from a health care provider, or the desire to break the routine. Unfortunately, because of issues with malingering, youth correctional officers will occasionally fail to investigate the cause of a youth's complaints of pain or distress, thus leading to tragedies. In addition, correctional officers do not always cooperate with the health care providers. They may fail to abide by treatment plans, follow-up on medical advice or ensure that youths receive their medications. As a result, tensions may exist between the security and medical staff (Roush 1996).

A nutritionally sound diet is an important component for all individuals, especially juveniles. For example, improper diets can lead to health problems, exacerbate existing medical conditions, and may be associated with acting-out behaviors. Youths with chronic illnesses such as diabetes, prenatal care, or obesity may require special diets. Some residents, however, may be reluctant to comply with such diets and nutritionists or nurse-educators can provide counseling to them. Adding to the problem, correctional food is also notorious for being unhealthy, and many facilities provide meals that are high in fat and starch content, and offer few fresh fruits or vegetables.

Other factors associated with healthy conditions in juvenile corrections, include cleanliness and taking precautions to reduce the transmission of infectious diseases (Bick 2005). This is worsened by the fact that juveniles often resist efforts to increase their hygiene. In some cases, youths might have very poor social skills, and must be educated about hygiene and healthy lifestyles. Providing youths with clean clothing, bedding and showers is typically a responsibility of the correctional staff as access to these amenities is often restricted. Moreover, the control over access to daily recreation, exercise, and fresh air rests with the security staff, and idleness often results in higher rates of misconduct.

Incarcerated juveniles tend to have high rates of asthma, hypertension, diabetes, tuberculosis, and dental problems (Committee on Adolescence 2001). These youths also exhibit higher rates of risk behaviors, including alcohol and tobacco use, assaultive behavior, gang membership, and sexual activity (Roush 1996). A sample of detained youth in Maryland found that 45 percent reported having a medical condition, with the majority suffering physical abuse, while many had reported having previous injuries, including stab and gunshot wounds, and more than a tenth never received treatment for these injuries (Shelton 2000).

Confidentiality

Little privacy exists in a secure detention facility. Staff work very closely with one another, and some may be privy to confidential health care information. Roush (1996) reports that this can cause problems if juveniles are fearful of discussing health care issues, such as their HIV status, when correctional staff are present. The Health Insurance Portability and Accountability Act of 1996 (HIPAA) resulted in significant changes in the manner that health-related information can be disseminated within a youth detention or correctional facility. In some cases, health care providers are not legally able to disclose to other facility staff or parents about the health status of the juveniles in their care (Nicoletti 2003). Bizzell (2003) suggests that even though some of the HIPAA guidelines are relaxed in correctional facilities, staff members who disclose the confidential health information of inmates without proper authorization may be placing themselves in jeopardy of being sued or prosecuted.

Despite the fact that some medical care information cannot be shared, it is critical that facilities develop comprehensive information systems that track health-related issues and that medical staff have access to this information. Some state correctional systems have developed quality management and peer review processes where health care is monitored to ensure that it is consistent with national standards. In California, for instance, the Division of Juvenile Justice within the California Department of Corrections and Rehabilitation (CDCR) has implemented Quality Management Committees to review the medical care delivered to juveniles in their care (CDCR 2006). Under their guidance, physicians working within this correctional system engage in peer review of practice to ensure that quality care is maintained.

Dental Care

Providing appropriate dental care in juvenile correctional facilities is challenged by a number of factors. Many youth fear dental exams, have poor dental hygiene, and may ignore what appear to be minor dental problems. The emergence of "meth mouth," a condition brought on by methamphetamine abuse, raises considerable concern for dentists who practice in correctional facilities (American Dental Association 2006; Rhodus and Little 2005). Dental emergencies such as impacted wisdom teeth or injuries resulting from recreational activities, unintentional causes, or assaults also occur behind bars. Because incarcerated youths are unlikely to have received any kind of comprehensive dental care in the community, it is important that juveniles who reside in these facilities for longer periods of time receive some preventative care, and if possible, health education about proper dental care.

Medical Care Expenditures

Providing appropriate correctional health care for juveniles is costly. According to a study that examined these expenditures, fixed costs, such as medical staff contracts and laboratory supplies, represent the greatest portion of health care outlays (Tennyson 2003). But intermediate costs (e.g., emergency care, dentistry) and variable costs (e.g., prescriptions) are also rising, and are less predictable than fixed costs. Mental health care expenditures are also costly, and can be three times the amount of general medical expenses (Tennyson 2003). Variable costs represented 11 percent of the budgets in Tennyson's (2003) study, and as items such as prescriptions increase in cost, the ability of administrators to adequately budget for medical expenditures decreases. A single case of HIV/AIDS, for example, represents a cost of $13,900 to $36,500 for HIV/AIDS medication per year (Infectious Diseases in Corrections Report 2006).

Juvenile correctional facilities must provide comprehensive health care treatment that tackles the problems of chronic medical conditions, past injuries, psychological problems, as well as dental and optometric services. Residents of these facilities also require emergency care, including access to nursing or health care staff at sick call (the term used when an inmate requests medical care). Not all juvenile correctional facilities provide appropriate care. At a minimum, juvenile correctional facilities must treat the most obvious or emergent conditions, bring immunizations up-to-date, and provide educational information about risk behaviors affecting the minor. The short-term nature of juvenile detention, for instance, may be an ideal place to deliver basic health education and promotion information to high-risk populations. One problem with delivering these educational programs, however, is that many juvenile halls have failed to partner with local public health agencies to deliver such courses.

The Challenges of Blood Borne Pathogens and Infectious Diseases

Controlling the spread of blood borne pathogens and infectious diseases are key issues in the operation of youth facilities. Communicable diseases such as sexually transmitted infections (STIs), HIV/AIDS, and hepatitis must be detected and treated. Because inmates are usually housed in close quarters, the likelihood of transmission is increased. In addition, some of the negative behaviors of youths in custody, such as engaging in consensual sex or assaults and rape, increase the risk of transmitting diseases.

Chlamydia trachomatis (CT) and gonorrhea are two common STIs that affect sexually active juveniles. In a study of juvenile detention facilities that screened for these infections, researchers found that females experienced significantly higher rates than males, and that both males and females tested positive for both over 50 percent of the time (Kahn et al. 2005). A cross-sectional survey of incarcerated juveniles, aged 13 to 18 years, investigated the risk factors for STI contraction, specifically CT and gonorrhea (Robertson et al. 2005). Females experienced higher rates of infection for both diseases, with demographic characteristics such as age and race accounting for over half of the variation, and behavior accounting for one-third of the variance (Robertson et al. 2005). Screenings for CT are more common for female detainees (Lofy et al. 2006), but expanding screenings to sexually active male adolescents has increased the success rate in identifying and treating CT (Tebb et al. 2005).

Rates of hepatitis are higher in correctional populations than in the community. This is a problem because the illness is associated with long-term rates of adult liver failure (Murray et al. 2003). A variety of risky behaviors increase one's exposure to hepatitis and these include engaging in unprotected sex and having multiple sexual partners. Additionally, intravenous drug use, tattooing, or body piercing are adding to these numbers. One study of incarcerated juveniles found relatively low rates of hepatitis infection, with the greatest rate among intravenous drug users (Feldman et al. 2004). The study's authors advocated increased testing and intervention in order to keep hepatitis infections at a low level (Feldman et al. 2004). Murray and colleagues (2003) confirmed that incarcerated juveniles have lower hepatitis infection rates than the adult population, but have a higher hepatitis prevalence rate than the non-incarcerated juvenile population, and are more likely to engage in high-risk behaviors.

The risks associated with spreading blood-borne pathogens and communicable diseases are significant for the youths who reside in juvenile facilities, as well as the staff who work within them. As a result, in most jurisdictions staff members receive orientation training about blood-borne pathogen containment as well as annual training updates. Further, some juvenile correctional systems have established infection-control committees and hired public health practitioners to investigate, control, and prevent the spread of infections (CDCR 2006). Unfortunately, many correctional systems have been slow to implement these types of interventions.

Special Health Needs of Female Juveniles

Females present unique challenges for the juvenile justice system, and as their numbers increase, the demand for female-specific programming has also grown (Budnick and Shields-Fletcher 1998). One long-standing concern is that correctional health care has typically been delivered on models created for male populations, but females require a greater degree of services. One cross-sectional survey of incarcerated female juveniles found high percentages of sexual transmitted diseases (Robertson et al. 2005), past pregnancies, suicide attempts, and substance abuse (Crosby et al. 2004). Reproductive health care and pregnancy are female-specific conditions that require significant health care treatment (Fitzgibbon 2004). In addition, some disorders, such as anorexia, bulimia, suicide attempts, and depression, disproportionately affect incarcerated females (Roush 1996).

A recent survey examined the lifestyle characteristics of detained females (Lederman et al. 2004). Respondents admitted for the first time indicated the presence of the following family problems: mental health (21 percent), alcohol abuse (27 percent), drugs (26 percent), and criminal justice system involvement (58 percent). Respondents who had been admitted more than once, by contrast, reported higher percentages of the same problems. In addition to coming from dysfunctional families, Lederman and colleagues (2004) also found that a vast majority of sampled female detainees experienced a major trauma, such as witnessing a death or being threatened with a weapon. High percentages of respondents also reported having mental health or substance abuse problems and being sexually active. Last, youths admitted for the first-time (22 percent) and minors admitted more than once (29 percent) also reported being the victims of sexual abuse.

Assessing and Treating the Mental Health Needs of Juveniles

The physical well-being of detained youths is an important component of juvenile correctional health care, but of critical importance, both during their incarceration and after their release, is the mental health of juveniles. Rogers and colleagues (2002) report that as many as 60 percent of incarcerated youth have some type of mental health disorder. In contrast, only 22 percent youth in the community population are estimated to suffer from similar disorders (National Mental Health Association 2004). Teplin (2001) found that as many as two-thirds of incarcerated youth have alcohol, drug or mental health disorders, and that females are much more likely to experience these problems. After excluding persons with conduct disorders, 59.7 percent of males, and 68.2 percent of detained females were diagnosed with emotional disorders (Teplin et al. 2002).

One of the foremost issues facing juvenile justice systems is accurately assessing and diagnosing mental health functioning. Mental health professionals use a variety of assessment instruments that have been developed specifically for juvenile populations. Some of the most commonly encountered instruments within juvenile corrections are the Minnesota Multiphasic Personality Inventory-Adolescent (MMPI-A), the Massachusetts Youth Screening Instrument (MAYSI), the Massachusetts Screening Indicator 2 (MAYSI-2), and different versions of the Diagnostic Interview Schedule for Children (DISC). The following paragraphs briefly outline the strengths of these instruments.

There is increasing interest in evaluating the effectiveness of these different assessment instruments in adolescent populations. Research indicates that the MMPI-A is effective at differentiating various mental health disorders among male juveniles, allowing juvenile justice professionals to develop appropriate interventions for these delinquents (Archer et al. 2003). The MAYSI-2, by contrast, is an effective instrument for assessing a variety of disorders. Investigators suggest that pairing it with elements of the MMPI-A can lead to greater diagnostic success (Archer et al. 2004). The same study also indicated that females are more likely to report depression and anxiety (Archer et al. 2004). Other research has supported the effectiveness of employing the MAYSI-2 (Grisso et al. 2001), although Wasserman et al. (2004) argue that it does a poor job of identifying some disorders, and they suggest that multiple assessment tools be used for each case.

Co-occurring disorders—when adolescents have both a mental health and an addictions problem—are a significant obstacle for many juveniles. The National Mental Health Association (2004) reported that between 75 and 80 percent of youth receiving substance abuse treatment also suffered from another mental disorder. The Practical Adolescent Dual Diagnostic Interview (PADDI) helps determine the presence of co-occurring disorders in juveniles (Abrantes et al. 2004). The PADDI alerts mental health staff to the presence of potential problems, and promises to increase our understanding of how co-occurring disorders develop. Also, it enables practitioners to formulate more effective treatment plans that look at holistic options, rather than disorder-specific, treatment alone.

Proper mental health assessments are important because the prevalence of persons with mental health needs within a correctional facility is incumbent upon types of definitions that are used. For example, a high percentage of youths with cognitive disabilities such as Attention Deficit Disorder reside in correctional facilities. While youths with severe mental health problems require more comprehensive care, both groups require special attention. As a result of the Individuals with Disabilities Education Improvement Act (IDEIA) of 2004, for example, all youths with cognitive disabilities must have a specialized Individualized Educational Program (Stenhjem 2005). This legislation has a significant impact on correctional facilities that place juveniles in long-term educational programs.

Behavioral Interventions

Juvenile correctional facilities provide educational, recreational, vocational, and life skills programming for their residents, but the design of the curriculum can lead to what Abrams et al. (2005) terms the "paradox of treatment." The authors contend that the overall correctional approach—one that emphasizes discipline even for minor infractions—often conflicts with behavioral, psychological, cognitive-behavior approaches (Abrams et al. 2005). They suggest that juvenile correctional staff need to "distinguish more clearly the treatment aspects of a program from the aspects that are more control-oriented" (Abrams et al. 2005: 22). By doing so, the varieties of programming will make more sense to youth, leading to long-term behavioral changes.

Research on various programs and interventions provides a basis for making informed judgments about juvenile correctional programs. The types of programs that are delivered in these facilities are often dictated by the following: the mission of the correctional facility (e.g., whether they hold youths on a short- or long-term basis), the priorities of the facility superintendents, state standards, accreditation with organizations such as the NCCHC, existing consent decrees, and the threat of future litigation. The following paragraphs outline some of the current "best practices" in managing the conduct of juveniles in correctional facilities.

The planning for a juvenile's release to the community begins early in the youth's incarceration. On this, the National Mental Health Association (NMHA) has recommended a two-pronged approach to improving the mental health of the juvenile delinquent population. First, they suggest that significant increases in community alternatives—including prevention and assessment, family support groups, residential, outpatient, and inpatient treatments, and wrap-around services—be developed to manage mental health issues outside the confines of secure detention facilities. Second, they propose to employ juvenile justice advocates who will create an atmosphere of accountability (NMHA n.d.).

Stroul and Friedman (1986) presented a model of care which called for a holistic treatment plan that encompasses all of the youth's psychological and physical needs. As a comprehensive method, this approach includes the treatment of families, occurs in the least restrictive environment, and relies upon the coordination of services to the family. The community treatment movement used Stroul and Friedman's model as a framework for several promising types of treatment. The foundation of the framework is the service continuum, where community- and institutional-based therapies are integrated for seamless delivery. Four closely related areas of the juvenile justice system are critical in this model: prevention and early intervention programs; diversion programs; mental health screening and treatment; and aftercare services (NMHA 2004). Several specific practices developed from this framework appear promising to reduce recidivism, and these interventions are reported in Table 3.1.

There are a number of promising approaches to delivering services to families of youths at-risk. Multisystemic Therapy (MST) is a family-based approach designed to provide families with internal discipline, stressing education and positive social ties (NMHA 2004). Another family-based intervention is Functional Family Therapy (FFT), which is shorter in length than MST. FFT equips families with specific and targeted tactics to deal with substance abuse, poor conduct, and disorders like oppositional defiant disorder and disruptive behavior disorder (NMHA

2004). The final family-based practice is Wraparound, which integrates service delivery for both the youth and family, through an overall assessment of the family, and the development of a total treatment plan. While this process has proved to a challenge to implement, there are examples of successful Wraparound programs in some U.S. cities (NMHA 2004).

Table 3.1 Treatment Interventions and Success Indicators

Interventions	Success Indicators
Multisystemic Therapy	70% reduction in recidivism; 64% reduction in out-of-home placements
Functional Family Therapy	50% reduction in recidivism; lower costs per juvenile
Wraparound	Improvements in social functioning
Cognitive-Behavioral Therapy	50% reduction in recidivism
Multidimensional Treatment Foster Care	Lower Recidivism; Three times less likely to run away; significantly less hard drug use
Moral Dilemma Discussion Groups	Evidence of significant moral-stage growth
Just Community	Gains in moral reasoning; awareness of democratic decision-making
Positive Peer Culture	Higher positive self-concept
EQUIP	Improved institutional and post-release conduct; decreased recidivism

Sources: National Mental Health Association. 2004. *Mental Health Treatment for Youth in the Juvenile Justice System: A Compendium of Promising Practices.* Arlington, VA: National Mental Health Association. Moody, Edward E. Jr. and Helen S. Lupton-Smith. 1999. "Interventions with Juvenile Offenders: Strategies to Prevent Acting Out Behavior." *Journal of Addictions and Offender Counseling* 20:1-13.

Other, non-family-based treatment programs also show promise. Cognitive-Behavioral Therapy helps youth think through situations where they would typically react emotionally. Among the techniques it provides are anger management and social skills, to improve decision-making skills (NMHA 2004). Multidimensional Treatment Foster Care (MTFC) supplies an alternative to other forms of placement. Youth are placed with specially trained foster families for periods of six to nine months, and intensive supervision, combined with various therapies, offers youth the opportunity for self-improvement and the ultimate goal of reunification (NMHA 2004).

Decades of managing behavioral disorders within juvenile corrections has led to several promising programs. *Moral Dilemma Discussion Groups* is one such approach. For example, it often takes place in school settings where a facilitator leads participants through a process that is intended to create a greater sense of self-awareness while encouraging cooperative and altruistic behavior to grow (Moody and Lupton-Smith 1999). Another program, *Just Community*, by contrast, integrates personal growth with institutional change by installing a democratic disciplinary system in juvenile facilities: allowing participants to perceive their misconduct from a number of perspectives, as well as to be an active learner (Moody and Lupton-Smith 1999). A third program, *Positive Peer Culture* uses peer groups to make the juveniles partners in the treatment process through discussion groups and modeling positive behavior (Moody and Lupton-Smith 1999). Finally, the *EQUIP* program combines elements from Moral Dilemma Discussion Groups and Positive Peer Culture to empower antisocial youth to work with one another to learn problem solving techniques and social skills (Moody and Lupton-Smith 1999).

Post-Release

After spending time in these highly structured environments, juveniles who are released from custody experience a vast array of choices, many of which contribute to high rates of recidivism. Youths often return to the same dysfunctional family, school, and community environments. While these juveniles are usually required to participate in a structured activity as part of their rehabilitation, such as attending alternative schools, home monitoring, or parole supervision, this does not compare to the level of structure they experienced during confinement.

Familial support is of key importance during the post-release period. A survey of juvenile detainees confirms that positive family functioning leads to higher post-release success rates (Brown et al. 2003). To reduce the chance of failure, the Intensive Aftercare Program (IAP) model is used to facilitate a more successful community reintegration for the juvenile. The cornerstones of IAP are risk classification, case planning, and linking the youth to appropriate recreational, treatment, educational or vocational services in the community (Gies 2003). Research indicates that participants in programs using this holistic model have shown significant, positive behavioral change (Gies 2003).

It is important that health care needs be considered before youths are reintegrated into the community. Youths may receive high levels of services while confined, but very little follow-up care in the community. If the correctional facility does not provide the discharged youth with enough prescription medications, for example, they will have poor medication compliance—which is a serious problem if they are receiving psychotropic medications. Moreover, juveniles with physical disabilities may require specialized housing or other forms of accommodation (such as assistive devices). Many youths with cognitive disabilities will need a comprehensive Individualized Educational Program that will be followed in community schools. Last, even though youths often have the best of intentions to abide by the law and engage in healthy lifestyles before leaving the facility, many have trouble following through on their commitments. As a result, it is important that they receive comprehensive aftercare, such as therapeutic support, as well as educational, recreational, and vocational opportunities.

Conclusions

Providing physical and mental health care is a critical responsibility within the entire continuum of juvenile corrections, from detention to placement in state correctional facilities. The effort is often costly, but strategies that focus on prevention are cost effective if viewed over the long-term. By taking a proactive health promotion approach with incarcerated juveniles, serious health problems may be avoided over the long term. Some health education programs, for instance, are short in duration and could be delivered to groups of residents, even those detained for a few days.

Accreditation standards place clear timeframes for medical professionals working within juvenile justice facilities to complete initial and ongoing physical and psychological assessments. Careful attention should be paid by regulatory bodies to ensure that these standards are met in all types of facilities. In reality, Gallagher and Dobrin (2007) find, however, that only a small percentage of youth facilities comply with NCCHC accreditation standards. Again, compliance with these national standards may prove expensive in the short-term, but once a facility has developed an accredited program, it is much easier to maintain.

Delivering constitutionally appropriate juvenile correctional health care is challenged by a number of issues. Concerns about privatization, confidentiality of health care information, changes in drug markets (e.g., the rising use of methamphetamine), the disproportionate population of minority youth in correctional facilities, growing numbers of females admitted to detention, and long-term periods of incarceration each represent unique challenges for the juvenile justice system. Yet, each of these issues is also an opportunity for health promotion strategies and public health interventions that may have a significant long-term impact on the mental and physical well-being of the residents in juvenile correctional facilities.

Delivering health care interventions in juvenile correctional settings is a complicated and costly endeavor, and providing services that comply with the Americans with Disabilities Act, the IDEIA, HIPAA, as well as the Constitution are a challenge to cash-strapped juvenile halls as well as state correctional systems where youths sometimes become lost in the shuffle. DeMuro (2003) writes about the importance of using "best practices" and observes how it is easier to deliver services in a well-operated and managed facility. Research about these best practices provides the juvenile justice system with an array of successful programs that can aid in the assessment of the mental health, the treatment and control of infectious diseases, controlling institutional behavior, treatment of chronic health care, and providing services and support for the youth once they are returned to the community.

References

Abrams, Laura S., Kyoungho Kim, and Ben Anderson-Nathe. 2005. "Paradoxes of Treatment in Juvenile Corrections." *Child and Youth Care Forum* 34:1:7-25.

Abrantes, Ana M., Norman G. Hoffman, Ronald P. Anton, and Todd W. Estroff. 2004. "Identifying Co-Occurring Disorders in Juvenile Justice Populations." *Youth Violence and Juvenile Justice* 2:329-341.

American Dental Association. 2006. "Meth Mouth Can Leave Users Toothless." Retrieved April 14, 2007 from: (http://www.ada.org/public/media/releases/0609_release03.asp)

Anderson, Britt and James A. Farrow. 1998. "Incarcerated Adolescents in Washington State." *Journal of Adolescent Health* 22:363-367.

Archer, Robert P., P. Kevin Bolinskey, Todd L. Morton, and Kelly L. Farris. 2003. "MMPI-A Characteristics of Males Adolescents in Juvenile Justice and Clinical Treatment Settings." *Assessment* 10:400-410.

Archer, Robert P., Rebecca Vauter Stredny, John A. Mason, and Randolph C. Arnau. 2004. "An Examination and Replication of the Psychometric Youth

Screening Instrument-Second Edition (MAYSI-2) Among Adolescents in Detention Settings." *Assessment* 11(4):290-302.

Belenko, Steven. 2001. *Research on Drug Courts: A Critical Review 2001 Update*. New York, NY: The National Center on Addiction and Substance Abuse at Columbia University.

Bick, Joseph. 2005. "Infection Control in the Correctional Setting." *Infectious Diseases In Corrections Report* 8:1-6.

Bizzell, Wesley D. 2003. *The Protection of Inmate's Medical Records: The Challenge of HIPAA Privacy Regulations*. Retrieved April 14, 2007 from: (www.corrections.com).

Brown, Randall, Eric Killian, and William P. Evans. 2003. "Familial Functioning as a Support System for Adolescents' Post-Detention Success." *International Journal of Offender Therapy and Comparative Criminology* 47:529-541.

Budnick, Kimberly J. and Ellen Shields-Fletcher. 1998. "What About Girls?" *OJJDP Fact Sheet*. Washington, DC: Office of Juvenile Justice and Delinquency Prevention.

California Department of Corrections and Rehabilitation. 2006. *Division of Juvenile Justice Health Care Remedial Plan*. Sacramento, CA: Author.

Committee on Adolescence. 2001. "Health Care for Children and Adolescents in the Juvenile Correctional Care System," *Pediatrics* 107:799-803.

Cooper, Caroline S. 2002. "Juvenile Drug Treatment Courts in the United States: Initial Lessons Learned and Issues Being Addressed." *Substance Use and Abuse* 37:1689-1722.

------. 2001. "Juvenile Drug Court Programs." *JAIBG Bulletin*. Washington, DC: Office of Juvenile Justice and Delinquency Prevention.

Crosby, Richard, Laura F. Salazar, Ralph J. DiClemente, William Yarber, Angela M. Caliendo, and Michelle Staples-Horne. 2004. "Health Risk Factors Among Detained Adolescent Females." *American Journal of Preventive Medicine* 27:404-410.

DeMuro, Paul. 2003. "Good News From Toledo: Real Improvements in Detention." *Journal for Juvenile Justice and Detention Services* 18(2):79-91.

Ericson, Nels. 2001. "Addressing the Problem of Juvenile Bullying." *OJJDP Fact Sheet*. Washington, DC: Office of Juvenile Justice and Delinquency Prevention.

Feldman, Gary M., Frank Sorvillo, Barbara Cole, William Lawrence, and Rebecca Mares. 2004. "Seroprevalence of Hepatitis C Among a Juvenile Detention Population." *Journal of Adolescent Health* 35:505-508.

Fitzgibbon, James J. 2004. "Health care for Adolescents in Juvenile Facilities: Increasing Needs for Adolescent Families." *Journal of Pediatric and Adolescent Gynecology* 17:3-5.

Gallagher, Catherine A. and Adam Dobrin. 2007. "Can Juvenile Justice Detention Facilities Meet the Call of the American Academy of Pediatrics and National Commission on Correctional Health Care? A National Analysis of Current Practices." *Pediatrics* 119: 991-1001.

Gies, Steve V. 2003. "Aftercare Services." *Juvenile Justice Bulletin*. Washington, DC: Office of Juvenile Justice and Delinquency Prevention.

Grisso, Thomas, Richard Barnum, Kenneth E. Fletcher, Elizabeth Cauffman, and Dawn Peuschold. 2001. "Massachusetts Youth Screening Instrument for Mental Health Needs of Juvenile Justice Youth." *Journal of the American Academy of Child and Adolescent Psychiatry* 40:541-548.

Hora, Peggy Fulton, William G. Schma, and John T. A. Rosenthal. 1999. "Therapeutic Jurisprudence and the Drug Treatment Court Movement: Revolutionizing the Criminal Justice System's Response to Drug Abuse and Crime in America," *Notre Dame Law Review* 74:439-538.

Infectious Diseases in Corrections Report. 2006. News and Literature Reviews: HIV Costs Have Decreased. *Infectious Diseases in Corrections Report* 9:8.

Kahn, R. H., D. J. Mosure, S. Blank, C. K. Kent, J. M. Chow, M. R. Boudov, J. Brock, and S. Tulloch. 2005. "Chlamydia trachomatis and Neisseria gonorrhoeae Prevalence and Coinfection in Adolescents Entering Selected U. S. Juvenile Detention Centers, 1997-2002." *Sexually Transmitted Diseases* 32:255-259.

Kurlychek, Megan, Patricia Torbet, and Melanie Bozynski. 1999. "Focus on Accountability: Best Practices for Juvenile Court and Probation." *JAIBG Bulletin.* Washington, DC: Office of Juvenile Justice and Delinquency Prevention.

Lederman, Cindy S., Gayle A. Dakof, Maria A. Larrea, and Hua Li. 2004. "Characteristics of Adolescent Females in Juvenile Detention." *International Journal of Law and Psychiatry* 27:321-337.

Lofy, Kathryn H., Jo Hofmann, Debra J. Mosure, David N. Fine, and Jeanne M. Marrazzo. 2006. Chlamydial Infections Among Female Adolescents Screened in Juvenile Detention Centers in Washington State, 1998-2002. *Sexually Transmitted Diseases* 33:63-67.

Molidor, Christian E., Laura B. Nissen, and Ted R. Watkins. 2002. "The Development of Theory and Treatment with Substance Abusing Female Juvenile Offenders." *Child and Adolescent Social Work Journal* 19:209-225.

Moody, Edward E. Jr. and Helen S. Lupton-Smith. 1999. "Interventions with Juvenile Offenders: Strategies to Prevent Acting Out Behavior." *Journal of Addictions and Offender Counseling* 20:2-14.

Murray, Karen F., Laura P. Richardson, Chihiro Morishima, James W. M. Owens, and David R. Gretch. 2003. "Prevalence of Hepatitis C Virus Infection and Risk Factors in an Incarcerated Juvenile Population: A Pilot Study." *Pediatrics* 111:153-157.

National Mental Health Association. 2004. *Mental Health Treatment for Youth in the Juvenile Justice System: A Compendium of Promising Practices.* Alexandria, VA: National Mental Health Association.

------. n.d. *Checking Up On Juvenile Justice Facilities: A Best Practices Guide.* Alexandria, VA: National Mental Health Association.

Nicoletti, Angela. 2003. "Teens, Confidentiality, and HIPAA." *Journal of Pediatric and Adolescent Gynecology.* 16: 113-114.

Office of Justice Programs. 1998. "Juvenile and Family Drug Courts: An Overview," *Drug Court Clearinghouse and Technical Assistance Project.* Washington, D.C.: Office of Justice Programs.

Parent, Dale G., Valerie Lieter, Stephen Kennedy, Lisa Livens, Daniel Wentworth, and Sarah Wilcox. 1994. "Conditions of Confinement: Juvenile Detention and Corrections Facilities," Research Report. Washington, DC: Office of Juvenile Justice and Delinquency Prevention.

Rhodus, Nelson and James W. Little. 2005. "Methamphetamine Abuse and "Meth Mouth." *Northwest Dentistry:* 84:29,31,33-37.

Robertson, Angela A., Connie Baird, Janet S. St. Lawrence, and Robert Pack. 2005. "Predictors of Infection with Chlamydia or Gonorrhea in Incarcerated Adolescents." *Sexually Transmitted Diseases* 32(2):115-122.

Robertson, Angela A., Patricia L. Dill, Jonelle Husain, and Cynthia Undesser. 2004. "Prevalence of Mental Illness and Substance Abuse Disorders Among Incarcerated Juvenile Offenders in Mississippi." *Child Psychiatry and Human Development* 35:55-74.

Rogers, Kenneth M., Bonnie Zima, Elaine Powell, and Andrew J. Pumariega. 2002. "Who Is Referred to Mental Health Services in the Juvenile Justice System?" *Journal of Child and Family Studies* 10:485-494.

Roush, David W. 1996. "Desktop Guide to Good Juvenile Detention Practice," Research Report. Washington, DC: Office of Juvenile Justice and Delinquency Prevention.

Sandel, Mark H. 2004. "Therapeutic Gardening in a Long-Term Detention Setting." *Journal for Juvenile Justice Services* 19:123-131.

Shelton, Deborah. 2000. "Health Status of Young Offenders and Their Families." *Journal of Nursing Scholarship* 32:173-178.

Sprague, Jeffrey, Hill M. Walker, Steve Stieber, Brandi Simonsen, and Vicki Nishioka. 2001. "Exploring the Relationship Between School Discipline Referrals and Delinquency." *Psychology in the Schools* 38:197-206.

Stenhjem, Pam. 2005. Youth With Disabilities in the Juvenile Justice System: Prevention and Intervention Strategies. Retrieved April 24, 2006 (http://www.edjj.org/Publications/NCSETIssueBrief_4.1.pdf).

Stroul, Beth A. and Robert M. Friedman. 1986. *A System of Care for Severely Emotionally Disturbed Children and Youth.* Washington, DC: Georgetown University Child Development Center.

Tauber, Jeff and C. West Huddleston. 1999. *Development and Implementation of Drug Court Systems.* Washington, DC: National Drug Court Institute.

Tebb, Kathleen P., Robert H. Pantell, Charles J. Wibbelsman, John M. Neuhaus, Ann C. Tipton, Samantha C. Pecson, Meaghan Pai-Dhungat, Timothy H. Ko, and Mary-Ann B. Shafer. 2005. "Screening Sexually Active Adolescents for Chlamydia trachomatis: What About the Boys?" *American Journal of Public Health* 95:1806-1810.

Teplin, Linda A. 2001. "Assessing Alcohol, Drug, and Mental Disorders in Juvenile Detainees." *OJJDP Fact Sheet.* Washington, DC: Office of Juvenile Justice and Delinquency Prevention.

Teplin, Linda A., Karen Abram, Gary M. McClelland, Mina K. Dulcan, and Amy A. Mericle. 2002. "Psychiatric Disorders in Youth in Juvenile Detention." *Archives of General Psychiatry* 59:1133-1143.

Tennyson, Debra H. 2003. "The High Cost of Health Care Within the Juvenile Justice System." *Journal of Correctional Health Care* 10:89-108.

Turner, Susan, Douglas Longshore, Suzanne Wenzel, Elizabeth Deshenes, Peter Greenwood, Terry Fain, Adele Harrell, Andrew Morral, Faye Taxman, Martin Iguchi, Judith Greene, and Duane McBride. 2002. "A Decade of Drug Treatment Court Research." *Substance Use and Misuse* 37:1489-1527.

Wasserman, Gail A., Jennice S. Vilhauer, Larkin McRenolds, Rebecca Shoal, and Reni John. 2004. "Mental Health Screening in the Juvenile Justice System: A Comparison Between the Voice-DISC-IV and the MAYSI-2." *Journal for Juvenile Justice Services* 19:7-17.

CHAPTER FOUR

Communicable Diseases: Correctional and Community Health

Cortney A. Franklin, Noelle E. Fearn and Travis W. Franklin

Rapidly expanding prison and jail populations that suffer disproportionately from communicable diseases have created a critical public health concern. Prevalence rates for infectious diseases such as HIV/AIDS, hepatitis, and tuberculosis are many times greater among jail and prison inmates than the general population (Hammett 1998; Hammett, Harmon, and Maruschak 1999; Rosen, Schoenbach, and Kaplan 2006). Crowded jail and prison conditions, inadequate ventilation, and poor medical care in many correctional facilities exacerbate the problem (see Allwright et al. 2000; Koehler 1994; Weild et al. 2000). The disproportionate prevalence rates and institutional obstacles, in combination with high-risk life choices—before, during, and after incarceration—present unique challenges to correctional and public health care providers and public health safety. This chapter focuses on the major communicable diseases (HIV/AIDS, tuberculosis, and hepatitis) prevalent in correctional settings with special attention to correctional and public health strategies that reduce the transmission of serious illness through diagnosis, treatment, and prevention among institutionalized offenders.

HIV/AIDS in Correctional Settings

The prevalence of HIV/AIDS among jail and prison inmates is cause for public health concern. The most recent data indicate that the rate of HIV/AIDS is more than three times higher among jail and prison inmates than among the general population (Maruschak 2006). While the rate of infection among inmates has varied over the past decade or so, prisons have experienced a slight reduction in the prevalence of HIV/AIDS, despite the increasing prevalence of infection among the general population—with 1.9 percent of state prison inmates and roughly one percent of federal prison inmates reporting HIV infection (Maruschak 2006). It is quite possible that the reliability of these estimates is somewhat limited depending on the method through which infection is detected and reported (Rosen, Schoenbach, and Kaplan 2006). For example, studies have documented a wide variation in testing methods across jurisdictions (Hammett et al. 1999; Harlow 1993). When correctional systems test all inmates for HIV/AIDS infection as opposed to testing samples of prisoners or testing inmates on a voluntary basis, it is likely that they may come up with different results (Amankwaa, Bavon, and Amankwaa 2001). Even so, it appears that the rate of HIV-infected inmates has been declining since 1999.

The declining infection among inmates has been accompanied by a significant drop (79 percent from the years 1995-2003) in the number of AIDS-related deaths in prison (Maruschak 2005). This reduction may be partially due to advances in the treatment of the HIV/AIDS virus. This decrease may also be a consequence of compassionate leave policies that release sick and dying inmate patients to their families so that they can live out their final days at home or in a community hospice (Franklin, Fearn, and Franklin 2005). Nonetheless, any indication of a decline in AIDS-related mortality among inmates is promising in terms of viral transmission and treatment. Further research indicates that HIV/AIDS prevalence varies by geographic region with higher rates of infection among inmates in the Northeastern part of the country (Muraschak 2005).

Sex Differences in Prevalence Rates

Although the concentration of HIV/AIDS in prisons poses a serious threat to inmates in general, HIV infection poses an increasingly serious threat to female inmates (Jacob Arriola, Braithwaite, and Newkirk 2006; Hammett et al. 1999; Kassira et al. 2001). In comparing the prevalence rates of AIDS-infected inmates over a twelve-year period, the rate of infected women remains consistently higher than their male counterparts. The most recent data indicates that women are infected at a rate that is approximately 50 percent higher than men (see also Franklin et al. 2005; Gellert et al. 1993; Kassira et al. 2001; Maruschak 2006).

Infection/Transmission

The HIV/AIDS virus is a blood-borne pathogen which means it is transmitted through the exchange of bodily fluids. HIV/AIDS can be transmitted through sexual contact, sharing needles and/or syringes, receiving tattoos, and through blood transfusions. Additionally, infected mothers can transmit the HIV/AIDS virus to their unborn babies or through breast milk after an infant is born (Hammett et al. 1999).

Pre-incarceration Infection

The ways that offenders contract HIV/AIDS prior to their incarceration reflect their relative lack of information and education related to the infection and spread of HIV/AIDS. Offenders have a tendency to engage in behaviors that put them at high risk for infection (see Franklin et al. 2005; Pollock 2004). For example, intravenous (IV) drug use, needle sharing, and unprotected sex with multiple partners (Berman and Brown 1990; Decker and Rosenfeld 1992; Hammett et al. 1999; Leigh 1990; Tewksbury, Vito, and Cummings 1998) all contribute to the transmission of HIV/AIDS. Female offenders report higher rates of pre-incarceration drug addiction, and research indicates that women are more likely than men to use drugs prior to their incarceration (Morash and Schram 2002; Pollock 2002; Zaitzow and West 2003) putting them at higher risk for antisocial behaviors and activities related to increased exposure to HIV/AIDS (Guyon et al. 1999; Leh 1999; Lurigio, Swartz, and Jones 2003; Marquart et al. 1999). Research also indicates that women engaged in prostitution are at higher risk for contracting the HIV/AIDS virus (Jacob Arriola, Braithwaite, and Newkirk 2006). Finally, low socioeconomic status and reduced access to health and medical care are additional factors that influence the prevalence of HIV/AIDS infection among male and female offenders prior to their admission to jail or prison (see Ehrmann 2002; Franklin et al. 2005 for reviews).

Contracting HIV/AIDS in Prison

A relatively large number of inmates enter correctional confinement HIV/AIDS positive (Zack, Flanigan, and DeCarlo 2000). There are, however, inmates who are infected while under correctional supervision (Hammett et al. 1999). This occurs as a result of engaging in high-risk behaviors while confined. Studies indicate that inmates transmit HIV/AIDS through sexual activity in prison where inmates participate in both consensual and coerced sex (Mahon 1996; Struckman-Johnson et al. 1996). In addition, some inmates engage in intravenous drug use (Darke, Kaye, and Finlay-Jones 1998; Rotily et al. 2001) often times sharing needles (see

Hammett et al. 1999), further increasing their risk of HIV transmission. Finally, inmates who receive tattoos while in prison face an increased risk of contracting communicable diseases if they use contaminated needles and take inadequate protections against blood-borne transmission (Frost and Tchertkov 2002; Hammett et al. 1999).

Diagnosis

HIV/AIDS testing policies vary by jurisdiction. Two-thirds of state and federal prison systems and 80 percent of city and county jails test inmates voluntarily or when there are clinical indications of seropositive symptoms (Amankwaa et al. 2001; Hammett et al. 1999). Other testing policies target inmates who have been involved in incidents that may put them at risk for contracting the virus. Some jurisdictions test all incoming inmates, while others focus on high-risk groups, or random samples of inmates. Some jurisdictions conduct blind or unlinked studies where blood is tested but there is no identifying information that links the inmate to the results of the test (Hammet et al. 1999). This form of testing provides aggregate numbers of infected inmates but does not allow for any type of medical treatment or educational follow-up. According to a review of prison system testing policies in 2003, Rosen and colleagues (2006: 4) found that 20 prison systems had mandatory testing polices, "11 targeted 'high risk' inmates (e.g., injection drug users, commercial sex workers) for HIV testing" and the remaining systems had voluntary testing policies. The degree to which testing is done in a correctional system seems to be dependent upon organizational factors such as a greater number of staff, more training and staff development, a higher budget, and a decentralized power structure (Oser, Tindall, and Leukefeld 2007).

Screening inmates for HIV/AIDS on a voluntary basis presents special challenges in terms of encouraging inmates to request testing. Many prisoners harbor misconceptions about what constitutes high-risk behaviors for contracting and transmitting HIV, are fearful of HIV testing, or are in denial about their particular risk status and may not request testing (Behrendt et al. 1994). Confidentiality concerns also complicate voluntary HIV/AIDS testing. Inmates are less likely to request HIV/AIDS testing if they fear that their test results will be disclosed to correctional staff and others who may discriminate against or mistreat them (Hammett et al. 1999; Zaitzow and West 2003). Moreover, finding that an inmate is HIV positive might result in stigma, segregation in some prison systems, and reduced educational or vocational opportunities within a prison (Rosen et al. 2006).

Treatment and Prevention Strategies

The 1996 introduction of protease inhibitors and combination drug therapies brought forth changes in the treatment of HIV/AIDS, providing the potential to seriously delay disease progression in infected inmates (Deeks et al. 1997). According to recent survey data gathered by the National Institute of Justice (NIJ) and the Centers for Disease Control and Prevention (CDC), these new drugs and combination therapies are widely available to correctional systems but are costly (Infectious Diseases in Corrections Report 2006). Despite widespread availability, staff and inmate interviews indicate that soaring medical costs, inmate reluctance, clinical incompetence, and lack of uniform treatment standards across correctional jurisdictions, have limited the extent to which these treatment regimens are made available to infected inmates (Hammett et al. 1999).

Mandatory Admissions Screening

Correctional settings have the potential to prevent the spread and transmission of HIV/AIDS infection. One of the primary ways in which this is accomplished is through some form of mandatory admissions screening. As of 2003, twenty prison systems employed mandatory HIV/AIDS testing (Rosen et al. 2006). Proponents of mandatory screening policies argue that identifying infected inmates allows correctional staff to address the health and medical needs of these individuals by providing them with early treatment intervention (Zaitzow and West 2003). Identifying inmates with positive HIV status upon admission to the facility provides staff the opportunity to target education and counseling to these prisoners regarding the types of behaviors that put them at high risk for transmitting infection. Early identification also allows correctional staff to segregate infected inmates, limiting the potential for spreading infection (Blumberg and Laster 1999), although only a few state prison systems utilize this approach (Rosen et al. 2006).

Opponents of mandatory admissions screening argue that because medical technology is not without error, inmates may have a false sense of security regarding who does and who does not have HIV/AIDS. Other arguments against mandatory testing include concerns dealing primarily with confidentiality and segregation issues—that mandatory screening could create a "class of outcasts" in the prison who are faced with harassment, mistreatment, and discrimination related to educational, employment, and other programming opportunities (Blumberg and Laster 1999; Zaitzow and West 2003).

Segregation

While housing HIV-positive inmates apart from the general correctional population may make sense in terms of prevention, this practice has declined in recent years (Hammett et al. 1999; Rosen et al. 2006). In 1997, for instance, only three state correctional systems had policies that called for segregating HIV-infected inmates. Further, 17 state and federal prisons had "no restrictions" housing policies and one facility housed infected inmates in the general population with minor precautions. Inmates are segregated only on a case-by-case basis in the remaining prison systems (Hammett et al. 1999). Rosen and colleagues (2006) reported similar findings in their survey of state and federal prison systems.

Nonetheless, segregation is supported on the basis of a number of claims. For example, proponents argue that segregating inmates enables correctional staff to prevent the spread of HIV/AIDS by limiting high-risk behaviors—such as unprotected sexual contact, tattooing, and needle sharing—with uninfected inmates (Blumberg and Laster 1999; Zaitzow and West 2003). Others have argued that since infected inmates have weakened immune systems segregating them from the general inmate population reduces their chances of contracting diseases and/or becoming ill.

Opponents argue that segregating HIV-infected inmates undermines the public health message that HIV is not transmitted through casual contact but instead, through high-risk behaviors. Further concern arises because these inmates may be placed in substandard housing with less than adequate living conditions, and experience exclusion from work and educational programming (Blumberg and Laster 1999; Rosen et al. 2006; Zaitzow and West 2003). As a result, inmates may be less likely to request voluntary testing if they fear segregation or other restrictions as a consequence of seropositive HIV status (Hammett et al. 1994).

Public Health Education

Health education programs are a promising strategy toward reducing the spread of HIV/AIDS in correctional settings, particularly among inmate populations who are likely unaware of the ways in which the disease is transmitted. While correctional institutions in virtually every state provide some type of HIV/AIDS education program (Hammett et al. 1999), vast differences exist in terms of delivery and content (see Zaitzow and West 2003). Further, jurisdictions vary in the quality of service and types of programs they provide. As of 1997, only ten percent of state and federal prison systems and five percent of jails offered comprehensive HIV/STD education that included instructor-led education, peer-led programs, pre- and post-test counseling, and multi-session prevention counseling (Hammett et al. 1999).

Research indicates that many programs supply questionable material or inaccurate information. Institutions also fail to deliver information that addresses issues relevant to prison populations and to do so in a way that is easily understood by inmates (Zaitzow and West 2003). According to the National Survey of AIDS in Correctional Facilities (1992), HIV/AIDS information is provided in correctional settings related specifically to safer sex practices, cleaning drug injection equipment, STDs, perinatal transmission, and drug treatment/medication (see Franklin et al. 2005). More recent data indicate however, that although all jurisdictions cover basic HIV information and the interpretation of HIV test results in HIV/STD education sessions, only 67 percent of jurisdictions discuss safe sex practices, 41 percent cover negotiation skills for safe sex, 45 percent explore the risks associated with injection hygiene and discuss safer injection practices, and 82 percent cover the risks associated with tattooing (Hammett et al. 1999).

Condom Distribution Programs

Despite the obvious risk-reduction and practical health implications of distributing condoms in correctional settings, most U.S. jails and prisons do not distribute condoms and actually prohibit inmates from possessing them. Reasons behind this prohibition policy include safety—correctional management believe that inmates will use condoms to fashion weapons and hide contraband—as well as discouraging sexual activity in prison (Hammett et al. 1999). Finally, there are issues as to whether or not the use of condoms actually prevents the transmission of HIV/AIDS, especially when used incorrectly (Blumberg and Laster 1999). Wohl (2006) suggests that condom distribution policies be reviewed in light of a recent Georgia study that found that inmate sex leads to the transmission of HIV.

A very limited number of U.S. prison (Vermont and Mississippi) and jail systems (Los Angeles, New York City, San Francisco, Philadelphia, and Washington, D.C.) make condoms available to inmates. To date, there have been few reports of malicious or antisocial behavior stemming from the distribution of condoms. Some of these jurisdictions have had their condom policies in place since 1990 (see Hammett et al 1990), but they do not distribute them in a standardized manner. Mississippi, for instance, makes an unlimited number available for purchase at the canteen (or commissary) while New York and Vermont limit condoms to one per inmate per medical visit. Jails in San Francisco and Washington,

DC, by contrast, make condoms available as part of their AIDS education programs and the Philadelphia jail provides condoms during counseling sessions related to HIV testing (Blumberg and Laster 1999; Hammett et al. 1994; Lipton 2002). Despite U.S. concerns about misuse, condoms are distributed in prisons located in Australia, Canada, and many Eastern and Western European nations and they have seldom been linked with inappropriate behavior (MacDonald 2005).

Bleach and Needle/Syringe Exchange Programs

Research indicates that cleaning needles and syringes with full-strength bleach may be an effective method of HIV disinfection. The Centers for Disease Control and Prevention (CDC) provides procedures for sterilizing injection equipment. This method however, is far less desirable than exchanging used needles for new ones. Hammett and colleagues (1999) found that approximately 20 percent of correctional systems made bleach available to inmates "for any purpose" but more current information is unavailable. Similar to condom distribution programs, bleach availability for the purpose of cleaning injection equipment is a prevention strategy that is widely used outside of, but not within, U.S. correctional systems (see MacDonald 2005).

Currently, there are no U.S. correctional systems that provide needle and/or syringe exchange programs for inmates as an HIV/AIDS prevention strategy. In fact, possessing a needle or a syringe in U.S. prisons and jails is a violation of the law and of correctional regulations (Hammett et al. 1999). However, as of 2000, there have been seven needle exchange programs identified in Swiss jurisdictions, seven programs in Germany, and five in Spain (Dolan, Rutter, and Wodak 2003). Reports indicate that drug consumption has not increased as a result of these exchange programs; and there have been no reports of the needles being used as weapons. Instead, needle sharing showed a marked decline with no cases of HIV or hepatitis infection among program participants (Dolan et al. 2003).

Methadone Maintenance

Methadone maintenance programs may be another way to prevent the spread of HIV infection by reducing needle use or sharing between infected and uninfected inmates. These are controversial programs as they are often seen as supporting drug use, but supporters of methadone maintenance argue that a controlled methadone program reduces heroin use within correctional facilities and the associated harms from using illegal drugs. Methadone maintenance programs are rarely encountered within the United States, but are found in Australia, Canada and Europe (MacDonald 2005). These programs have been used in New York State for some time and another was recently introduced in a New Mexico jail (Grimm 2006). Research about the effectiveness of methadone maintenance programs in reducing high-risk behavior in inmate populations has shown some tentative empirical support (see Heimer et al. 2005; Warren et al. 2006). Despite promising findings, it is doubtful that such programs will be widely introduced in U.S. facilities in the near future.

Inmate Peer Education Project

While public health education provided in correctional settings may fall short on a number of different counts, the Inmate Peer Education Project shows promise for successfully delivering HIV/AIDS-related information in an audience-appropriate manner. The program trains, educates, and employs inmate peers to teach HIV prevention strategies to incoming inmates and provide counseling and support for newly diagnosed inmates (Ehrmann 2002; Grinstead, Zack, and Faigeles 1999). The peer education program is set up to reduce high-risk behaviors among inmates by offering the opportunity for open and honest dialogue between program participants. Peer educators have been instrumental in encouraging inmates to request voluntary HIV/AIDS testing. Research indicated that 44 percent of inmates involved in a peer-led program volunteered for HIV testing despite the lack of anonymity and the fact that seropositive inmates were placed in segregated housing (Grinstead et al. 1999).

Simmons (2004:6), himself an inmate educator, outlines some of the benefits of these peer education programs:

> Peer educators are able to "speak the language" of other inmates, and may share similar experiences—thus having more inherent credibility than those who represent "the system" (often distrusted or even ignored). Peer educators can be quite successful in winning the trust of the inmate population.

Peer educators are given comprehensive training to undertake these roles and are supervised by prison staff. Simmons (2004:7) notes that "peer-based programs have four key advantages: credibility, range of services, benefits to inmates and peer educators, and cost-effectiveness." Martin Medical Services (2002) observed that these programs exist throughout the nation, and are used in both jails and prisons.

Utilizing inmates as peer educators not only provides an innovative and credible method of delivering information, but peer education is also cost effective and thus, sustainable, especially when budget cuts influence the availability of quality prison programming (Ehrmann 2002; Grinstead et al. 1999). Additionally, inmates trained as peer educators report improvements in their self-esteem and increased chances for post-release employment. A 1994 survey indicates that, despite the positive feedback and potential for disseminating information to a wide and captive audience, only 35 percent of state and federal prison systems in the United States operated peer-led HIV/AIDS prevention programs in at least one of their facilities (Grinstead et al. 1999).

Discharge Planning—Empowerment Through HIV/AIDS Information, Community, and Services (ETHICS)

Most individuals contract HIV prior to confinement, typically though inmates are made aware of their seropositive status while under correctional supervision. Discharge planning is designed to provide HIV/AIDS-infected inmates with community resources and ensure a smooth post-release transition. Discharge planning also attempts to deal with the medical, pharmaceutical, insurance, financial, housing, and social support needs of inmates who are being released from custody (Ehrmann 2002). Because many inmates are not familiar with HIV treatment in general or their individual drug therapy regimen in particular, discharge planning also attempts to educate inmates regarding their specific health and medical needs. Currently, 76 percent of jails and 92 percent of state and federal prisons report some form of discharge planning for HIV/AIDS-infected inmates (Hammett et al. 1999).

The Empowerment through HIV/AIDS Information Community and Services (ETHICS) program is an innovative, community-based effort funded by the Fortune Society in New York and is designed to provide discharge planning for inmates with HIV/AIDS who are housed at the Rikers Island Jail in New York City and New York State prisons. The ETHICS program provides outreach staff and volunteers to aid inmates with the difficult transition into the community. They do this by accompanying released inmates to prescheduled appointments and temporary housing. Further, ETHICS staff visit New York State correctional facilities and eligible inmates meet with planners to obtain information regarding the program. Reentry planning begins six months prior to release so that inmates can attend sessions with discharge planners to make appointments and get referrals related to the specific concerns of inmates with HIV/AIDS. The ETHICS program is a collaborative effort involving institutional and field parole officers, correctional facility medical staff, and counselors and service providers in the New York

City area that offer housing, substance abuse treatment, and medical care (Ehrmann 2002).

Tuberculosis (TB) in Correctional Settings

While tuberculosis (TB) is typically thought of as being eradicated several generations ago, this disease remains a public health priority given the nature of its transmission (airborne contagion), and because there have been numerous TB outbreaks in U.S. jails and prisons. Like other communicable diseases, offenders are at higher risk for being infected with Mycobacterium tuberculosis, the bacterium that that causes TB, than community members (Wilcock et al. 1996). This disease presents a significant treatment challenge as the therapy requires a prolonged period of taking medication. Further complications arise because the persons who are at highest risk for the disease are often the least likely to comply with taking their prescribed medications.

Prevalence Rates

TB cases are more prevalent among inmate populations as compared to their citizen counterparts (MacNeil, Lobato, and Moore 2005). Inmate TB cases represented almost four percent of the incidence in the U.S. population. According to Gadkowski and Stout (2006:1):

> [O]ver half (53.7%) of the inmates with TB disease were housed in local jails, and compared to non-inmates, they were younger, more likely to be male, U.S. born, and from racial and ethnic minorities. Not surprisingly, inmates more often had a history of excess alcohol use, illicit drug use and homelessness during the year prior to TB diagnosis.

The close quarters and overcrowding of correctional facilities are ideal for the transmission of TB. The high rates of admission and discharges in jails might make this problem more prevalent in local correctional institutions. For example, Bick (2004:3) observed that "the rate of active tuberculosis in jails is fifteen times that seen in the general population."

Correctional staff and health workers are also at risk for contracting TB (Mitchell et al. 2005; Wilcock, Hammett, and Parent 1995). According to the CDC, 18 correctional personnel were diagnosed with TB during 1997 (Hammett et al. 1999). Occupational hazards such as close contact with infected arrestees and offenders, as well as personal demographic characteristics may put correctional staff and health workers at risk for contracting TB (see Ashkin and Malecki 2005)

Tuberculosis Risk Factors

Tuberculosis is more prevalent among jail and prison inmates as a result of a variety of individual and institutional factors. First, a high proportion of jail and prison inmates experience poor overall health, communicable disease (HIV/AIDS and hepatitis B and C), and substance abuse problems—including IV drug abuse—all of which increase the chances of infection. Research indicates that a great proportion of the increase in the number of TB cases can be attributed to co-infection with HIV/AIDS (Barnes et al. 1992). More specifically, inmates infected with HIV/AIDS are susceptible to the active form of TB due to their weakened immune systems. Intravenous drug users also face increased risk as intravenous drug use is associated with TB infection (Hammett et al. 1999). Further, a high percentage of inmates come from distressed economic conditions with limited access to medical care, an increased chance of malnourishment, and many are members of racial and ethnic minorities —all potential correlates of active TB (Fearn and Parker 2005; Hammett et al. 1999; Hammett 1998). In addition to these individual risk factors, TB is more easily spread when persons share smaller living spaces such as the overcrowded conditions in prisons or jails. Inadequate ventilation, a poor diet, limited access to quality care in prison—including treatment and preventative therapy—short-term jail stays, and confidentiality concerns all exacerbate the problem of TB infection and transmission (Wilcock et al. 1996).

Infection/Transmission

Tuberculosis is spread when an infected host coughs up airborne droplets containing M. tuberculosis. When M. tuberculosis are inhaled, infection can result (Koehler 1994). If a healthy person becomes infected, it is likely that he/she will not develop the active and contagious form of TB, as a strong immune system should inactivate M. tuberculosis. Persons with compromised immune systems, however, are less able to fight off the active disease once inhaled. The latter is generally the case among jail and prison inmates who represent a high-risk population as a result of multiple factors related to TB exposure.

There is also a more dangerous form of tuberculosis known as multiple drug resistant tuberculosis (MDR-TB). Typically, a person infected with TB is treated with medication that is taken for six months to one year (Koehler 1994). If the patient discontinues their medication before the treatment regime is complete, the infection can reappear. When TB recurs, it is often resistant to medication and extremely difficult to treat. This form of tuberculosis infection is transmitted in the same manner as non-MDR-TB. It is for this reason that timely treatment and proper follow-up care is necessary for TB patients in general and inmate populations in particular. Special challenges arise when inmates are diagnosed and begin treatment upon entering the correctional system if their institutional stay is short. It is likely that they will have limited access to health/medical care upon release, thus increasing the chances of contracting and transmitting MDR-TB and endangering the health of those with whom they come into contact.

Treatment and Prevention Strategies

The initial treatment of TB is addressed by administering a course of drug therapy for at least six months (Ridzon 2004). Completion of drug treatment is necessary to ensure that inmates do not experience a recurrence of TB, continue to transmit the infection, and/or develop a drug-resistant form of tuberculosis (MDR-TB) (Hammett et al. 1999). Since inmates are confined while in custody, and nursing staff typically administer medication to each inmate, this treatment follows the World Health Organization's method of Directly Observed Therapy (DOTS) whereby TB patients are watched by the practitioner to assure they are taking their medicines. As mentioned earlier, however, administering drug treatment to jail inmates whose length of stay is relatively short may be problematic, as many may not complete the drug therapy once released. In addition to medication non-compliance, inmates are sometimes shuffled between jails or prisons, worsening the situation. And, in some cases medical information may not be transferred. As a result, treatment is delayed. Also, there may not be a coordinated effort by the correctional facility with the local public health department to assure the discharged inmates continue to take the prescribed TB medication. TB is a reportable disease in the U.S. (a disease that must be reported to authorities after detection), and it is a crime not to take the full course of treatment. Individuals not taking their medications may be quarantined. Riccardi (2007) reports about a Maricopa County, Arizona man with a drug-resistant form of TB who had been jailed for nine months because he was not complying with treatment.

Tuberculosis Screening and Interventions

In some cases, infection control staff within correctional facilities may attempt to prevent the spread of TB. This is accomplished by screening inmates, utilizing preventative drug therapy, and isolating symptomatic TB-infected inmates. Other prevention strategies include discharge planning and public health education (Hammett et al. 1999; Wilcock et al. 1996). Screening strategies—symptom screening, PPD skin test, and chest x-rays—are effective tools for identifying inmates with TB infection. Screening inmates upon admission to the jail/prison facility allows correctional staff to identify and contain potential health threats as soon as possible (Gadkowski and Stout 2006). When TB-contagious inmates are admitted and are not identified as infected, the health of other inmates and correctional staff is at risk.

Inmates who have TB, but do not show symptoms of the disease, are given preventative drug therapy to reduce the likelihood of developing active TB (Wilcock et al. 1996). If the infected asymptomatic inmate is not HIV positive, they are given a six-month course of treatment. Seventy-six percent of state and federal prison systems report using preventative drug therapy for inmates with TB infection who do not show signs of disease in order to prevent and contain the spread of tuberculosis (Wilcock et al. 1996).

Once an inmate is diagnosed with TB, they will likely be isolated in a ventilated or reverse air pressure cell so that the potential for transmission is reduced (Hammett et al. 1999). Isolation serves the interests of other inmates as well as correctional workers who are in continuous contact with inmates. A TB-infected inmate may remain in isolation until he/she begins treatment and shows signs of improvement. Isolating inmates with TB can be a costly prevention method, but, as TB is transmitted in an airborne fashion, it is a necessary strategy to limit these outbreaks in crowded correctional settings.

New guidelines on tuberculosis treatment have placed more importance on the role of correctional health care providers. Ridzon (2004: 1) observed that the American Thoracic Society guidelines:

> Strongly emphasizes that 1) the responsibility of successful treatment of TB rests with the provider rather than the patient and 2) case management should be patient-centered, with direct observation of therapy as the strongly preferred method of administration of medicines.

These guidelines suggest patients need considerable support and supervision to ensure that they comply with treatment. It is possible these guidelines were established because one significant hazard with TB treatment is that noncompliance may increase the prevalence of drug resistant strains of TB.

Discharge Planning

Ensuring continuity of care between the correctional facility and the community is often difficult. As a result, medical officials engage in discharge planning prior to the inmate's release from confinement (Hammett et al. 1999). Correctional personnel refer inmates to the public health department, providing the names, locations, and contact information of inmates released from the facility with active TB (Wilcock et al. 1996). These referrals provide important information to public health officials in order to prevent TB and MDR-TB outbreaks in the community. Additionally, notification allows public health departments to follow up with inmates once they are released from correctional supervision. In order to increase medication compliance, medical staff arrange appointments for inmates with community health providers. Referrals to these health providers set up community ties so that infected inmates in need of medical attention related to their TB infection know who to contact for assistance—all of which promotes adherence to TB treatment regimens (Wilcock et al. 1996). Residential instability or homelessness, high rates of addictions and dysfunctional lifestyles will, however, reduce the likelihood that ex-inmates will comply with treatment.

Public Health Education

Like HIV/AIDS, many inmates are unaware of their TB-infection status. Research indicates that inmates also hold misconceptions about the ways in which TB is transmitted, prevented, and treated (Hammett et al. 1999). Misconceptions about airborne transmission may exacerbate the potential for tuberculosis outbreaks both in the confinement facility as well as among the citizen population. Further, when inmates do not understand the differences between TB infection, active TB disease, and drug resistant tuberculosis (MDR-TB), and are not aware of proper treatment/prevention methods, they will be unable to take necessary health and treatment precautions.

Correctional staff have confronted these issues by educating inmates about the lifestyle risks, infection/transmission factors, and drug treatment and prevention strategies related to tuberculosis (Hammett et al. 1999). Because correctional populations are a captive audience, educational programs related to communicable diseases are a surefire way to improve adherence to treatment both during confinement and after inmates are released. Health education or promotion programs for inmates should be sensitive to literacy levels as well as gender and cultural differences. Successful health education will facilitate behavioral change among inmates and reduce the spread of and potential for TB and MDR-TB outbreaks among correctional populations.

Controlling tuberculosis outbreaks in correctional settings is accomplished by paying careful attention to the infected and at-risk populations, providing effective health education, responding quickly to outbreaks, and reinforcing adherence to treatment among inmate populations.

Hepatitis B and C (HBV/HCV) in Correctional Settings

Concern over the hepatitis virus increases as the prison population continues to grow. This is primarily the result of increased infection risks associated with IV drug use, risky sexual behavior, and a rising population of IV drug-using offenders (Macalino et al. 2004; Samuel et al. 2001). Cassidy, Guidry, and Colton (2005:1) reported that rates of the hepatitis C virus HCV among U.S. inmate populations are estimated at 16 to 43 percent of correctional populations and "nearly one-third of all HCV-infected persons pass through correctional facilities each year." There are, however, no national or systematically collected data on the prevalence of hepatitis in U.S. correctional systems—making it difficult to estimate the true rate of infection (Hammett, Harmon, and Rhodes 2002a). Instead, prevalence estimates are derived from studies conducted in specific correctional systems (see Hammett et al., 2002a for a review; Ruiz and Mikanda 1996).[1]

A recent study by the Bureau of Justice Statistics revealed that 31 percent of the 57,018 state prison inmates who were tested were HCV positive (Beck and Maruschak 2004). National prevalence estimates of jail and prison populations indicate that between 17 and 25 percent of inmates are infected with HCV, with some estimates as high as 40 percent (Boutwell, Allen, and Rich 2005; Hammett et al. 2002a, 2002b). Estimates on the prevalence of the hepatitis B virus (HBV) among the incarcerated population ranges from eight to 43 percent (Barry et al. 1990; Crofts et al. 1995; Weild et al. 2000). Additional reports indicate that HBV prevalence is higher among women than among men (see Gondles 2005), especially among those women who have been re-incarcerated (Macalino et al. 2005).

Infection/Transmission

As with other communicable diseases, high-risk infection and transmission behavior is common among inmate populations. The hepatitis B and hepatitis C viruses are highly contagious blood-borne pathogens, meaning they are transmitted through the exchange of infected blood and other bodily fluids. Hepatitis is spread by sharing drug injection equipment such as needles and syringes (Butler et al. 2004; Goldstein et al. 2002; Hammett et al. 2002a; Hammett et al. 1999). This is especially problematic considering the degree to which inmates were drug users prior to their incarceration or engage in IV drug use while in custody and remain unaware of the connection between their high-risk behaviors and viral infection. Further, hepatitis contraction risks include tattooing, body piercing and sexual contact with infected partners[2] (Beck and Maruschak 2004; Goldstein et al. 2002; Kahn et al. 2005), all of which occur at high rates amongst offender populations. Assaults that result in cuts, lacerations, and skin abrasions are also potential transmission risks (Gondles 2005).

Hepatitis B and hepatitis C are both viral diseases that attack the liver and can result in infection, cirrhosis of the liver, cancer, liver failure, and death (Beck and Maruschak 2004). HBV is deemed less serious than HCV because it causes an infection that a healthy body may fight off in a few weeks. If a person is exposed to HBV without contracting an infection, they develop immunity to the virus. Approximately five to ten percent of people infected with HBV develop chronic hepatitis B (Beck and Maruschak 2004). The risk of developing chronic HBV may be higher for jail/prison inmates given their low socioeconomic backgrounds, potential for malnourishment, general lack of good health, and limited access to medical care—all of which influences a body's ability to fight off infection. Fortunately, HBV can be treated with immunization as long as two weeks after exposure. HCV, however, is more threatening, as roughly 80 percent of people infected will develop chronic hepatitis C. HCV is also treatable with antiviral medications and boasts a success rate of 30 to 40 percent (Beck and Maruschak 2004), despite some negative and potentially severe side effects (Allen et al. 2003).

Diagnosis

Screening policies for hepatitis infection vary by institution, and prison systems follow state or federal guidelines. The most common way to diagnose for HCV is by testing a targeted group of inmates such as those who are at high risk, upon inmate request, or as a result of clinical indications that lead medical staff to believe inmates are infected carriers of this disease (Beck and Maruschak 2004). It is less common for correctional institutions to screen all inmates upon admission to the facility or to employ some other type of universal screening—a policy which may prevent the spread of viral infection to other inmates and correctional staff. Serological testing is available for diagnosing the presence of HBV infection. Little information exists regarding the extent to which correctional settings systematically screen inmates for hepatitis B. This may be the result of 1) the widespread availability of HBV vaccinations, 2) correctional system policies to vaccinate inmates (or at least inmates whom correctional staff believe to be at high risk for infection and viral transmission) (Beck and Maruschak 2004), or 3) a lack of funding limiting the routine use of HBV vaccinations (Charuvastra et al. 2001).

Treatment and Prevention Strategies[3]

Currently, hepatitis C can be treated with drug therapy which promises the potential for success, but medications may produce unwanted side effects (Bauman and DeWitt 2007). For example, psychiatric disorders such as depression and suicidal ideation have been reported as a consequence of taking HCV antiviral medications (Allen et al. 2003). Research is sparse regarding the extent to which correctional settings offer treatment regimens to HCV-infected inmates. A recent survey indicates that 70 percent of states operating adult correctional facilities have policies to treat inmates for HCV (Beck and Maruschak 2004), but provides no specific information on the treatment regimens or the number of inmates actually receiving drug therapy. Of those institutions that report having HCV treatment policies (1104), only 14 percent (155) treat all inmates with confirmed cases of HCV infection.

As with other infectious disease drug therapies, treatment for HCV imposes clinical and financial burdens on correctional facilities. Further, correctional medical staff may withhold treatment from inmates who have co-occurring disorders (e.g., HIV and HCV), existing psychiatric problems (depression, post traumatic stress disorder), and substance abuse problems. And, some factors may also influence compliance with treatment such as short-term stays, frequent inter-facility transfers, or unwillingness to cooperate. These factors serve as possible explanations for the lack of universal HCV treatment in correctional jurisdictions (Allen et al. 2003).[4]

Immunization Programs

The widespread availability of the HBV vaccine[5] and the increasingly serious risk of hepatitis infection in U.S. jails/prisons calls for the use of immunization programs in all facilities housing correctional populations as a preventative strategy to stop the spread of HBV (Gondles 2005). Currently, however, only two-thirds of correctional facilities have policies that ensure the immunization of inmates for HBV. Forty-four percent of facilities immunize high-risk inmates, 13 percent immunize inmates upon voluntary request, 12 percent provide universal immunizations or immunize all inmates in the facility, and one percent immunize inmates with sexually transmitted diseases (Beck and Maruschak 2004). As it stands, most correctional institutions do not offer routine or universal HBV vaccination. According to Charuvastra et al. (2001), a universal HBV immunization system is not in place primarily because state and federal prison systems lack adequate financial resources to provide all inmates with vaccinations. If the funds were available, correctional systems would have a better opportunity to prevent and control the spread of hepatitis B.

Admissions Screening

Another potentially effective strategy for controlling the spread of hepatitis C is through the use of admissions screening. Institutions that test inmates for HCV, whether through universal screening strategies or by screening targeted groups (inmate request, high-risk inmates, or through clinical indications), are better able to identify inmates in need of treatment and public education regarding transmission and high-risk behavior. This is especially important in a correctional setting for three reasons. First, most inmates are at high risk for communicable diseases which means jails/prisons are essentially breeding grounds for infections that may be transmitted to the general community when the inmates are released. Second, the majority of inmates have not had the relevant health education necessary to facilitate behavioral change or the health services appropriate for their general wellbeing. Finally, and as previously mentioned, inmates represent a captive audience and the correctional setting is a perfect opportunity to screen, treat, vaccinate, and educate (Fearn and Parker 2005; Franklin et al. 2005; Hammett et al. 1999; Zaitzow and West 2003).

Public Health Education

Public health education is an effective strategy for preventing the spread of communicable diseases in general and hepatitis in particular. Inmates usually have poor literacy skills and little knowledge of public health (see Fox et al. 2005; Franklin et al. 2005; Gondles 2005). More specifically, men and women under correctional supervision are likely unaware of the how viral transmission occurs, what symptoms are related to chronic hepatitis, how the disease progresses, and the long-term health consequences. Further, inmates are unfamiliar with the differences between HCV and HBV, the treatment and vaccination options available to them, and the risks associated with needle sharing, careless sexual practices, and other forms of related contact (Gondles 2005). Providing inmates with information related to safer needle use and sex practices and IV drug use counseling may minimize the risk of HBV transmission both in prison and in the community (Awofeso 2002). Without public health education, most inmates will continue to engage in the same high-risk behaviors that exposed them to disease either before or during their incarceration. Offering prisoners health education in a correctional setting empowers them to change risky behaviors and prepares them for the challenges they face as they reintegrate back into their communities.

Conclusions

Public concern related to the spread of communicable diseases (HIV/AIDS, TB, and HBV and HCV) in jail and prison settings is warranted to the degree that infection prevalence in inmate populations is higher than the general population. With that said, however, there are a host of diagnostic, treatment, and prevention strategies currently being utilized in U.S. correctional settings to stop the spread of communicable diseases. Nonetheless, correctional systems must raise the bar in terms of their treatment and prevention responses to this highly susceptible and potentially infectious population. In other words, current strategies are heading in the right direction, but there is significant room for improvement.

Collaborative programs that bring together state health and correctional agencies in addition to community-based organizations are working to create support systems that aid infected inmates in the transition from prison to community and assist in adherence to treatment once prisoners are released from custody. The health status of inmates and the interests of the general public demand that local and state correctional and health systems develop more of these collaborations.

As the prison population continues to grow, correctional institutions must persist in their efforts toward screening inmates for communicable diseases and providing treatment and health care for a population that would otherwise experience medical neglect—only furthering the spread of infectious diseases to the communities they return to once they are released. Inmates are in desperate need of public health education related to their high-risk behaviors and the potential for disease transmission. Jail and prison settings provide the perfect opportunity to empower these individuals and facilitate behavioral change.

Endnotes

1. California estimates that 41 percent of male and female inmates are carriers for HCV; Connecticut estimates 32 percent of females in Connecticut correctional systems are HCV positive; 38 percent of Maryland's male and female inmates are infected with hepatitis C; and approximately 30 to 40 percent of Washington's male and female inmates report the presence of HCV (see Hammett et al.

2002a for a review).

2. The risk of contracting/transmitting HCV through sexual contact is considered rare as compared to the other ways in which the virus is spread. HBV is contracted most commonly through sexual contact (Hammett et al. 2002a).
3. Other hepatitis prevention programs advocated by European countries and the World Health Organization (WHO) include condom distribution, needle exchange, and the availability of bleach for the purpose of sterilizing injection equipment (see Awofeso 2002). Refer to the above discussion of treatment and prevention strategies under the section discussing HIV/AIDS for more information about these programs.
4. Hepatitis B is treated with immunization (Beck and Maruschak 2004).
5. Currently, there is no vaccine for hepatitis C (Hunziker et al. 2001).

References

Allen, Scott A., Anne C. Spaulding, Albert M. Osei, Lynne E. Taylor, Asya M. Cabral, and Josiah D. Rich. 2003. "Treatment of Chronic Hepatitis C in a State Correctional Facility." *Annals of Internal Medicine* 138:187-190.

Allwright, Shane, Fiona Bradley, Jean Long, Joseph Barry, Lelia Thornton, and John V. Parry. 2000. "Prevalence of Antibodies to Hepatitis B, Hepatitis C, and HIV and Risk Factors in Irish Prisoners: Results of a National Cross Sectional Survey." *British Medical Journal* 328:78-82.

Amankwaa, Adansi A., Al Bavon, and Linda C. Amankwaa. 2001. "Gaps Between HIV/AIDS Policies and Treatment in Correctional Facilities." *Journal of Health and Human Service Administration* 24:171-198.

Ashkin, David and Jean Malecki. 2005. "Tuberculosis Outbreak Among Staff in Correctional Facilities, Florida, 2001-2004: Lessons Re-learned." *Infectious Diseases in Corrections Report* 8:1-4.

Awofeso, Niyi. 2002. "Hepatitis B Vaccination in Prisons." *Bulletin of the World Health Organization* 80:569-574.

Barnes, S. E., G. L. White Jr., P. W. Sharkey, and C. J. Parkman. 1992. "Pulmonary Tuberculosis Resurgence after Near Eradication." *Clinician Reviews* 3:69-93.

Barry, Michael A., D. Gleavey, Karen Herd, Pamela J. Schwingl, and Barbara G. Werner. 1990. "Prevalence of Markers for Hepatitis B and Hepatitis D in a Municipal House of Correction." *American Journal of Public Health* 80:471-473.

Bauman, Kay A. and Steven K. DeWitt. 2007. "Managing the Side Effects of Hepatitis C Treatment in a Correctional Environment." *Infectious Diseases in Corrections* Report 9: 1-5.

Beck, Allen J. and Laura M. Maruschak. 2004. Hepatitis Testing and Treatment in State Prisons, Special Report. Washington, DC: Department of Justice, Bureau of Justice Statistics.

Behrendt, C., N. Kendig, and C. Dambita. 1994. "Voluntary Testing for HIV in a Prison Population with High HIV Prevalence." *American Journal of Epidemiology* 139:918-926.

Berman-Davis, Jennifer and Debra Brown. 1990. "AIDS Knowledge and Risky Behavior by Incarcerated Females: IV and Non-IV Drug users." *Sociology and Social Research* 75:816.

Bick, Joseph. 2004. "Letter From The Editor." *HIV & Hepatitis Education Prison Project 3.*

Boutwell, Amy E., Scott A. Allen, and Josiah D. Rich. 2005. "Opportunities to Address the Hepatitis C Epidemic in the Correctional Setting." *Clinical Infectious Diseases* 40:S367-S372.

Blumberg, Mark and J. Dennis Laster. 1999. "The Impact of HIV/AIDS on Corrections." Pp. 574-591 in *The Dilemmas of Corrections: Contemporary Readings*, edited by K. C. Haas and G. P. Alpert. Prospect Heights, IL: Waveland Press, Inc.

Butler, Tony, Azar Kariminia, Michael Levy, and John Kaldor. 2004. "Prisons are at Risk for Hepatitis C Transmission." *European Journal of Epidemiology* 19:1119-1122.

Charuvastra, Anothony, Julie Stein, Beth Schwartzapfel, Anne Spaulding, Evalyn Horowitz, Grace Macalino, and Josiah D. Rich. 2001. "Hepatitis B Vaccination Practices in State and Federal Prisons." *Public Health Reports* 116:203-209.

Crofts, Nick, Tony Stewart, Peter Hearne, Xin Yi Ping, Alan M. Breschkin, and Stephen A. Locarnini. 1995. "Spread of Bloodborne Viruses among Australian Prison Entrants." *British Medical Journal* 310:285-288.

Darke, Shane, Sharlene Kaye, and Robert Finlay-Jones. 1998. "Drug Use and Injection Risk-Taking among Prison Methadone Maintenance Patients." *Addiction* 93:1169-1175.

Decker, Scott H. and Richard Rosenfeld. 1992. "Intravenous Drug Use and the AIDS Epidemic: Findings from a 20 City Sample of Arrestees." *Crime & Delinquency* 38:492-509.

Deeks, Steven G., M. Smith, Mark Holodniy, and James O. Kahn. 1997. "HIV-1 Protease Inhibitors: A Review for Clinicians." *Journal of the American Medical Association* 277:145-153.

Dolan, Kate and Alex Wodak. 1996. "An International Review of Methadone Provision in Prisons." *Addiction Research* 4:85-97

Dolan, Kate, Wayne Hall, and Alex D. Wodak. 1996. "Methadone Maintenance Reduces Injecting in Prison." *British Journal of Medicine* 312:1162.

Dolan, Kate, Scott Rutter, and Alex D. Wodak. 2003. "Prison-Based Syringe Exchange Programmes: A Review of International Research and Development." *Addiction* 98:153-158.

Ehrmann, Tanya. 2002. "Community-Based Organizations and HIV Prevention for Incarcerated Populations: Three HIV Prevention Program Models." *AIDS Education and Prevention* 14:75-84.

Fearn, Noelle E. and Kelly Parker. 2005. "Health Care for Women Inmates: Issues, Perceptions, and Policy Considerations." *Californian Journal of Health Promotion* 3(2):1-22.

Fox, Rena K., Sue L. Currie, Jennifer Evans, Teresa L. Wright, Leslie Tobler, Bruce Phelps, Michael P. Busch, and Kimberly A. Page-Shafer. 2005. "Hepatitis C Virus Infection Among Prisoners in the California State Correctional System." *Clinical Infectious Diseases* 41:177-186.

Franklin, Cortney A., Noelle E. Fearn, and Travis W. Franklin. 2005. "HIV/AIDS among Female Prison Inmates: A Public Health Concern." *Californian Journal of Health Promotion* 3(2):99-112.

Frost, Lizz and Vladimir Tchertkov. 2002. "Prisoner Risk Taking in the Russian Federation." *AIDS Education and Prevention* 14:7-23.

Gadkowski, L. Beth and Jason E. Stout. 2006. "Tuberculosis in Corrections." *Infectious Diseases in Corrections Report* 9:1-6.

Gellert, G., R. Maxwell, K. Higgins, T. Pendergast, and N. Wilker. 1993. "HIV Infection in the Women's Jail, Orange County, California, 1985-1991." *American Journal of Public Health* 83:1454-1456.

Goldstein, Susan T., Miriam J. Alter, Ian T. Williams, Linda A. Moyer, Franklyn N. Judson, Karen Mottram, Michael Fleenor, Patricia L. Ryder, and Harold S. Margolis. 2002. "Incidence and Risk Factors for Acute Hepatitis B in the United States, 1982-1998: Implications for Vaccination Programs." *The Journal of Infectious Diseases* 185:713-719.

Gondles, Elizabeth F. 2005. "A Call to Immunize the Correctional Population for Hepatitis A and B." *The American Journal of Medicine* 118:845-895.

Grimm, Julie A. 2006. "Stop the Revolving Door: Program Helps Those Behind Bars Cope With Heroin Addiction." *The Santa Fe New Mexican*, March 17, 2006.

Grinstead, Olga A., Barry Zack, and Bonnie Faigeles. 1999. "Collaborative Research to Prevent HIV among Male Prison Inmates and their Female Partners." *Health Education and Behavior* 26:225-238.

Guyon, Louise, Serge Brochu, Isabelle Parent, and Lyne Desjardins. 1999. "At-Risk Behaviors with regard to HIV and Addiction among Women in Prison." *Women and Health* 29:49-66.

Hammett, Theodore M. 1998. *Public Health/Corrections Collaborations: Prevention and Treatment of HIV/AIDS, STDs, and TB: Research in Brief.* Washington, DC: U.S. Department of Justice, Office of Justice Programs, National Institute of Justice.

Hammett, Theodore, Mary Patricia Harmon, and Laura M. Maruschak. 1999. 1996-1997 *Update: HIV/AIDS, STDs, and TB in Correctional Facilities.* Washington, DC: U.S. Department of Justice, Office of Justice Programs, National Institute of Justice.

Hammett, Theodore, Lynne Harold, Michael Gross, and Joel Epstein. 1994. 1992 *Update: HIV/AIDS in Correctional Facilities: Issues and Options.* Washington, DC: U. S. Department of Justice, National Institute of Justice and Centers for Disease Control Prevention.

Hammett, Theodore, Mary Patricia Harmon, and William Rhodes. 2002a. "The Burden of Infectious Disease Among Inmates and Releasees from Correctional Facilities." Pp. 13-37 in *The Health Care Needs of Soon-To-Be Released Inmates: Report to the U.S. Congress.* National Institute of Justice. Chicago, IL: National Commission on Correctional Health Care.

------. 2002b. "The Burden of Infectious Disease Among Inmates of and Releasees from U.S. Correctional Facilities, 1997." *American Journal of Public Health* 92:1789-1794.

Harlow, Catherine W. 1993. *HIV in U.S. Prison and Jails.* Washington, DC: U.S. Department of Justice, Bureau of Justice Statistics, Special Report.

Heimer, Robert, Holly Catania, Robert G. Newman, John Zambrano, Arlyn Brunet, and Arturo Marti Ortiz. 2005. "Methadone Maintenance in Prison: Evaluation of a Pilot Program in Puerto Rico. *Drug and Alcohol Dependence* 83:122-129.

Hunziker, I. P., R. Zurbriggen, R. Glueck, O. B. Engler, J. Reichen, W. J. Dai, W. J. Pichler, and A. Cerny. 2001. "Perspectives: Towards a Peptide-Based Vaccine Against Hepatitis C Virus." *Molecular Immunology* 38:475-484.

Infectious Diseases in Corrections Report. 2006. "News and Literature Reviews: HIV Costs Have Decreased." *Infectious Diseases in Corrections* 9:8.

Jacob Arriola, Kimberly R., Braithwaite, Ronald L., and Cassandra Newkirk. 2006. "At the Intersection Between Poverty, Race, and HIV Infection: HIV-Related Services for Incarcerated Women." *Infectious Diseases in Corrections* Report 9:1-5.

Kahn, Amy J., Edgar P. Simard, William A. Bower, Health L. Wurtzel, Marina Khristova, Karla D. Wagner, Kathryn E. Arnold, Omana V. Nalnan, Madeleine LaMarre, and Beth P. Bell. 2005. "Ongoing Transmission of Hepatitis B Virus Infection among Inmates at a State Correctional Facility." *American Journal of Public Health* 95:1793-1799.

Kassira, Edward N., Robert L. Bauserman, Naomi Tomoyasu, Ellen Caldeira, Anthony Swetz, and Liza Solomon. 2001. "HIV and AIDS Surveillance among Inmates in Maryland Prisons." *Journal of Urban Health: Bulletin of the New York Academy of Medicine* 78:256-263.

Koehler, Richard J. 1994. "HIV Infection, TB, and the Health Crisis in Corrections." *Public Administration Review* 54:31-35.

Leh, Sandra K. 1999. "HIV Infection in the U.S. Correctional Systems: Its Effect on the Community." *Journal of Community Health Nursing* 16:53-63.

Leigh, B.C. 1990. "Venus gets my Thinking: Drinking and Female Sexuality in the Age of AIDS." *Journal of Substance Abuse* 2:129-145.

Lipton, Douglas S. 2002. "HIV/AIDS and the Correctional System." Pp. 86-95 in *Correctional Perspectives: Views from Academics, Practitioners, and Prisoners,* edited by L. F. Alarid and P. F. Cromwell. Los Angeles, CA: Roxbury.

Lurigio, Arthur J., James A. Swartz, and Ciuinal Jones. 2003. "HIV Disease and Women Offenders." Pp. 152-171 in *It's a Crime: Women and Justice,* edited by R. Muraskin. Englewood Cliffs, NJ: Prentice Hall.

Macalino, Grace E., David Vlahov, Brian P. Dickinson, Beth Schwartzapfel, and Josiah D. Rich. 2005. "Community Incidence of Hepatitis B and C among Reincarcerated Women." *Clinical Infectious Diseases* 41:998-1002.

Macalino, Grace E., David Vlahov, Stephanie Sanford-Colby, Sarju Patel, Keith Sabin, Christopher Salas, and Josiah D. Rich. 2004. "Prevalence and Incidence of HIV, Hepatitis B Virus, and Hepatitis C Virus among Males in Rhode Island Prisons." *American Journal of Public Health* 94:1218-1223.

MacDonald, Morag. 2005. *Study of the Health Care Provision, Existing Drug Services and Strategies Operating in Prisons in Ten Countries From Central and Eastern Europe*. Helsinki, Finland: United Nations European Institute for Crime Prevention and Control.

MacNeil, Jessica R., Mark N. Lobato, and Marisa Moore. 2005. "An Unanswered Health Disparity: Tuberculosis Among Correctional Inmates, 1993-2003." *American Journal of Public Health* 95:1800-1805.

Mahon, N. 1996. "New York Inmates' HIV Risk Behaviors: The Implications for Prevention Policy and Programs." *American Journal of Public Health* 86:1211-1215.

Marquart, James M., Victoria E. Brewer, Janet Mullings, and Ben M. Crouch. 1999. "The Implications of Crime Control Policy on HIV/AIDS Related Risk among Women Prisoners." *Crime & Delinquency* 45:82-98.

Martin Medical Services. 2002. "Peer Education Programs Reach Far Beyond Correctional Walls, Benefiting Offenders, Ex-offenders and Public Health." *Positive Populations* 3:1-12.

Maruschak, Laura M. 2006. HIV in Prisons, 2004. Washington, DC: U.S. Department of Justice, Office of Justice Programs.

Mitchell, Clifford S., Robyn R.M. Gershon, Mary Kathleen Lears, David Vlahov, Sarah Felknor, Rebecca A. Lubelczyk, Martin F. Sherman, and George W. Comstock. 2005. "Risk of Tuberculosis in Correctional Healthcare Workers." *Journal of Occupational and Environmental Medicine* 47:580-586.

Morash, Merry and Pamela J. Schram 2002. *The Prison Experience: Special Issues of Women in Prison*. Prospect Heights, IL: Waveland Press, Inc.

Oser, Carrie B., Michele Staton Tindall, and Carl G. Leukefeld. 2007. "HIV Testing in Correctional Agencies and Community Treatment Programs: The Impact of Internal Organizational Structure." *Journal of Substance Abuse Treatment* 32: 301-310.

Pollock, Jocelyn M. 2004. *Prisons and Prison life: Costs and Consequences*. Los Angeles, CA: Roxbury.

------. 2002. Women, Prison, and Crime. Belmont, CA: Wadsworth Thompson Learning.

Reichard, Audrey A., Mark N. Lobato, Cheryl A. Roberts, Lauri B. Bazerman, and Theodore M. Hammett. 2003. "Assessment of Tuberculosis Screening and Management Practices of Large Jail Systems." *Public Health Reports* 118:500-507.

Riccardi, Nicholas. 2007 "TB patient jailed after not following doctor's orders." *Los Angeles Times*. Retrieved May 5, 2007 (www.latimes.com)

Rosen, David L., Victor J. Schoenbach, and Andrew H. Kaplan. 2006. "HIV Testing in State Prisons: Balancing Human Rights and Public Health. *Infectious Disease In Corrections Report* 9:1-5.

Rotily, Michel, Caren Weilandt, Sheila M. Bird, Kerstin Kall, Harry J.A. Van Haastrecht, Emma Landolo, and Sylvette Rousseau. 2001. "Surveillance of HIV Infection and Related Risk Behavior in European Prisons." *European Journal of Public Health* 11:243-250.

Ruiz, Juan D. and John Mikanda. 1996. *Seroprevalence of HIV, Hepatitis B, Hepatitis C, and Risk Behaviors Among Inmates Entering the California Correctional System*. California Department of Health Services, Office of AIDS, HIV/AIDS Epidemiology Office.

Samuel, M. C., P. M. Doherty, M. Bulterys, and S. A. Jenison. 2001. "Association between Heroin Use, Needle Sharing and Tattoos Received in Prison with Hepatitis B and C Positivity among Street-Recruited Injecting Drug Users in New Mexico, USA." *Epidemiology and Infection* 127:475-484.

Simmons, Thomas M. 2004. "Inmate Peer Education Programs: 101." *Infectious Diseases In Corrections Report* 7:6-7.

Struckman-Johnson, Cindy, David Struckman-Johnson, Lila Rucker, Kurt Bumby, and Stephen Donaldson. 1996. "Sexual Coercion Reported by Men and Women in Prison." *Journal of Sex Research* 33:67-76.

Tewksbury, Richard, Gennaro F. Vito and Scott Cummings. 1998. "Injection Drug Users and HIV Risk Behaviors: Criminal Justice Professionals' Role in Identifying and Responding to Risk Behaviors." *Journal of Crime and Justice* 21:1-22.

Warren, Emma, Rosalie Viney, James Shearer, Marian Shanahan, Alex Wodak, and Kate Dolan. 2006. "Value for Money in Drug Treatment: Economic Evaluation of Prison Methadone." *Drug and Alcohol Dependence* 84:160-166.

Weild, A. R., O. N. Gil, D. Bennett, S. J. M. Livingstone, J. V. Parry, and L.Curran. 2000. "Prevalence of HIV, Hepatitis B, and Hepatitis C Antibodies in Prisoners in England and Wales: A National Survey." *Communicable Diseases in Public Health* 3:121-126.

Wilcock, Karen, Theodore M. Hammett, and Dale G. Parent. 1995. *Controlling Tuberculosis in Community Corrections.* Washington, DC: U. S. Department of Justice, Office of Justice Programs.

Wilcock, Karen. Theodore M. Hammett, Rebecca Widom, and Joel Epstein. 1996. *Tuberculosis in Correctional Facilities, 1994-1995.* Washington DC: U. S. Department of Justice, Office of Justice Programs.

Wohl, David A. 2006. "Special Report: Transmission of HIV Within a State Prison." *Infectious Diseases in Corrections Report* 9:1-2.

Young, Vernetta D. and Rebecca Reviere. 2001. "Meeting the Health Care Needs of the New Woman Inmate: A National Survey of Prison Practices." *Journal of Offender Rehabilitation* 34:31-38.

Zach, Barry, Timothy Flanigan, and Pamela DeCarlo. 2000. *What is the Role of Prisons in HIV, Hepatitis, STD and TB Prevention?* San Francisco, CA: Center for AIDS Prevention Studies.

Zaitzow, Barbara H. and Angela D. West. 2003. "Doing Time in the Shadow of Death: Women Prisoners and HIV/AIDS." Pp. 73-90 in *The Incarcerated Woman: Rehabilitative Programming in Women's Prisons,* edited by S. Sharp. Upper Saddle River, NJ: Prentice Hall.

CHAPTER FIVE

Civil Liability When Dental Care Is Denied to Inmates in Correctional Facilities

Clarissa F. Dias and Michael S. Vaughn

While dental care is a critical component of overall quality health care, many prisoners enter correctional facilities in the United States with little history of good dental hygiene and even less history of access to dentists for routine dental examinations. As a result, the incarceration experience presents opportunities for inmates to receive quality dental care, often for the first time in their lives. Care delivered by correctional dentists is complicated, however, by the array of serious dental conditions and difficult to treat cases in clinical settings. These conditions exist within a legal environment that mandates the state provide adequate dental care to prisoners. This chapter examines prisoner lawsuits, claiming that denying of dental care violates inmates' statutory and constitutional rights. The discussion focuses on what the courts in the U.S. have required of correctional officials in the form of dental care and when officials are most likely to be held liable for issues associated with dental care lawsuits.

The American Dental Association (2002) sets minimal standards for basic dental care, including preventative maintenance, pain relief, infection control, and preservation and restoration of natural teeth. In free-world dentistry, preservation and restoration of natural teeth are paramount (Lewis 1996). Preservation of natural teeth shows a commitment to overall oral health as part of a comprehensive approach to individuals' well-being and health (Friedman 1990). Routine care includes regular cleanings, consultations with oral hygienists, filling cavities as early as possible and early diagnostic and treatment of dental problems (Doring 2004).

Previous research shows little standardization across prison systems regarding the level of dental care provided to prisoners (Boyer, Nielsen, Thompson, and Hill 2002). The care that exists is primarily determined by a patchwork of national court decisions, consent decrees at the state and local levels, government officials contracting out medical services, professionals working within correctional systems, and accrediting bodies that develop guidelines and standards of professional practice (National Commission on Correctional Health Care [NCCHC] 2003a, 2003b). This individualized case-by-case approach has not resulted in correctional dental care being the subject of large-scale examination by scholarly studies; however, adequate dental care, similar to medical care, is a guaranteed constitutional right under *Estelle v. Gamble* for pretrial detainees and prison inmates.

In modern prisons, many of the most systemic problems with delivery of dental care have been remediated by court decisions, professionalism within the corrections field, and responsible administrators (James 2004). Standards of practice articulated by the NCCHC (2003a, 2003b), American Correctional Association (2003), and the American Public Health Association (2003) require mandatory preventive oral hygiene, periodic check-ups, and regular prophylactic care. Despite the existence of such guidelines, when inmates with poor oral health are sent to correctional environments, limited dental care is the norm because many of their oral health conditions are irreversible. In fact, previous research indicates inmates often have little history of preventive dental care and teeth that are in borderline condition are not considered salvageable (Ormes, Carolyn, Thompson, and Brim 1997). Presented with inmates that have little real commitment to their oral health and few assurances inmates will have access to routine dental care upon release, as a solution to these problems, correctional dentists frequently either extract teeth or provide limited restorative intervention to borderline salvageable teeth (Frencken, Pilot, Songpaisan and Phantumvanit 1996; Ramos-Rodriguez, Schwartz, Rogers, and Alos 2004).

As a result, research shows that correctional dental practice extracts too many teeth and generally does not adhere to national standards of care established by accrediting agencies (Vaughn and Smith 1999). Indeed, dentists have been accused of being unsympathetic to disadvantaged groups who have not had access to preventative dental care (Balsa and McGuire 2003). In 2005, United States District Court Judge Thelton E. Henderson visited the "broken medical system" at San Quentin Prison. Judge Henderson personally observed that the "main medical examining room lacked any means of sanitation—there was no sink and no alcohol [cleaning solution]—where roughly 100 men per day undergo medical screening." Judge Henderson was particularly shocked when he saw that the prison dentist neither washed his hands nor changed gloves after treating patients into whose mouths he had placed his hands" (*Plata v. Schwarzenegger*). If this sort of dysfunctional dental care system becomes institutionalized, resulting in salvageable teeth being denied legitimate dental care, the practice can result in more litigation and lawsuits filed by inmates, seeking to remedy perceived dental indifference.

This chapter explores correctional dental care lawsuits filed by inmates under Section 1983.[1] It focuses on denying dental care for inmates, the consequences of such denial, and the harms associated with such practices. After discussing the methodology employed to find and record the cases from the U.S. Court of Appeals from 1980 to 2005, the article applies the U.S. Supreme Court's legal standard of deliberate indifference established in 1976 by *Estelle v. Gamble* to Federal Circuit Court of Appeals cases involving serious dental needs. Case outcomes are organized into different sections, depending on whether the plaintiff or the defendant prevailed in the litigation.

The chapter shows that the care provided to detainees and inmates must be defensible by the dental profession. Care must be grounded in the professional dental judgment of the correctional health care provider. Correctional officials and dentists cannot deny prisoners supplies for basic oral hygiene, care by retaliating against inmates for exercising their constitutional rights to file grievances or lawsuits. Also, they cannot deny care that was ordered or prescribed by a physician or by a dentist, and/or deny treatment for serious dental injuries or illnesses. Dental care may sometimes be inadequate because prisoners have no rights to pick their own dental care provider, to have their teeth cleaned on a routine schedule, or to object to policies that lead to tooth extraction as long as those policies are defensible in the dental profession.

Methods

Under federal law, the Eighth Amendment to the United States Constitution prohibits cruel and unusual punishment. Inmates may seek remedies for violations of federal law pursuant to Title 42 U.S. Code Section 1983. Under *Estelle v. Gamble*, for example, the U.S. Supreme Court established the standard of deliberate indifference to serious medical needs for Section 1983 liability for all medical care lawsuits, including dental care causes of action. Cases in this article were found by searching the Westlaw online computerized database. Cases from the U.S. Circuit Courts of Appeals from January 1, 1980 to March 9, 2005 were identified by using the following search strategy "dental or dentist with prison or jail," resulting in the identification of 144 relevant cases pertaining to Section 1983 lawsuits. The 21 cases in this article pertaining to denial of dental care were drawn from the larger pool of 144 cases.

U.S. Supreme Court Precedent Pertaining to Prison Medical Care

In *Estelle v. Gamble*, J. W. Gamble, an inmate in the Texas Department of Corrections, filed a Section 1983 lawsuit against prison officials, alleging that his Eighth Amendment rights were violated because the defendants failed to provide adequate medical care. Gamble was injured while unloading a prison truck full of cotton. After Gamble received medical treatment, prison doctors prescribed medication, recommended work restriction for two days, and allowed him to eat in his cell.

Because he was not satisfied with his treatment, Gamble sued; where upon the district court dismissed the lawsuit, ruling that Gamble failed to state a cause of action. The U.S. Court of Appeals for the Fifth Circuit reversed the lower court's decision, reinstating Gamble's lawsuit. The U.S. Supreme Court also reversed, holding that the district court properly dismissed Gamble's complaint because he failed to show that prison officials acted with deliberate indifference to his serious medical needs. According to the Supreme Court, only inadequate medical care that rises to deliberate indifference violates the cruel and unusual punishment clause of the Eighth Amendment. The Court also held that medical malpractice is not deliberate indifference; therefore, medical negligence or the lack of adherence to national standards of care is not a constitutional violation that can be litigated under Section 1983. Only prison officials' acts or omissions that are sufficiently harmful to evidence deliberate indifference to serious medical needs run afoul of evolving standards of decency (*Trop v. Dulles*) triggering an Eighth Amendment violation.

While the Supreme Court adopted the deliberate indifference standard in Gamble, it took 18 years for them to precisely define the concept in *Farmer v. Brennan*. In this case the Court clarified the level of culpability needed to hold officials liable via deliberate indifference. Deliberate indifference occurs when prison officials have knowledge of a substantial risk of harm and recklessly disregard that risk. To prove prison officials acted with deliberate indifference, inmates must show that prison officials had knowledge of a substantial risk of harm and recklessly disregarded that awareness. The Court limited deliberate indifference allegations to prison officials' response to a substantial risk, but cautioned that merely to find that a reasonable person would have known, or should have known, does not constitute deliberate indifference. In sum, prison administrators are liable if they know of a risk to inmate health or safety and intentionally ignore that risk through their acts or omissions.

Section 1983 Cases on Denial of Dental Care Litigated in the U.S. Courts of Appeals: The Inmate Prevails

The cases below highlight the failure of correctional personnel to provide minimum conditions of confinement through the denial of dental care, thus leading to constitutional violations. Prison officials and health care providers are liable when they do not provide inmates with basic oral hygiene items, refuse to provide dental care in retaliation of inmates' filing grievances and lawsuits, deny inmates dental care prescribed by a physician or by a dentist, and decline inmates' requests to be treated from serious dental injury or illness.

Denial of Basic Oral Hygiene Supplies

Basic hygiene is an important part of oral health (Danner 2003; Schwartz 2003). One of the most fundamental daily hygiene activities involves the use of fluoride-based toothpaste while brushing teeth (ADA 2004). Prison officials have a legal duty to provide pretrial detainees and prison inmates' basic dental hygiene items such as toothpaste and soft round-bristle toothbrushes (NCCHC 2003a, 2003b). Failure to do so may lead to constitutional deprivations. Such was the case in *Penrod v. Zavaras*, in which an inmate brought a Section 1983 lawsuit against prison officials, alleging he was denied toothpaste for two months. Inmate Donald Penrod asserted that his constitutional rights were violated because the denial of toothpaste caused his gums to bleed and recede, and eventually contributed to tooth decay that had to be treated by a dentist.

The U.S. Court of Appeals for the Tenth Circuit held that conditions of confinement must be guided by "contemporary standards of decency" (*Estelle v. Gamble*); therefore, prison officials can be held liable under the Eighth Amendment for denying "humane conditions of confinement" (*Farmer v. Brennan*). Although the constitution is only violated if the inmate can show deliberate indifference, meaning that the alleged deprivations were objectively and sufficiently serious, and that prison officials disregarded the seriousness of the inmate's dental needs, the Tenth Circuit opined that the plaintiff raised a genuine issue of material fact with respect to whether prison officials caused plaintiff serious harm by failing to satisfy his basic hygienic needs.

Brushing the teeth at least twice a day—after breakfast and before bed—with fluoride toothpaste that is approved by the National Dental Association is the basis of dental hygiene that prevents caries (tooth decay) or erosions (Cameron, Moss, Till, Johnsen, and Douglas 1997). As a result, correctional facilities must provide sufficient oral hygiene supplies under the Eighth Amendment. In *Board v. Farnham*, plaintiffs Hebert and Jerome Board filed a lawsuit under Section 1983, alleging that they were deprived of basic hygiene supplies during their incarceration in the Edgar County (Illinois) Jail. Jerome Board claimed that he did not have toothpaste during most of his period of detention. Similarly, Hebert Board claimed that he too was also denied toothpaste for three-and-a-half weeks, although several requests for toothpaste were made. The plaintiff Hebert Board also claimed that this deprivation caused him to incur tooth decay, which resulted later in the removal of several of his teeth.

Citing *Helling v. McKinney*, the U.S. Court of Appeals for the Seventh Circuit ruled that "the Eighth Amendment protects a detainee not only from deliberate indifference to his or her current health problems, but also from deliberate indifference to conditions posing an 'unreasonable risk of serious damage to future health'" (*Board v. Farnham*). In addition, the Seventh Circuit disagreed with the defendant, who claimed that the detainees were not protected under the Eighth Amendment. The court stated that "although the Eighth Amendment does not apply to pre-trial detainees, pretrial detainees are entitled to at least as much protection as the constitution provides convicted prisoners" (*Board v. Farnham*). In fact, the Eighth Amendment protects an inmate from governmental deliberate indifference to his or her basic dental needs. The court concluded that a jury could find that Farnham had knowledge of plaintiff Herbert Board's lack of toothpaste and was "aware of the damage that such a deprivation was causing" (*Board v. Farnham*).

The U.S. Supreme Court in *Rhodes v. Chapman* held that prison officials are required to provide inmates with the "minimum civilized measure of life's necessities," and, when prison officials fail to provide toothpaste and a toothbrush for extended time periods they deny inmates their basic rights to sanitation and hygiene. In another case, *James v. O'Sullivan,* an inmate brought a Section 1983 action against prison officials, alleging that he was denied personal hygiene items, such as a toothbrush and toothpaste, thus violating his constitutional rights. The plaintiff claimed that he spent 49 days in segregation. While in isolation, James made several requests to correctional officers for the provision of toothpaste and a toothbrush, although none of the requests were granted. Ruling on the lawsuit filed by James, the U.S. Court of Appeals for the Seventh Circuit held that there was a genuine issue of material fact of whether withholding a toothbrush and toothpaste over an extended period of time—in this case 49 days—jeopardized basic sanitation and hygiene. The court vacated the dismissal of the plaintiff's cruel and unusual punishment claims, and remanded the case back to the district court for further proceedings.

Summary of Denial of Basic Oral Hygiene Supplies

Research shows that brushing teeth with fluoride-based toothpaste is one of the most effective ways to fight dental decay (Chrisman 1989). In addition, bad oral hygiene is responsible for unleashing bacteria into the body, thus promoting the occurrence of other problems, such as diabetes, stroke, heart disease, and even early delivery and low birth weight (Gura 1998). Subsequently, courts have ruled that basic oral hygiene supplies are a constitutional requirement of correctional dental care, which prison officials and health care providers are obligated to provide.

Denying Dental Care in Retaliation of Inmates' Filing Complaints, Grievances, and/or Lawsuits

Courts have ruled that it is an unconstitutional form of retaliation when prison officials threaten inmates with punishment when prisoners file grievances complaining about a lack of dental care *(Badea v. Moran)*. Inmates have a constitutional right to inform staff of their need for dental care (*Hoptowit v. Ray*). The U.S. Supreme Court in Estelle v. Gamble ruled that medical decisions based on the professional judgment of the health care providers are not actionable under Section 1983. Hence, if an inmate can prove that a dental treatment decision was not based on clinical indicators or dental expertise, the inmate may then be able to sue for constitutional violations. Such was the case in *Mitchell v. Duckworth,* in which James Mitchell, an inmate at Pendleton Correctional Facility, brought a Section 1983 action, alleging that the prison dentist had violated his Eighth Amendment right by refusing to prescribe a soft mechanical diet (SMD) as retaliation for a state-court malpractice action filed against the prison dentist.

At the time of his admission into the correctional facility, Mitchell lacked several teeth, he had sore and bloody gums, and he was not capable of chewig regular food. After reviewing his condition, the prison dentist prescribed a SMD of boiled and baked foods. Mitchell was told that because of his lack of mouth bones, he could not be fitted with a lower denture. The prison dentist recommended keeping the inmate on the SMD. After Mitchell filed a tort claim for malpractice, the prison dentist threatened to discontinue the SMD unless Mitchell withdrew the tort claim. In return, Mitchell filed grievances against the prison dentist, who in response stopped the SMD. The U.S. Court of Appeals for the Seventh Circuit reversed the district court's initial ruling siding with the prison dentist, saying that the dentist acted outside his professional medical judgment, which was in violation of the Eighth Amendment.

Research shows that inmates complain about every aspect associated with their incarceration experience (Lombardo 1989). These complaints often take the form of filing lawsuits and prison grievances, and actions such as contacting media representatives to expose prison conditions (Farkas 1999). In some situations, prison officials and dental providers retaliate against inmates who have complained about their dental care (Maeve and Vaughn 2001). Retaliation in the form of denying inmates dental care for exercising their constitutional rights has been recognized by courts as a cause of action under Section 1983 (Vaughn 1995; Vaughn and Carroll 1998). Courts rule that prison officials who deny "necessary treatment to a prisoner for non-medical reasons may exhibit deliberate indifference" (*Farrow v. West*). Such was the case in *Kinney v. Kalfus*, where a Section 1983 lawsuit was brought against the prison dentist because the dentist had denied the inmate dental care in retaliation for a malpractice lawsuit previously filed by the inmate Kinney. During his release on parole, Kinney consulted a free world dentist who diagnosed his serious dental needs. The free world dentist recommended that the patient's upper left molar be extracted, his cavities be filled, and his gum disease be treated. After violating parole and being returned to prison, the inmate reported to the prison dentist his dental needs as diagnosed by the free world dentist.

Despite having knowledge about the inmate's decayed tooth, the prison dentist extracted the wrong tooth. Then the dentist refused the plaintiff's request to pull the correct tooth and complete the treatment because the inmate was "uncooperative." In addition, the prison dentist refused to follow the free world dentist's treatment plan. Six months after the inmate's initial dental visit to the prison dentist, the prison dentist relented and filled the inmate's cavity; however, another dentist had to remove the inmate's decayed tooth as the prison dentist refused to do so.

The U.S. Court of Appeals for the Eighth Circuit affirmed the district court's denial of the prison dentist's motion for summary judgment, ruling that the "refusal to provide follow-up dental care..., despite... knowledge that an inmate is suffering severe pain, could support a Section 1983 violation" (*Kinney v. Kalfus*). The court also opined that even though the plaintiff does not have a constitutional right to choose his own dentist, or dental care, the prison dentist should had referred the inmate to another dentist. Since the prison dentist refused to provide the inmate with the necessary treatment, according to the court, this denial of treatment constituted deliberate indifference.

The difference between pretrial detainees and convicted inmates is that detainees cannot be punished, while convicted inmates can be subject to punishment (*Bell v. Wolfish*). Detainees are subject to protections under the due process clause of the Fourteenth Amendment (*Bell v. Wolfish*). Alternatively, the state must not subject convicted inmates to cruel and unusual punishment pursuant to the Eighth Amendment (*Estelle v. Gamble*). In *Brownlee v. Conine*, a pretrial detainee brought a civil rights action against jail personnel, alleging that jail officials refused to allow him to see the jail dentist. The detainee was in jail awaiting trial and needed dental care for severe tooth pain. In retaliation for the detainee's prior complaint, the jailer refused to allow the plaintiff to obtain dental care, which according to the U.S. Court of Appeals for the Seventh Circuit was a violation of the detainee's right to due process. The court said denial of dental care for persons in jail awaiting trial is tantamount to punishment, a practice forbidden by the Fourteenth Amendment.

Summary of Denial of Dental Care in Retaliation against Inmates for Filing Complaints, Grievances, and Lawsuits

Courts rule that when inmates' dental care is denied for exercising their free speech rights, it constitutes a form of retaliation that is actionable under Section 1983. Inmates have the right to file grievances, complain internally using the prison or jail grievance system, and bring lawsuits about the denial of dental care. In these circumstances, prisoners need to demonstrate they were penalized for exercising their First Amendment rights (*Farrow v. West*). This requires a showing that speech was a substantial or motivating factor in the retaliatory behavior of prison officials or dental care providers (*Mt. Healthy City School District Board of Education v. Doyle*).

Denial of Physician or Dentist-Prescribed Dental Care

In *Hoptowit v. Ray*, the U.S. Court of Appeals for the Ninth Circuit established the minimum level of medical care constitutionally required in state prisons. Namely, prisoners are entitled 1) to have access to competent medical personnel, 2) to receive medical care ordered by medical officials, and 3) to receive adequate emergency care.

Traumatic injuries of teeth, their supporting structures, and the maxilla-facial complex are very common in correctional facilities. (Poland 2003). Because dental injuries are likely to become serious, and result in complications, early diagnosis can increase a satisfactory outcome and prevent permanent damages (Cameron et al. 1997). Tooth fracture or loss may result in long-term disability, poor patient self image, as well as reducing the ability to chew properly, which has been linked to defective nutritional intake (Bos, Hoogstraten, and Prahl-Andersen 2003). Treatment of facial fractures involves medication and repair with arch bars or wires (Poland 2003). Inmates subject to those surgical procedures require special treatment, such as adequate nutrition, oral hygiene maintenance, and especially post-fixation monitoring by trained personnel. If they disregard recommendations and orders, denying treatment to an inmate needing special dental care, prison officials may be liable under Section 1983

Prison officials and health care providers must ensure that inmates receive diagnostic and other health services ordered by clinicians (Van Steenkiste 2004). The NCCHC (2003a, 2003b) indicates that correctional personnel should provide continuity of care throughout detention and incarceration to guarantee that detainees and inmates are being treated according to clinicians' orders. When the dentist prescribes a specific type of care, jailers and prison officials have no authority to refuse to implement the recommendation, if they do not have the expertise to do so. In *Lopez v. Smith*, a prisoner brought a Section 1983 lawsuit against prison officials, alleging that they violated his civil rights by denying him follow-up care prescribed by the dentist.

The case emerged from the following events: Lopez broke his jaw and was taken to a hospital for surgery. After the surgery, Lopez returned to prison under the care of the prison's medical staff. The dentist who performed the plaintiff's surgery recommended a clear liquid diet of 2,500 to 3,000 calories daily, drinking it through a straw. In addition, the attending dentist ordered that the plaintiff return to the hospital's clinic for follow-up care once a week for the next four weeks. However, Lopez was not permitted to return to the hospital until three months after his surgery. Moreover, his liquid diet was not properly administered. Instead, he was provided with a thick liquid diet that could not be sucked through a straw. Consequently, Lopez lost 22 pounds, and his jaw did not properly heal because of a lack of proper nutrition. Ruling on Lopez's lawsuit, the U.S. Court of Appeals for the Ninth Circuit reversed the district court, holding that there was sufficient evidence to establish that prison officials acted with deliberate indifference when they intentionally interfered with the plaintiff's dentist-prescribed treatment.

Some courts have ruled that there is no distinction between a prison dentist's and a community dentist's treatment order. Orders for dental treatment based on the professional and medical judgment made by free world dentists must be followed by prison dentists, unless the prison dentists can prove that their own recommended changes to these procedures are based on sound professional dentistry. In *Creech v. Nguyen,* Jimmie Creech, an inmate at the Powhatan Correctional Facility, filed a civil rights action under Section 1983, alleging that the prison dentist acted with deliberate indifference to his serious dental needs for post-operative care recommended by a free world dentist. To recap, on October, 1990, Creech underwent oral surgery at the Medical College of Virginia Oral Surgery Clinic (MCV) to immobilize his jaw, so it could properly heal from a mandibular fracture. A free world dentist performed the surgery and was treating Creech for his serious dental needs. The dentist ordered that the plaintiff return to the clinic for regular evaluations and check-ups, thus attending to his post-operative progress. Despite the order, Creech did not return to the clinic until January, 1991, four months following his operation.

A jury found in favor of Creech, and awarded him $60,000 in damages. The defendant appealed, and the trial judge granted his motion for a new trial. Creech appealed to the U.S. Court of Appeals for the Fourth Circuit, who concluded that the trial judge erred by entering a judgment for the defendant. The Fourth Circuit held that the prison dentist disregarded the plaintiff's serious dental needs by not allowing him to return to the clinic for post-operative care. In addition, the court stated that, during the trial, testimony showed that the prison dentist's deliberate indifference resulted in permanently damaging Creech's jaw.

In *Wilkins v. Correctional Medical System,* Earl Wilkins, a prisoner at the Maryland State Penitentiary, appealed the district court's grant of summary judgment for the defendants. Wilkins sued officials for denying him the proper treatment for a mouth infection. In August 1989, Wilkins was examined by a prison dermatologist. During the examination, the dermatologist recommended that the plaintiff's mouth infection be treated at the University of Maryland Hospital (UMH), because the hospital could treat the infection in a more efficacious manner. Despite this doctor's multiple referrals for treatment, the prison medical director overruled his recommendation, saying that the infection could be managed properly at the prison.

Since the prison infirmary didn't provide appropriate treatment for the mouth infection, the inmate filed an administrative grievance several months later. The prison medical director again refused to authorize the dermatologist's treatment plan. The district court dismissed Wilkins' Section 1983 lawsuit. On appeal, the U.S. Court of Appeals for the Fourth

Circuit reversed, noting that failure to provide the care that the physician recommended exceeded negligence and constituted deliberate indifference. Also, the court ruled that the prison medical director's refusal to comply with the prison doctor's professional medical opinion could be the basis of Section 1983 liability.

Summary of Denial of Physician or Dentist-Prescribed Dental Care
Courts rule that prison officials and correctional health care providers may be liable if they intentionally disregard physician or dentist-prescribed dental care. Dental care ordered by treating physicians or dentists cannot be denied by non-treating custody officers, non-treating correctional doctors, or other correctional health care personnel who are not exercising their professional medical or dental opinions. Denying detainees or inmates the care that is medically indicated violates the constitution. In clinical settings, the treating and/or examining dentist or physician who orders the treatment is the medical or dental professional whose orders should be implemented.

Denial of Care for Serious Dental Injury or Illness
Based on rulings in the cases of *Chance v. Armstrong* and *Cooper v. Schriro* prison officials must provide inmates with dentures because teeth are needed to eat and chew food. Living for an extended time without dentures can seriously undermine an inmate's health (*Hunt v. Dental Department*). In *Wynn v. Southward*, inmate Sylvester Wynn was housed in the Indiana Department of Corrections. After a disciplinary infraction, Wynn was moved from the general population to punitive isolation. As part of prison protocol, Wynn's non-contraband personal property was to be transferred to his segregated living quarters. Wynn's dentures, however, were lost in the move. Wynn alleged that two prison guards intentionally lost his dentures, forged his name on the property receipt records, and then refused to replace his dentures for seven months. Wynn sued the guards, claiming deliberate indifference to his serious dental needs. For example, without his dentures, Wynn "suffered bleeding, headaches, inability to chew his food, humiliation, shame, and disfigurement." The U.S. Court of Appeals for the Seventh Circuit later reversed the district court's dismissal of the inmate's Section 1983 lawsuit, saying that Wynn's lawsuit was valid because without his dentures, he could not chew food or eat properly, which led to "bleeding, headaches, and disfigurement" (*Wynn v. Southward*).

Healthy teeth are considered essential to a quality life (*Wynn v. Southward)*. Because adequate dental care is essential for health, prison dentists are required to provide basic dental treatment. When treatment is denied, several problems can result, including the failure to attend to and diagnose serious dental conditions as well as other health care problems that are frequently diagnosed by dentists, which can lead to tooth loss (Dolatowski 2002). Denial of dental treatment that results in loss of several of teeth is actionable under Section 1983 for deliberate indifference. In *Dellier v. Williams*, an inmate brought a civil rights action, under Section 1983, against the prison dentist, alleging that he lost several teeth because of the denial of dental treatment. The U.S. Court of Appeals for the Ninth Circuit held that the plaintiff alleged more than mere negligence, and the defendant acted with deliberate indifference when disregarding Dellier's dental treatment.

Correctional facilities and health care administrators are required to have emergency services available to provide 24-hour medical, mental, and dental services (NCCHC 2003a). An inmate who suffers from an immediate dental need cannot be denied treatment because health care staff were unavailable at the time of the incident, if it occurs after hours or on a weekend, especially when the inmate is suffering from excruciating pain. Courts have reached this conclusion because severe pain is recognized as a serious dental need (Kugelmann 2003). In addition, not intervening when inmates suffer from excruciating pain may show that prison officials were deliberately indifferent to inmates' serious dental needs. In *Harris v. Hegmann*, a prisoner brought a Section 1983 lawsuit against a physician and nurses for failing to treat a serious dental condition that caused excruciating pain.

The case was inspired by the following events. Harris had a broken jaw and received dental treatment to heal the fracture. Twenty days after his surgery, the retaining wires used to set Harris' jaw were removed at the clinic. Immediately after the wires were removed, Harris's jaw fell out of place, causing him extreme pain. Harris therein requested to be returned to the hospital's oral surgery clinic. Correctional officers said that would not be possible because no health care providers were available at the clinic. Harris subsequently returned to the Hunt Correctional Center without receiving treatment. Back at the correctional facility's infirmary, Harris again requested emergency dental treatment. The nurse denied his request. Instead she made an appointment for Harris to be examined by the prison dentist on a non-emergency basis. When Harris finally saw the prison dentist, the dentist performed a perfunctory examination, discharging him from the infirmary. In addition, the prison dentist ordered that Harris could return to his prison work assignment and resume eating a normal diet. After filing several complaints, Harris was finally transported to the hospital's oral surgery clinic, where an x-ray verified that his jaw was still broken (had never healed). The U.S. Court of Appeals for the Fifth Circuit reversed the district court, ruling that the defendants disregarded a substantial risk to Harris' serious dental needs when they denied him treatment. The Fifth Circuit said that prison officials and health care providers were deliberately indifferent when they failed to reset Harris' broken jaw after he requested treatment, thus leaving him to suffer excruciating pain.

Prisons and jails must make available an appropriate system that provides detainees and inmates medical and dental care and/or assessment of their medical and dental needs (*Murphy v. Bray*). When inmates are deprived of medications that are required for a severe toothache it is a constitutional violation under the Eighth Amendment. In *Mallette v. Dunning*, for example, Mallette appealed from the district court's dismissal of his Section 1983 lawsuit, alleging denial of medication for a severe toothache. Despite his pain, the nurses refused to give Mallette his prescribed pain medication, and instead gave him an over-the-counter substitute. Two days later, Mallette requested stronger pain medication, prompting the nurse to cancel all of Mallette's medication. The U.S. Court of Appeals for the Fourth Circuit ruled that the district court incorrectly dismissed Mallette's complaint, saying that the allegations of denial of pain medication for the purpose of inflicting pain raised a valid Section 1983 lawsuit.

Summary of Denial of Care for Serious Dental Injury or Illness

Courts rule that prison officials are deliberately indifferent when they disregard inmates' serious dental injuries and/or illnesses, letting them suffer wanton and unnecessary pain. When inmates or detainees need dentures to avoid cutting their mouth and to chew food properly, prison staff must provide them as part of the inmates' or detainees' essential dental care. Courts have also ruled that denial of dental care that results in loss of multiple teeth or causes the inmate or detainee severe pain is deliberate indifference under Section 1983.

Section 1983 Cases on Denial of Dental Care Litigated in the U.S. Courts of Appeals: The Defendant Prevails

Not all Section 1983 lawsuits pertaining to denial of prison dental care result in the inmate plaintiff prevailing. For inmates to win Section 1983 cases, they must show deliberate indifference to their serious dental needs. The cases below show that prison officials and correctional dentists are not required to provide routine teeth cleaning, may reject an inmate's request for a specific therapy, and may adopt policies that lead to extraction of teeth as long as those policies are medically defensible.

Denial of Prophylactic Oral Hygiene

According to the American Dental Association (2004) periodic teeth cleaning by a dental hygienist is recommended to maintain overall health. The courts have ruled, however, that regular teeth cleanings by correctional dentists are not a constitutional requirement. In *Hallett v. Morgan,* inmates at the Washington Corrections Center for Women filed a class action lawsuit, alleging that routine oral health care at the prison was customarily denied. The U.S. District Court for the Western District of Washington held that inmates failed to demonstrate that officials' actions violated the Eighth Amendment. On appeal, the U.S. Court of Appeals for the Ninth Circuit ruled that a lack of regular teeth cleaning was not deliberately indifferent to serious dental needs, as long as inmates with periodontal disease were referred to a dental hygienist if their condition required such treatment. This practice, according to the court, followed the dental standards established by the National Commission on Correctional Health Care.

Pursuant to the U.S. Supreme Court precedent of *Estelle v. Gamble,* the constitution only requires treatment for serious dental needs. Prophylactic dental care is beyond the scope of this constitutional mandate. In other words, correctional dentists are only required to provide immediate and emergency oral treatment. In *Taylor v. Christain,* for example, Taylor brought a Section 1983 lawsuit against prison officials, alleging he was denied routine dental cleaning. The district court granted summary judgment to defendants, and the U.S. Court of Appeals for the Seventh Circuit affirmed, stating that Taylor's complaint did not allege any serious dental problems needing immediate and emergency treatment. The court concluded that the denial of routine dental care does not constitute a constitutional violation because the inmate is not entitled to routine teeth cleaning.

Summary of Denial of Prophylactic Oral Hygiene

While routine oral hygiene defined as regular teeth cleaning is recommended to maintain oral health, courts do not require regular teeth cleaning. Prison dentists are constitutionally mandated to refer inmates to dental hygienists only when periodontal disease or other serious dental conditions exist. The constitutional floor at which treatment must commence for prison dental care is seriousness of the dental condition, which is determined on a case-by-case basis.

Denial of Desired/Requested Dental Therapies

Courts have held that prisoners do not have a constitutional right to dental treatment by free world dentists (see *Wilson v. Wilkinson*), to the services that are commonly available to individuals living in the free world (*Hallett v. Morgan*), or even to the services being provided by another correctional facility (*Shepherd v. Malan*). For the most part, courts consistently rule that inmates do not get to decide what kind of dental treatment they will receive. Inmates do not state a cause of action when a warden at their newly transferred facility refuses to continue the same dental treatment the inmate received at their previous prison (*Allen v. Hemingway*), especially if it is medically justifiable to stop the treatment. Moreover, inmates are not entitled to cosmetic dental care if the care is not medically required (*Poirier v. Casperson*).

Also, inmates cannot refuse reasonable dental care offered to them by a prison dentist and then sue the facility for denying them care. In *Foster v. Hori*, for example, Foster filed a lawsuit under Section 1983 against prison officials, alleging that the defendants were deliberately indifferent by denying his requested dental treatment. Foster suffered from periodontal disease, and most of his teeth were missing. The prison dentist recommended that Foster's remaining teeth be pulled and replaced with a full upper denture. Foster disagreed with the prison dentist because he wanted bridges and implants. Therefore, he did not consent to the prison dentist's recommendation; consequently, he received no treatment. The U.S. Court of Appeals for the Ninth Circuit affirmed the district court's ruling for the defendant, opining that the plaintiff's refusal to accept the prison dentist's recommendation prevented him from being treated. The court said that the plaintiff who suffered from gum disease was not entitled to bridges and implants when his remaining teeth were not salvageable.

Some inmates are concerned about the types of dental fillings that they might receive while incarcerated. Myths surround the use of mercury to fill cavities (Bailer et al. 2001). Research conducted by the U. S. Food and Drug Administration (FDA), American Dental Association, and U. S. Public Health Service shows, however, that there is no evidence that amalgams containing mercury cause harm except in the rare case of an allergic reaction (Verkler 2005). In fact, a three year clinical study comparing two different types of filling material—galloy and dispersalloy, a high mercury based filling—concluded that cavity fillings with dispersalloy are highly recommended for clinical use in moderate to large or multi-surface cavities because of its superior characteristics (Dunne, Abraham, and Pankhurst 2005).

Prison dentists are not liable if inmates cannot show that using mercury fillings resulted in serious injury or illness. In *Minniecheske v. Gudmanson*, an inmate sued prison officials under Section 1983, alleging that the prison dentist committed malpractice by providing inadequate dental care. Minniecheske claimed that the prison dentist used mercury fillings to treat him, which were considered by the plaintiff to be inadequate dental treatment. The U.S. Court of Appeals for the Seventh Circuit affirmed the district court's judgment for the defendants, concluding that the prison dentist, relying on his professional expertise, may use mercury fillings against an inmate's expressed wishes.

Summary of Denial of Desired/Requested Dental Therapies

Courts rule that inmates are not entitled to request specific dental therapies. Prison officials and health care providers can prescribe reasonable treatment that conflict with inmates' desires as long as the therapies are medically justifiable. Incarcerated prisoners have no right to be treated by their free world dentist, they are not entitled to continuity of care from one prison facility to another, and there is no constitutional right to cosmetic dentistry that is not a medical necessity.

Extraction Policies

Several factors enter into the decision to attempt to save or extract a tooth. When forming a correct treatment plan, dentists consider the likely success of aggressive treatment given the inmate's prior oral health history and likely future overall dental health (Davarpanah et al. 2000). Given the poor condition of many inmates' teeth, many correctional dentists are put in the position where pulling the inmates' teeth becomes a reasonable option. The U.S. Marshals Service policy, for example, of extracting teeth as the only treatment provided is constitutional (*Wagner v. United States*).

Dentists may disagree over the appropriate remedial care required to treat a serious dental condition (*Wagner v. United States*). The same can be true for a patient and a dentist, especially in a correctional facility when inmates frequently object to the treatment recommended by health care providers (*Wagner v. United States*). Courts rule that inmates' disagreement with correctional health care providers' professional medical judgment is not actionable under Section 1983 (Vaughn 1997). In *Davis v. Norris*, an inmate sued under Section 1983, alleging that he was denied a root canal for a serious dental need because the prison dentist would only perform an extraction. The U.S. Court of Appeals for the Eighth Circuit concluded that the summary judgment was properly granted to the defendants because a disagreement between a dentist's recommendation and an inmate's desired treatment does not amount to deliberate indifference, but merely a difference of opinion regarding legitimate treatment alternatives. Thus, disagreement over a particular type of dental procedure is not actionable under the Eighth Amendment.

Courts have ruled that correctional facilities may pull inmates' teeth instead of providing a root canal. In *Berry v. Lee,* Berry appealed the district court's grant of summary judgment for the defendants in his Section 1983 lawsuit. Berry claimed that he was denied dental care, when pursuing a root canal because jail custodial personnel instructed the prison dentist to pull Berry's tooth instead of providing a root canal. The U.S. Court of Appeals for the Ninth Circuit affirmed the district court, ruling that there was no deliberate indifference when the prison dentist pulled Berry's tooth.

Inmates have filed lawsuits claiming that some prison dentists are more apt to extract teeth rather than providing alternative treatments. The frequency with which some prison dentists extract teeth, however, is not per se evidence of deliberate indifference. In *Hallett v. Morgan,* inmates sued because Dr. Weaver, a prison dentist, had a record of pulling more teeth than other prison dentists. The U.S. Court of Appeals for the Ninth Circuit ruled that because of the division of labor among the dentists in the prison's dental clinic, Dr. Weaver extracted more teeth than other prison dentists. As a result, according to the court, he developed a reputation for pulling teeth unnecessarily, when in actuality that was his specialty. Other dentists in the prison dental clinic specialized in making dentures, while others worked exclusively on filling cavities. Because Dr. Weaver specialized in extractions, the court said he was not deliberately indifferent to inmates' serious dental needs.

Summary of Extraction Policies

At least one court has ruled that extraction only policies pass constitutional muster (*Wagner v. United States*). Courts hold that correctional facilities may extract teeth instead of providing complicated surgical procedures, especially when dentists could disagree over the most appropriate treatment for the particular condition. The constitution requires adequate dental care, which may not be the best or the most expensive, but any treatment provided must be grounded in the dentist's professional dental judgment. Prison dental clinics may assign specific dentists to perform extractions without violating the Eighth Amendment, as long as other dentists in the clinic perform restorative care.

Conclusion

Dental care is one of the most important medical needs in correctional facilities (Anno 2001). Because of poor hygiene, decayed teeth, and previous drug abuse, inmates and pretrial detainees are the most difficult type of patient to be treated (Vogt 2005). Despite those difficulties, prison officials and health care providers are legally required to offer adequate dental care to prisoners. Standards of practice are articulated by numerous associations, including the National Commission on Correctional Health Care, American Correctional Association, American Dental Association, and the American Public Health Association. When prison officials and prison dentists follow those standards, inmates and pretrial detainees are less likely to file lawsuits.

Within prison systems in the United States, there exists "little standardization of dental care." (Makrides and Shulman 2002). Levels of care currently are based on a piecemeal system devised primarily by court decisions, professional standards of care, accrediting guidelines, private providers, and committed individuals working in the field, in various jurisdictions across the nation. To move beyond the basic dental needs of prisoners, correctional systems need to establish a national standard for care. Ideally, a national standard centered on the principle of "elimination of dental disease" would serve the public health needs of all of society (Makrides and Shulman 2002).

This chapter has explored correctional dental care lawsuits filed by inmates and pretrial detainees under Section 1983. It focused on denying dental care to prisoners, and the consequences of such denial on their health. Under U.S. Supreme Court precedents *Estelle v. Gamble* and *Farmer v. Brennan*, prison dentists and prison officials are liable when they know of a risk to an inmate's health and intentionally or deliberately ignore the risk, which leads to injury. Prison officials and health care providers can be sued under Section 1983 when they deny basic oral hygiene supplies, deny dental care in retaliation of inmates' filing grievances and lawsuits, deny inmates dental care prescribed by a physician or by a dentist, and deny inmates' or pretrial detainees' requests to be treated for serious dental injury or illness.

Not all lawsuits under Section 1983 result in the inmate plaintiff prevailing. Prison officials and correctional dentists are not required to provide routine teeth cleaning, may reject an inmate's request for a specific dental therapy, and may adopt policies that lead to extraction of teeth as long as those policies are medically defensible. The constitutional floor at which treatment must commence for prison dental care is seriousness of the dental condition, which is determined on a case-by-case basis.

Future research should uncover more about dental care within prisons and jails. National surveys need to be undertaken to assess the extent of prisoners' dental needs. Incarceration presents an opportunity for correctional systems to address the poor dental conditions of prisoners, thus contributing to their overall health and possibly leading to early diagnosis of other serious medical conditions. Research also needs to uncover the state of correctional dentists, who practices dentistry in correctional facilities, what are the minimal requirements for employment, the extent to which care is contracted out to private dental providers, and the level of accreditation attainment within prison and jail dental clinics. Correctional dental care is an important element in the overall health care system provided to prisoners. More needs to be known so that the state of correctional dentistry can be assessed and improvements can be made to establish prison and jail dental clinics that adhere to national standards of care.

Endnote

1. Section 1 of the Civil Rights Act of 1871 is codified as Title 42 of the United States Code Section 1983 and states: Every person who, under color of any statute, ordinance, regulation, custom, or usage, of any State or Territory, subjects, or causes to be subjected, any citizen of the United States or other person within the jurisdiction thereof to the deprivation of any rights, privileges, or immunities secured by the Constitution and laws, shall be liable to the party injured in an action at law, suit in equity, or other proper proceeding for redress.

References

Allen v. Hemingway, WL 1480877 (6th Cir. 2001).

American Correctional Association. 2003. *Standards for Adult Correctional Institutions* 4th ed. Lanham, MD: Author.

American Dental Association. 2002. *Aging and Toothbrushes.* Retrieved May 26, 2006 (http://www.ada.org/public/media/videos/minute/adults_toothbrush.pdf).

American Dental Association. 2004. P*racticing Good Oral Hygiene is Top Oral Health Issue.* Retrieved May 26, 2006 (http://www.ada.org/public/media/releases/0403_release01.asp).

American Public Health Association. 2003. *Standards for Health Services in Correctional Institutions.* Washington, DC: Author.

Anno, B. Jaye. 2001. *Correctional Health Care: Guidelines for the Management of an Adequate Delivery System*. Chicago, IL: National Commission on Correctional Health Care.

Badea v. Moran, 894 F.2d 409 (9th Cir. 1990).

Bailer, Josef, Fred Rist, Anton Rudolf, Hans J. Staehle, Peter Eickholz, Gerhard Triebig, Michael Bader, and U. Pfeifer. 2001. "Adverse Health Effects Related to Mercury Exposure from Dental Amalgam Fillings: Toxicological or Psychological Causes?" *Psychological Medicine* 31:255-63.

Balsa, Ana I. and Thomas G. McGuire. 2003. "Prejudice, Clinical Uncertainty, and Stereotyping as Sources of Health Disparities." *Journal of Health Economics* 22:89-116.

Bell v. Wolfish, 441 U.S. 520 (1979).

Berry v. Lee, WL 387626 (9th Cir. 1992).

Board v. Farnham, 394 F.3d 469 (7th Cir. 2005).

Bos, Annemieke, Johan Hoogstraten, and Birte Prahl-Andersen. 2003. "Expectations of Treatment and Satisfaction with Dentofacial Appearance in Orthodontic Patients." *American Journal of Orthodontics and Dentofacial Orthopedics* 123:127-32.

Boyer E. Marcia, Nancy J. Nielsen-Thompson, and Tracy J. Hill. 2002. "A Comparison of Dental Caries and Tooth Loss for Iowa Prisoners with Other Prison Populations and Dentate U. S. Adults." *Journal of Dental Hygiene* 76:141-50.

Brownlee v. Conine, 957 F. 2d 353 (7th Cir. 1992).

Cameron, Angus, C., Stephen J. Moss, Michael Till, David C. Johnsen, and D. Stephen Douglas. 1997. "Roundtable: Dental Care and Injury Prevention in Athletes." *Sports Science Exchange* 8:1-6.

Chance v. Armstrong, 143 F.3d 698 (2nd Cir. 1998).

Chrisman, Noel J. 1989. "Dental Difficulties: Americans' Explanations of Periodontal Disease." *Anthropology Today* 5:14-16

Cooper v. Schriro, 189 F.3d 781 (8th Cir. 1999).

Creech v. Nguyen, WL 486354 (4th Cir. 1998).

Davis v. Norris, WL 1006437 (8th Cir. 1999).

Danner, Valerie. 2003. "Oral Health Trends in the U.S." *International Journal of Dental Hygiene* 1:78-83.

Davarpanah, Mithridade, Henry Martinez, Jean Francois Tecucianu, Olivier Fromentin, and Renato Celletti. 2000. "To Conserve or Implant: Which Choice of Therapy?" *International Journal of Periodontics and Restorative Dentistry* 20:412-22.

Dellier v. Williams, WL 10005 (9th Cir. 1994).

Dolatowski, Thomas J. 2002. "Buying Dental Benefits." *Compensation and Benefits Review* 34:45-48.

Doring, Katrin. 2004. "Treating the Whole Patient Builds the Practice." *Dentistry Today* 23:66-8.

Dunne, Stephen M., R. Abraham, and Caroline L. Pankhurst. 2005. "A 3-Year Longitudinal, Controlled, Clinical Study of a Gallium-based Restorative Material." *British Dental Journal* 198:355-9.

Estelle v. Gamble, 429 U.S. 97 (1976).

Farkas, Mary A. 1999. "Correctional Officer Attitudes Toward Inmates and Working With Inmates in a Get Tough Era." *Journal of Criminal Justice* 27:495-506.

Farmer v. Brennan, 114 S.Ct. 1970 (1994).

Farrow v. West, 320 F.3d 1235 (11th Cir. 2003).

Foster v. Hori, WL 22214 (9th Cir. 1993).

Frencken, Jo E., Taco Pilot, Yupin Songpaisan, and Prathip Phantumvanit. 1996. "Atraumatic Restorative Treatment: Rationale, Technique, and Development." *Journal of Public Health Dentistry* 56:135-40.

Friedman, Shimon. 1990. "Endodontic Retreatment." *Alpha Omegan* 83:32-37.

González-Vallejo, Claudia, Paul C. Sorum, Thomas R. Stewart, John B. Chessare, and Jaryl L. Mumpower. 1998. "Physicians' Diagnostic Judgments and Treatment Decisions for Acute Otitis Media in Children." *Medical Decision Making* 18:149-62.

Gura, Trisha. 1998. "Infections: A Cause of Artery-clogging Plaques?" *Science* 281:35-37.

Hallett v. Morgan, 296 F.3d 732 (9th Cir. 2002).

Harris v. Hegmann, 198 F.3d 153 (5th Cir. 1999).

Helling v. McKinney, 509 U.S. 25 (1993).

Hoptowit v. Ray, 682 F.2d 1237 (9th Cir. 1982).

Hunt v. Dental Department, 865 F.2d 198 (9th Cir. 1989).

James v. O'Sullivan, 62 Fed.Appx. 636 (7th Cir. 2003).

James, Doris J. 2004. *Profile of Jail Inmates, 2002*. Washington, DC: Bureau of Justice Statistics.

Jayanti, Rama K. and Alvin C. Burns. 1998. "The Antecedents of Preventive Health Care Behavior: An Empirical Study." *Journal of the Academy of Marketing Science* 26:6-15.

Kinney v. Kalfus, 25 F.3d 633 (8th Cir. 1994).

Kugelmann, Robert R. 2003. "Pain as Symptom, Pain as Sign." *Health* 7:29-50.

Lewis, S. 1996. "Treatment Planning: Teeth Versus Implants." *International Journal of Periodontics and Restorative Dentistry* 16:366-77.

Lombardo, Lucien. 1989. *Guards Imprisoned* 2nd ed. Cincinnati, OH: Anderson.

Lopez v. Smith, 203 F.3d 1122 (9th Cir. 2000).

Maeve, M. Katherine and Michael S. Vaughn. 2001. "Nursing with Prisoners: The Practice of Caring, Forensic Nursing, or Penal Harm Nursing." *Advances in Nursing Science* 24:47-64.

Makrides, Nicholas S. and Jay D. Shulman. 2002. "Dental Health Care of Prison Populations." *Journal of Correctional Health Care* 9:291-306.

Mallette v. Dunning, 896 F.2d 546 (4th Cir. 1990).

Mendonca, Teresa C. 2001. "Dental Mutilation: Rural Workers' Concepts of Responsibility for Tooth Loss." *Caderno de Saude Publica* 17:1545-47.

Minniecheske v. Gudmanson, WL 203806 (7th Cir. 1992).

Mitchell v. Duckworth, WL 6201 (7th Cir. 2000).

Mt. Healthy City School District Board of Education v. Doyle, 429 U.S. 274 (1976).

Murphy v. Bray, 51 F.Supp.2d 877 (S.D. Ohio 1999).

National Commission on Correctional Health Care. 2003a. *Standards for Health Service in Prisons*. Chicago, IL: Author.

National Commission on Correctional Health Care. 2003b. *Standards for Health Services in Jails*. Chicago, IL: Author.

Noble, A. 2005. *Dental Triage for Nursing*. Presented at Clinical Updates in Correctional Health Care Conference, April 2005, Las Vegas (NV).

Ormes, Walter S., Dean Carolyn, W. Foster Thompson, and Melanie Brim. 1997. "The Measurement of Dental Disease in a Correctional Setting and its Importance to Functional Service Delivery." *Journal of Correctional Health Care* 4:105-19.

Penrod v. Zavaras, 94 F.3d 1399 (10th Cir. 1996).

Plata v. Schwarzenegger, Lexis 8878 (N.D. Cal. 2005)

Poirier v. Casperson, WL 950875 (7th Cir. 2001).

Poland, M.J. (2003). "Dental Emergencias: A Primer for Non-Dental Health Professionals in Correctional Settings." In Jacqueline Moore (Ed.) *Management and Administration of Correctional Health Care* (pp. 1-13). Kingston NJ: Civic Research Institute.

Ramos-Rodriguez, C, Schwartz, MD, Rogers, V, Alos, V. 2004. "Institutional Barriers to Providing Oral Health Services for Underserved Populations in New York City." *Journal of Public Health Dentistry* 64:55-7.

Rhodes v. Chapman, 452 U.S. 337, 348 (1981).

Schwartz, Steven. 2003. "It's Magic: A Unique Practice Management Strategy." *Journal of Contemporary Dental Practice* 4:121-26.

Shepherd v. Malan, WL 727320 (9th Cir. 2001).

Taylor v. Christain, WL 684028 (7th Cir. 1994).

Trop v. Dulles, 356 U.S. 86 (1958)

Van Steenkiste, Marc. 2004. "Access to Oral Care and Attitudes Toward the Dentist by German and Turkish Parents." *Gesundheitswesen* 66:93-101.

Vaughn, Michael S. 1995. "Section 1983 Civil Liability of Prison Officials for Denying and Delaying Medication and Drugs to Prison Inmates. *Issues in Law and Medicine* 11:47-76

Vaughn, Michael S. 1997. "Civil Liability Against Prison Officials for Prescribing and Dispensing Medication and Drugs to Prison Inmates." *Journal of Legal Medicine*, 18:315-44.

Vaughn, Michael S. and Leo Carroll. 1998. "Separate and Unequal: Prison Versus Free-World Medical Care. *Justice Quarterly* 15:3-40.

Vaughn, Michael S. and Linda G. Smith 1999. "Practicing Penal Harm Medicine in the United States: Prisoners' Voices from Jail." *Justice Quarterly* 16:175-231.

Verkler, Erin. 2005. *Mercury and Cavities: Are Your Children's Fillings Scary or Safe?* Retrieved May 26, 2006 (http://www.prevention.com/article/0,5778,s1-5-89-191-2445-1,00.html).

Vogt, Robert P. 2005. "When an Inmate Refuses Medical Care." *Correct Care* 19:8.

Wagner v. United States, WL 464281 (8th Cir. 1994).

Wilkins v. Correctional Medical System, 928 F.2d 400 (4th Cir. 1991).

Wilson v. Wilkinson, 62 Fed.Appx. 590 (6th Cir. 2003).

Wynn v. Southward, 251 F.3d 588 (7th Cir. 2001)

CHAPTER SIX

Violence Reduction: Incarceration Shouldn't Be a Death Sentence

Travis W. Franklin and Cortney A. Franklin

Over the past several decades, both prisons and jails have faced the increasingly difficult challenge of housing a rapidly growing inmate population while ensuring a safe and orderly environment for these inmates and the staff. Between 1980 and 2005, the prison population more than quadrupled, steadily outpacing the construction of new institutions (Harrison and Beck 2006). The growing inmate population has significantly increased the number of staff, and consequently, a greater quantity of people—both prisoners and non-prisoners —are affected by what occurs behind prison walls (Jiang and Fisher-Giorlando 2002). Thus, jail and prison administrators hold as a primary objective the maintenance of safety and order within correctional institutions (Cullen et al. 1993; Flanagan 1980).

Although levels and forms of prison violence vary widely from institution to institution, particularly across levels of security (such as minimum versus maximum security facilities), recent trends indicate that the most serious offense—inmate homicide—has steadily declined in both prisons and jails, with the largest effects within state prison systems. Suicide rates have also demonstrated a similar downward trend (Mumola 2005). Despite the apparent improvement in prison and jail safety, violence reduction remains a primary focus within correctional institutions, and methods to effectively achieve this goal are critical to successful institutional management.

The purpose of this chapter is to answer the "what works?" question with regard to preventing acts of inmate violence. To effectively answer this question, it is helpful to first understand the factors that lead to prison violence. This is accomplished by exploring the theoretical context in which prison violence occurs. Moreover, the development and implementation of successful strategies for reducing violence is dependent upon a solid understanding of the nature, extent, and long-term impacts of the violence problem. Once these issues are addressed, we explore what is currently known about effective strategies for violence reduction in prisons and jails.

Explaining Prison Violence

Over the course of several decades, researchers have developed a number of explanations of the causes of prisoner violence. These propositions generally focus on four broad factors related to inmate behavior: 1) conditions of the prison environment, 2) personal characteristics of the inmates within the institution, 3) situational factors surrounding specific acts of violence, and 4) prison management techniques. While each of these factors is helpful for understanding inmate violence, it should be noted that our primary focus is to explain acts of individual inmate violence as opposed to collective inmate violence or prison riots (violence perpetrated by large groups). While prison riots are important in their own right, it is notable that they have decreased in a pattern similar to individual-level prison violence (Useem and Piehl 2006). It is likely that the factors that successfully decreased individual violence also had a positive influence on prison riots, although this question is beyond the scope of this chapter. The following sections outline the four theoretical models that explain inmate-on-inmate and inmate-on-staff violence.

Deprivation Model

The primary assumption underlying the deprivation model is that inmate behavior is influenced by the conditions of the prison environment. Researchers had historically focused on examining the unique characteristics of the prison environment that they believed would produce negative impacts on inmates' attitudes, values, and methods of social interaction. These characteristics, they presumed, ultimately forced prisoners to reenter the community in a less capable state than when they began their sentence (Goodstein and Wright 1989). This condition, Sykes (1958) argues, is the result of being exposed to five "pains of imprisonment" that are intrinsic to all prisons. These deprivations—loss of social acceptance, material possessions, personal security, heterosexual relations, and personal autonomy—shape the social organization of the prison and the behavior of the inmates.

Researchers have since expanded the focus of the deprivation model to include factors related to the "fixed institutional environment" (Huebner 2003:108). Deprivation in this sense has been explained through various environmental conditions such as jail or prison overcrowding, high levels of security and surveillance, poor medical and food services, and a lack of meaningful rehabilitative programs. In sum, the deprivation model argues that specific conditions of the jail and prison environment inevitably lead to prisoner violence. While it is not possible to eliminate all sources of deprivation (part of the prison experience is purposefully designed to deprive inmates of basic freedoms), many aspects of the prison environment are dynamic, allowing for the possibility to improve conditions. Changes may lead to decreased levels of inmate stress and frustration, resulting in less violence.

Importation Model

The importation model introduced the idea that prisoners do not develop violent subcultures, modes of social interaction, and value systems purely as a response to the deprivations of incarceration. Rather, Irwin (1970) and Irwin and Cressey, (1962) argue that these developments are an extension of street cultures or community environments and that negative personal characteristics are imported into prisons and jails. In this sense, Goodstein and Wright (1989:234) suggest that inmate behavior can be explained by looking "no further than the street for the origins of prisonization."

Researchers have explored the assumptions of the importation model based on a multitude of inmate factors that are arguably brought into the correctional facility from the outside. For example, studies have examined demographic characteristics such as age, race, level of education, (Jiang and Fisher-Giorlando 2003; Wooldredge 1991) socioeconomic and employment status prior to incarceration (Wooldredge 1991), marital status, number of prior convictions, type of crime, gang membership, drug use, area of residence, and various personality variables (Goodstein and Wright 1989). In sum, the importation model primarily looks to the imported characteristics of the inmate population as opposed to the prison environment to explain inmate behavior.

Situational Model

While the deprivation and importation models focus on the prison environment and inmate characteristics, they neglect to consider the situational variables surrounding acts of violence and misconduct (Steinke 1991). While the situational model has been afforded less attention, it has increased our knowledge of the sources of prison violence. These factors are grouped into three categories referred to as "where," "when," and "with whom" (Jiang and Fisher-Giorlando 2003). The first category considers the location of the incident and the inmates' specific housing situation (such as a cell block or dormitory). This factor is of particular concern since inmate violence often occurs where there is little supervision and surveillance or where opportunities for assault are higher, such as areas where inmates congregate. The second category considers the time of day when incidents occur and ask questions such as, "Do acts of inmate violence tend to occur during hours when fewer staff are present?" Finally, the third category considers who was involved in the incident and whether other inmates were present or participating (Kratcoski 1988; Steinke 1991).

One significant change that may influence the situational nature of correctional violence is the introduction of new architectural designs that increase the ability of staff to supervise the inmates, reduce the number of "blind spots" (where inmate activities are hidden from staff scrutiny) and increase the ability of staff to intervene before problems escalate. Prior to the 1980s, most jails and prisons were built on the "linear" model, where inmates were housed in cells in long corridors. These corridors were often stacked in tiers, and in most places, the inmates were locked behind actual bars. Most facilities today, however, are constructed using the "podular" or new generation design where the cells are constructed around a common area—where inmates have their recreation, educational programming, and dine. This change enables an individual officer to supervise inmates more effectively and it has been proposed that this architectural change (and philosophical change in inmate management) has been instrumental in reducing violence (Wener 2006).

Administrative Control Model

The administrative-control model stems from DiIulio's (1987) comparative analysis of prison systems in Texas, Michigan, and California. Three managerial frameworks representing administrative approaches to prison control were identified: 1) control model, 2) responsibility model, and 3) consensual model. Administrators prescribing to the control model hold that inmates must be subjected to a highly regimented environment where formal restraints closely control their activities. On the other end of the continuum, administrators adopting the responsibility model claim that prisons should maintain order with minimal formal controls while allowing opportunities for inmate self-governance. Finally, the consensual model describes a more flexible management style, extracting features from both the control and responsibility models.

Reviews of these models have resulted in disagreement as to what type of control should be employed (DiIulio 1987; Reisig 1998). Two specific types of control, coercive control and remunerative control, have been discussed at length (Colvin 1992; Huebner 2003). Coercive control assumes the need for threats and sanctions, but remunerative control emphasizes rewarding prisoners and offering incentives for good behavior. A recent review of misconduct and violence in prison revealed that managerial control weighed heavily in the increased "order" in state and federal prisons since the 1980s (Useem and Piehl 2006). What is most important is that order increased at the same time that prison populations grew four-fold and the number of high-risk or disruptive populations increased (e.g., gang members and inmates with mental illnesses).

Ultimately the administrative-control model posits that inmate misconduct is a direct result of weak or poor management practices. Even the most troublesome inmate populations, typically younger inmates with violent histories, can be successfully managed in ways that minimize inmate violence, misconduct, and other forms of disturbances. While the prison environment fosters deprivations, managerial shortcomings—such as insufficient staff training, high staff turnover, and poor security practices—produce higher rates of inmate misconduct in prison. Properly managed prisons, despite their unavoidable deprivations, will be safer institutions for both inmates and staff.

The Extent of Prison and Jail Violence

One the most unfortunate characteristics of many jails and prisons is the existence of an inmate subculture where prisoners are forced to choose between victimizing or becoming the targets of victimization. This is not surprising, given the nature of prisons and the populations they hold. Grouping large numbers of violent and non-violent offenders into crowded and under-staffed institutions is sure to create a dangerous and volatile environment. The following sections shed light on the degree to which various forms of violence occur in U.S. correctional settings.

Homicide and Suicide

Recent data compiled by the Bureau of Justice Statistics (BJS) indicates that correctional homicide and suicide rates have been on a decline since the early 1980s (Mumola 2005). Suicide rates in American jails underwent a dramatic decrease between 1983 and 2002, falling from 129 to 47 per 100,000 inmates (63 percent decrease). While suicide was once the leading cause of death in jails, the most common form of death has shifted to natural causes (Mumola 2007). Over the past two decades, suicide rates in state prisons have remained more stable, declining from a high of 34 per 100,000 prisoners in 1980 to 16 per 100,000 prisoners in 1990 (53 percent decrease). Since 1990, suicide rates in state prisons have experienced less change, declining from 16 per 100,000 prisoners to 14 per 100,000 prisoners in 2002. Based on this evidence it is safe to conclude that suicide remains far more probabilistic in local jails as compared to state prisons—in 2002, the suicide rate was more than three times higher in jails (Mumola 2005).

An examination of prison and jail homicide trends reveals similar findings, although in this instance, homicide rates appear more stable in jails than prisons. Between 1980 and 2002, homicide rates declined from 54 to four per 100,000 prisoners, a 93 percent decrease. From 1983-2002, by contrast, jails experienced a comparatively stable homicide rate, ranging from a high of five to a low of three murders per 100,000 jail inmates. Though homicide rates were nearly ten times higher in prisons than jails in the early 1980s, recent trends indicate that the homicide trends in jails and prisons have converged.

In sum, two of the most serious forms of institutional violence appear to have undergone substantial decreases over the past two decades. Of particular concern, however, are the underlying causes for such a dramatic change. It is likely that multiple factors are responsible. For example, architectural design improvements, increased use of surveillance technology, improved management techniques, increased academy and annual staff training may have all played a role in lowering suicide and homicide rates. An additional factor that may have increased the safety of correctional facilities is the increasing sophistication of inmate classification.

Inmate classification refers to the practice of placing inmates in housing units within prisons (or jails) that provide the appropriate levels of security for that inmate. Most correctional facilities now classify an inmate based on their current offense, their prior criminal record, and history of conduct within institutions. Thus, an inmate with a history of violent offenses, attempted or successful escapes, gang-affiliation, and assaults within correctional facilities will be placed in a high security unit. Inmates with less serious offenses and no history of institutional misconduct are placed in less secure facilities. Inmates admitted to prison in most large systems first pass through a reception center, where they are classified and placed into the most appropriate prison or housing unit. Classification is also a cost-effective approach, as inmates who require less security can be housed in less "hardened" facilities, such as correctional camps rather than prisons.

It is also possible that the reduction in homicide and suicide rates have been influenced by the changing ratio of violent to non-violent inmates in prisons and jails. According to the BJS, the proportion of violent offenders in state prisons decreased from 57 percent of the total inmate population in 1980 (Beck and Gilliard 1995) to 51.7 percent in 2003 (Harrison and Beck 2006). During this same time period, non-violent drug offenders increased from 6.4 to 19.96 percent of all state prisoners, a trend that directly coincides with the decrease in lethal prison violence (Beck and Gilliard 1995; Harrison and Beck 2006). The percentage of drug offenders in federal prisons, by contrast, more than doubled during the same era. These changes in the prison population are helpful for understanding the decline in prison homicide and suicide rates for two key reasons: 1) a majority of prison homicides and suicides involve violent offenders, and 2) drug offenders have the lowest homicide and suicide rates of all state prisoners (Mumola 2005). Thus, decreasing levels of lethal prison violence is at least, in part, due to the shifting inmate population.

Jail populations underwent similar changes where the proportion of violent offenders declined significantly due to the influx of non-violent drug offenders. Specifically, between 1983 and 1993, the number of drug law violators in local jails increased fivefold, driving the proportion of violent offenders down from 31 to 22 percent of the total jail population (Beck and Gilliard 1995). This is particularly important in light of recent data indicating that violent offenders commit suicide at three times the rate of non-violent offenders in jails. Furthermore, drug law violators, the fastest growing segment of the jail population during the 1980s and early 1990s, tend to exhibit the lowest rate of jail suicides (Mumola 2005).

When examining suicide and homicide trends within correctional populations, it is critical to consider situational and contextual factors that may impact the numbers of incidents. While general trends indicate steep declines in prison homicide and jail suicide, both forms of violence remain a relatively serious problem among specific subgroups of the inmate population—particularly violent offenders. As a result, as long as prisons hold high numbers of these offenders, prison administrators will have to adopt strategies that specifically target violence reduction.

Violent Assault

Prison assaults, whether directed toward inmates or staff, are far more prevalent than that of murder or suicide, which are rare incidents. Unfortunately, uncovering the degree to which these incidents happen is a difficult task, as many assaults are undetected and the reporting of assaults by inmates is often shunned or avoided out of fear of further victimization. As Bottoms (1999) points out, the use of official prison reports is helpful for accurately determining levels of serious incidents, yet these same reports offer little in the way of constructing an accurate assessment of prison assaults (also see Light 1990a). Rather than relying on official records, a more appropriate source of information is the use of victimization surveys of prisoners. Widespread use of such surveys, however, has not been implemented, and thus, our understanding of violence in American prisons remains incomplete.

Table 6-1. Assault Rates in State and Federal Prisons.

	Year			
Type of Assault	1984	1990	1995	2000
Inmate-Inmate	45	31.3	27	28
Inmate-Staff	17.2	15.5	14.7	14.6

Note: Assault rates are based on the average daily population of the institution (Rates are the number of incidents per 1,000 inmates).

Despite this limitation, the use of officially reported information is helpful for examining national trends in assaults against both inmates and correctional staff. Though less information concerning jail assaults is accessible, national data for state and federal prisons is available from the Census of State and Federal Correctional Facilities from 1984 through 2000. As Table 6-1 indicates, the period between 1984 and 2000 has seen a decline in both inmate-inmate and inmate-staff assaults. More specifically, inmate-inmate assault rates in state and federal prisons decreased by 50 percent, from 45 per 1,000 prisoners in 1984 to 31.3 per 1,000 prisoners in 1990 and subsequently stabilized over the following ten years. During the same time period, inmate-staff assault rates have remained both lower and more stable than inmate-inmate assault rates. Between the years 1984 and 2000, the total inmate-staff assault rate declined from 17.2 per 1,000 to 14.6 per 1,000 prisoners representing a 15 percent decrease.

Overall it appears as if assaults, particularly acts of violence between inmates, are becoming less prevalent—an indication that prisons are becoming safer environments. As noted above, however, official records provide only partial insight to the true extent of violence (with the exception of lethal violence). Researchers comparing self-reported victimization to official records of victimization have discovered sharp discrepancies. For example, Cooley (1993) found that self-report surveys revealed nearly three times the number of assaults disclosed by official prison records. Moreover, as was the case with homicide and suicide trends, the observed decline in prison assaults may be partially explained by the increase of non-violent drug offenders behind bars, more effective classification, and better administrative control (Useem and Piehl 2006).

Sexual Assault

There is very little accurate information about the prevalence of sexual assaults that occur in correctional facilities. Researchers have primarily relied on the use of small scale studies (typically of a single institution) to determine the rates of sexual assault. Unfortunately, studies exploring sexual violence provide inconsistent findings, making it difficult to accurately determine the degree to which such events occur. For example, Struckman-Johnson and Struckman-Johnson (2000) found that 21 percent of the inmates surveyed across seven Midwestern prison facilities reported being forced or pressured to engage in sexual contact at some point during their sentence. Other researchers argue that the occurrence of prison rape is often exaggerated, thus perpetuating the idea that sexual assault is a common experience. To more accurately guage the prevalence of prison rape, Gaes and Goldberg (2004) conducted a meta-analysis of 19 prison rape studies and found that across all studies the average prevalence of prison rape was 1.91 percent. Based on this evidence, approximately two percent of prison inmates are raped sometime during their sentence.

Beck and Harrison (2006) recently conducted a national survey investigating the prevalence of sexual violence in correctional facilities. While the data are based on official reports of sexual violence, they provide the opportunity to compare sexual misconduct across various correctional agencies. Allegations of sexual violence were highest among state prisons (3.86 incidents per 1,000 inmates), followed by local jails (1.86 incidents), and federal prisons (1.71 incidents). Rates of substantiated incidents were less than the alleged assaults. Beck and Harrison (2006: 2) observe, "Due to a fear of reprisal from perpetrators, a code of silence among inmates, personal embarrassment, and a lack of trust in staff, victims are often reluctant to report incidents." As a result, the BJS hopes to use surveys of former inmates to get a better understanding of the true rate of these crimes.

Long-Term Impacts of Correctional Violence

While various forms of institutional violence—including physical threats, violent assault, homicide, and prison rape—clearly have immediate consequences for those involved, these incidents also have negative long-term effects on inmate quality of life and the ability to function in a pro-social manner. Incidents of severe violence or continued threats of violence have been linked to psychological disorders, including depression and post-traumatic stress disorder (PTSD) (Dumond 2000). Researchers have found that the threat of victimization significantly influences inmate well-being (McCorkle 1993), forcing many prisoners to make weapons for self-protection (McCorkle 1992). In fact there is good reason to expect exacerbated psychological effects of prison victimization, especially since victims are forced to live with their attackers for extended periods of time (Hochstetler, Murphy, and Simons 2004), and have no way of escaping the violence (Human Rights Watch 2001).

Incidents of sexual violence, particularly prison or jail rape, have devastating and long-lasting physical, social, and psychological effects on victims (Fagan, Wennerstrom, and Miller 1996). Some victims of sexual assault are subjected to psychological taunts and threats, leading to elevated levels of fear throughout the remainder of their sentence (Toch 1992). Further complicating the situation, victims are faced with severe consequences for reporting incidences of rape—stigmatization or labeling frequently occurs, resulting in further victimization (Donaldson 2001). In addition, rape victims often suffer from conditions such as rape trauma syndrome as well as PTSD and severe depression (Dumond 2000; Franklin and Lutze 2007; Robertson 2000). Prison rape may also lead to substance abuse as a method of self-medication, while in more extreme cases, rape victims may turn to suicide to escape feelings of self-hatred and fear (Dumond 1992; Roberts et al. 1991). Like victims of less serious violent assault, inmates suffering from the physiological effects of rape undergo similar challenges of successfully reintegrating into the broader community while suffering from psychological disorders.

There is considerable concern over releasing into the community inmates who have been brutalized by sexual assaults (McGuire 2005). Some researchers believe being raped in prison can lead to the development of extreme anger and aggressive behavior, which directly threatens communities after these victims are released from prison (Dumond 1992). Further, the interracial nature of many rape victimizations raises concern that racism will be perpetuated by victims upon release. According to McGuire (2005:76), "it would actually be very surprising if white victims of racialized sexual violence in prison did not develop attitudes of fear, hatred and loathing towards their assailants that could quite easily translate into racist attitudes toward black people in general." Though additional empirical evaluation is needed to confirm the direct impact of rape on post-release behavior, the enduring effects of such events pose significant concerns to the mental health of the inmates, the well-being of their families, and community safety.

Beyond the psychological impacts of sexual victimization, rape victims are exposed to various long-term health risks, including potential HIV/AIDS infection (see Franklin, Fearn, and Franklin 2005). This risk is elevated within the prison system where the rate of HIV/AIDS infected inmates is estimated to be over three times that of the general population (Maruschak 2006). In addition, rape victims also suffer the possibility of contracting other sexually transmitted infections, such as syphilis, gonorrhea, herpes, and hepatitis (McGuire 2005). Struckman-Johnson et al. (1996) found that the average prison rape victim in their sample experienced nine assaults. When combined with findings that a substantial proportion of prison sexual assaults are gang rapes (Robertson 2003; Struckman-Johnson et al. 1996), the health risks associated with such acts becomes clear.

The negative emotional, behavioral, and health effects of prison sexual violence are not confined to correctional communities. Many rape victims tend to be young, non-violent, first-time offenders (Human Rights Watch 2001) who are likely serving relatively short sentences and will be released into the community. The spread of infectious disease as a result of prison rape is a public health concern, as most infected offenders are unaware of both their infection status as well as the ways in which disease is spread (Franklin et al. 2005). These factors create the potential for higher levels of disease transmission to the community.

Reducing Violence Behind Bars

The prevalence of violence in prisons and jails has a profound influence on inmate populations. Moreover, the negative effects of these incidents extend beyond the prison, to the community. High levels of violence and uncertainty also contribute to correctional officer stress. As a result, despite the recent declines in serious incidents, jails and prisons can benefit from interventions to reduce harm. Correctional institutions currently rely upon classification systems to identify potentially dangerous individuals, yet additional inmate management strategies are still required to lessen violence. The following sections identify strategies aimed to reduce prisoner violence.

Prison Programming

Several studies have been conducted to determine the predictors of prison violence (e.g., Harer and Steffensmeirer 1996; Kratcoski 1988; Walters 1998). Many of these risk factors have been incorporated into inmate classification systems. Less attention, however, has been dedicated to developing and evaluating programs or management strategies aimed to specifically reduce inmate violence. The vast majority of jail and prison based programs are designed to reduce post-release recidivism. There is some empirical evidence, however, that programs developed to help inmates integrate into the community also reduce prison misconduct.

McCorkle, Miethe, and Drass (1995) analyzed prison programs in 371 state prisons. These investigators found that prisons with larger proportions of the inmate population enrolled in rehabilitative programs had lower levels of inmate-inmate and inmate-staff assaults. In addition, interventions aimed at behavioral change and self-improvement were more effective than programs designed only to keep the inmates occupied (e.g., vocational 'work-experience' programs such as mopping floors). This was the case even after controlling for institutional characteristics such as the security level of the facility.

French and Gendreau (2003) recently conducted a meta-analysis of 70 studies (involving a total of 21,370 inmates) to evaluate the effect of various prison programs on prison safety and order. These investigators discovered several findings of value to correctional administrators. First, results of the meta-analysis indicated that effective reduction of inmate misconduct varied by program type. For example, behavioral programs—such as those focusing on social learning and cognitive skills—had the most powerful effect on prison misconduct. These programs reduced reported institutional misconduct by 26 percent. Moreover, behavioral programs were found to be more effective than non-behavioral programs 68 percent of the time, and over three-quarters of these interventions were more effective than educational/vocational programs. Second, French and Gendreau (2003) found that programs with higher levels of therapeutic integrity (e.g., well-trained staff and targeting high risk inmates) significantly outperformed programs with lower levels of these characteristics, leading to less misconduct 63 percent of the time. Finally, programs that targeted a greater number of criminogenic needs (such as criminal thinking, antisocial attitudes, and substance abuse) were more effective than those targeting fewer criminogenic needs. Programs that addressed three to eight criminogenic needs were more effective at reducing levels of misconduct over one-half of the time when compared to programs addressing two or fewer needs, and 73 percent of the time when compared to programs that did not address criminogenic needs.

Overall, the results of French and Gendreau's (2003) meta-analysis provide strong support for the effectiveness of rehabilitative programs to enhance prison safety. This research provides useful information for identifying the components of successful programs. Evidence suggests that the implementation of well-planned behavioral programs designed to address inmates' various criminogenic needs is more effective than relying on traditional educational or vocational training alone. In fact, programs of this nature were not only shown to reduce inmate misconduct within prisons, but also to reduce rates of recidivism upon release. Last, the use of inmate classification systems enhances rehabilitative programs by targeting high-risk inmates who are most in need of treatment (and show the most success).

Situational Prevention Strategies

Recently, situational violence prevention strategies have gained more attention in the correctional literature. Advocates of these strategies suggest that modifying the prison environment will reduce opportunities for violence and are currently used in various forms (e.g., protective segregation, surveillance of inmates). Researchers have found some support for these methods, but, at the same time, they caution against an overly controlling prison regime. For example, reducing the time inmates spend outside their cells can produce an immediate reduction in the opportunity for violence against staff and other inmates. The long-term consequences of greater inmate control, however, may be antithetical, leading to increased violence (Bottoms, Hay, and Sparks 1995; McCorkle et al. 1995).

Less obstructive strategies, however, offer the potential to create safer prison environments without upsetting institutional social order. For example, as the average age of the inmate population decreases, inmate-inmate violence may rise (Light 1990b). Subsequently, increasing age heterogeneity within institutions may lead to lower levels of violence among inmates and reducing the need for coercive controls. Recent studies have provided empirical support for modifying the prison environment based on inmate age characteristics. In a meta-analysis of 16 prison crowding studies, Franklin, Franklin, and Pratt (2006) found that prison misconduct and violence were influenced by levels of institutional overcrowding, but only in samples of younger prisoners (aged 18 to 25 years). While crowding in general appears to have little or no effect on prison misconduct, reducing the level of crowding among younger inmates may produce a less violent environment.

National-level studies find that gangs (also called 'security threat groups') represent approximately 16 percent of all jail inmates and 13 percent of state prisoners (Wells, Minor, Angel, Carter, and Cox 2002), and their presence may contribute to correctional violence. Prior research has found that gang-involved inmates contribute to higher rates of prison violence (Camp and Camp 1985), and perpetuate racial tensions within prisons (Anti-Defamation League of B'nai B'rith 2002). In fact, these two factors may be related with disorder in some facilities. In January 2006, for instance, a number of uprisings occurred in the Los Angeles County jail system, and these conflicts were both gang and race-related. Ethnographic accounts of correctional life suggest that these groups are persistent, have a negative influence on the operation of jails and prisons, and make it difficult for an inmate to "do their own time" (see Ross and Richards 2002).

Ruddell, Decker, and Egley (2006) suggest that gang interventions might also lower the risk of disorder within some correctional facilities. In some jails and prisons, for instance, inmates are segregated on the basis of gang affiliation or involvement. The long-term impact of such interventions, however, is unknown and such practices are considered controversial. For example, segregating inmates on the basis of gang affiliation may be seen as surrendering to gangs or institutional racism.

Situational prevention strategies must be carefully monitored and evaluated because prevention strategies that are based on overly restrictive practices may lead to increased violence over the long-term. Conversely, less intrusive strategies may alter the inmate environment without disturbing the social order, providing safer conditions for inmates and correctional workers. To be effective, prison management strategies must maintain a balance between that of an overly coercive environment and one that provides inmates with an excess of freedoms.

Preventing Sexual Assault in Correctional Facilities

Sexual violence has been a perennial problem in jails and prisons. Recently, increased attention has been paid to defining the boundaries of the problem, and the most effectie responses to reduce prison rape. Local, state, and federal correctional agencies are developing harm reduction strategies in response to the Prison Rape Elimination Act of 2003 (PREA). Knowels (1999) for example, contends that inmate classification be used to identify and segregate potential sexual aggressors. Others suggest that permitting more conjugal visits (where family members can visit overnight with their spouses in self-contained units) may reduce the incidents of sexual assault. Yet many inmates are unmarried and and would not be eligible for such visits. Moreover, expanding the availability of conjugal visits is unlikely to have a significant impact on rape reduction as jail and prison rape is rarely about sexual gratification. Instead, sexual assault is motivated primarily by power and dominance (Rideau and Wikberg 1992). As a result of the complexity of the problem it is likely that correctional officials will have to develop rape reduction strategies that rely on a number of different approaches.

Historically, rape reduction was not seen as a priority by all correctional administrators, although these attitudes have shifted in the past few decades, and there has been much interest in preventing these acts. Beyond encouraging the continued use of classification systems and investigating such crimes when they occur, few interventions exist. With the recent enactment of the PREA, however, correctional agencies in conjunction with state and federal governments can channel resources towards the development of realistic solutions to the sexual violence problems in correctional facilities.

Discussion and Conclusions

Deaths from murder and suicide in jails and prisons have decreased over the last 25 years. Suicide rates have sharply declined in U.S. jails, and likewise, homicide rates have decreased in prisons. Though substantial positive changes have occurred, violence remains an ever-present reality in correctional settings. Violent interactions remain a significant part of the prison experience. As a result, many inmates live in constant fear (Hassine 2002). Given the long-term mental and physical effects of prison violence on inmates (e.g., post-traumatic stress disorder, depression, behavioral problems) and the potential threat to the public when these prisoners are released (e.g., post-release violence, spread of infectious diseases), violence reduction strategies to provide safer correctional environments are paramount.

The most effective strategies for dealing with and reducing prison violence appear to be comprehensive rehabilitative programs. Directing high-risk prisoners into interventions designed to address their specific criminogenic needs is a promising strategy to be pursued by correctional administrators. It should be noted, however, that few of the correctional programs evaluated by researchers were specifically designed for violence reduction. Instead these programs were developed for modifying inmate behaviors with the primary purpose of reducing post-release criminality. Fortunately these interventions have also produced lower levels of institutional violence. Thus, future programs designed specifically to reduce inmate violence will likely be even more effective.

Given the damaging effects of jail and prison rape, the lack of specific interventions and/or promising strategies focusing on the issue of inmate sexual violence is discouraging. Clearly, prisons and jails can take advantage of inmate classification systems to help prevent rape, but efforts must extend beyond this point. Interventions should be developed to address rape prevention specifically, along with the attitudes and behaviors (of both correctional officers and inmates) that perpetuate sexual assaults. In this regard, as is the case with programming aimed at reducing other forms of institutional violence, additional research is needed.

References

Anti-Defamation League of B'nai B'rith. 2002. *Dangerous Convictions: An Introduction to Extremist Activities in Prisons.* New York: Anti-Defamation League of B'nai B'rith.

Beck, Allen J. and Darrell K. Gilliard. 1995. *Prisoners in 1994.* Washington, DC: U. S. Department of Justice, Bureau of Justice Statistics.

Beck, Allen J. and Paige M. Harrison. 2006. *Sexual Violence Reported by Correctional Authorities, 2005.* Washington, DC: U.S. Department of Justice, Bureau of Justice Statistics.

Bottoms, Anthony E. 1999. "Interpersonal violence and social order in prisons." Pp. 205-281 in *Prisons: Crime and Justice, A Review of Research,* vol. 26, edited by M. Tonry and J. Petersilia. Chicago, IL: The University of Chicago Press.

Bottoms, Anthony E., William Hay, and J. Richard Sparks. 1990. "Situational and Social Approaches to the Prevention of Disorder in Long-Term Prisons." *The Prison Journal* 80:83-95.

Camp, George M. and Camile G. Camp. 1985. *Prison Gangs: Their Extent, Nature, and Impact on Prisons.* Washington, DC: U.S. Government Printing Office.

Colvin, Mark. 1992. *The Penitentiary in Crisis: From Accommodation to Riot in New Mexico.* Albany, NY: State University of New York Press.

Cooley, Dennis. 1993. "Criminal Victimization in Male Federal Prisons." *Canadian Journal of Criminology* 35:479-495.

Cullen, Frank, Edward Latessa, Velmer Burton, and Lucien Lombardo. 1993. "The Correctional Orientation of Prison Wardens: Is the Rehabilitation Ideal Supported?" *Criminology* 31:69-92.

DiLulio, John. 1987. *Governing Prisons.* New York: The Free Press.

Donaldson, Stephen. 2001. "A Million Jockers, Punks and Queens." Pp. 118-126 in *Prison Masculinities,* edited by D. Sabo, T. Kupers and W. London. Philadelphia, PA: Temple University Press.

Dumond, Robert W. 1992. "The Sexual Assault of Male Inmates in Incarcerated Settings." Sociology of Law 20:135-157.

------. 2000. "Inmate Sexual Assault: The Plague that Persists." *The Prison Journal* 80:407-414.

Fagan, Thomas J., Deborah Wennerstrom, and Jeanne Miller. 1996. "Sexual Assault of Male Inmates: Prevention, Identification and Intervention." *Journal of Correctional Health Care* 3:49-65.

Flanagan, Timothy J. 1980. "Time Served and Institutional Misconduct: Patterns of Involvement in Disciplinary Infractions among Long-Term and Short-Term Inmates." *Journal of Criminal Justice* 8:357-367.

Franklin, Cortney A., Noelle E. Fearn, and Travis W. Franklin. 2005. "HIV/AIDS Among Female Prison Inmates: A Public Health Concern." *Californian Journal of Health Promotion* 3(2):99-112.

Franklin, Cortney A. and Faith E. Lutze. 2007. "Home Confinement and Intensive Supervision as Unsafe Havens: The unintended consequences for women." Pp. 608-623. in *It's a Crime: Women and Justice*, edited by R. Muraskin. Upper Saddle River, NJ: Prentice Hall.

Franklin, Travis F., Cortney A. Franklin, and Travis C. Pratt. 2006. "Examining the Empirical Relationship between Prison Crowding and Inmate Misconduct: A Meta-Analysis of Conflicting Research Results." *Journal of Criminal Justice* 34: 401-412.

French, Sheila and Paul Gendreau. 2003. *Safe and Humane Corrections Through Effective Treatment.* Ottawa: Correctional Service Canada.

Gaes, Gerald G. and Andrew L. Goldberg. 2004. "Prison Rape: A Critical Review of the Literature." Working Paper. National Institute of Justice: Washington, DC.

Goodstein, Lynne and Kevin Wright. 1989. "Inmate Adjustment to Prison." Pp. 229-251 in *The American Prison: Issues in Research and Policy*, edited by L. Goodstein and D. MacKenzie. New York: Plenum Press.

Harer, Miles D. and Darrell J. Steffensmeier. 1996. "Race and Prison Violence." *Criminology* 34:323-355.

Harrison, Paige M. and Allen J. Beck. 2006. *Prisoners at Yearend 2005.* Washington, DC: U. S. Department of Justice, Bureau of Justice Statistics.

Hassine, Victor. 2002. "Prison Violence: From Where I Stand." Pp. 38-56 in *Turnstile Justice,* edited by Rosemary L. Gido and Ted Alleman. Upper Saddle River, NJ: Prentice Hall.

Hochstetler, Andy, Daniel S. Murphy, and Ronald L. Simmons. 2004. "Damaged Goods: Exploring Predictors of Stress in Prison Inmates." *Crime & Delinquency* 50:436-457.

Huebner, Beth M. 2003. "Administrative Determinants of Inmate Violence: A Multilevel Analysis." *Journal of Criminal Justice* 31:107-117.

Human Rights Watch. 2001. "No Escape: Male Rape in U. S. Prisons." Retrieved May 26, 2006 (http://www.hrw.org/reports/2001/prison/report.html#_1_2).

Irwin, John. 1970. The Felon. Englewood Cliffs, NJ: Prentice Hall.

Irwin, John. and Donald R. Cressey. 1962. "Thieves, Convicts, and the Inmate Culture." *Social Problems* 10:142-155.

Jiang, Shanhe, and Marianne Fisher-Giorlando. 2002. "Inmate Misconduct: A Test of the Deprivation, Importation, and Situational Models." *The Prison Journal* 82:335-338.

Knowles, James G. 1999. "Male Prison Rape: A Search for Causation and Prevention." *The Howard Journal* 38:267-282.

Kratcoski, Peter C. 1988. "The Implications of Research Explaining Prison Violence and Disruption." *Federal Probation* 52:27-32.

Light, Stephen C. 1990a. "Measurement Error in Official Statistics: Prison Rule Infraction Data." *Federal Probation* 54:63-68.

------. 1990b. "The Severity of Assaults on Prison Officers: A Contextual Study." Social

Maruschak, Laura M. 2006. HIV in Prisons, 2004. Washington, DC: U.S. Department of Justice, Bureau of Justice Statistics.

McCorkle, Richard C. 1992. "Personal Precautions to Violence in Prison." *Criminal Justice and Behavior* 19:160-173.

------. 1993. "Fear of Victimization and Symptoms of Psychopathology Among Prison Inmates." *Journal of Offender Rehabilitation* 20:73-91.

McCorkle, Richard C., Terance D. Miethe, and Kriss A. Drass. 1995. "The Roots of Prison Violence: A Test of the Deprivation, Management, and 'Not-So-Total' Institution Models." *Crime & Delinquency* 41:317-331.

McGuire, M. Dyan. 2005. "The Impact of Prison Rape on Public Health." *Californian Journal of Health Promotion* 3(2):72-83.

Mumola, Christopher. 2007. *Medical Causes of Deaths in State Prisons.* Washington, DC: U.S. Department of Justice, Bureau of Justice Statistics.

Mumola, Christopher. 2005. *Suicide and Homicide in State Prisons and Local Jails.* Washington, DC: U. S. Department of Justice, Bureau of Justice Statistics.

Nacci, Peter L. and Thomas R. Kane. 1982. *Sex and Sexual Aggression in Federal Prisons.* Washington, DC: U. S. Department of Justice, Federal Prison System.

Nacci, Peter L., Hugh E. Teitelbuam, and Jerry Prather. 1977. "Population Density and Inmate Misconduct Rates in the Federal Prison System." *Federal Probation* 41:26-31.

Reisig, Michael. 1998. "Rates of Disorder in Higher-Custody State Prisons: A Comparative Analysis of Managerial Practices." *Crime & Delinquency* 44:229-244.

Rideau, Wilbert and Ron Wikberg. 1992. *Life Sentences: Rage and Survival Behind Bars.* New York: Random House.

Roberts, Julian V., Michael Jackson, James Bonta, and Paul Gendreau. 1991. "Boats Against the Current: A Note of the Effects of Imprisonment." *Law and Human Behavior* 15:557-562.

Robertson, James E. 2003. "Rape Among Incarcerated Men: Sex Coercion and STDs." *AIDS Patient Care and STDs* 17:423-430.

Ross, Jeffrey I. and Stephen C. Richards. 2002. *Behind Bars: Surviving Prison.* Indianapolis, IN: Alpha Books.

Ruddell, Rick, Scott H. Decker, and Arlen Egley. 2006. "Gang Interventions in Jails: A National Analysis." Criminal Justice Review 31:33-46.

Steinke, Pamela. 1991. "Using Situational Factors to Predict Types of Prison Violence." *Journal of Offender Rehabilitation* 17:119-132.

Struckman-Johnson, Cindy and David Struckman-Johnson. 2000. "Sexual Coercion Rates in Seven Midwestern Prison Facilities for Men." *The Prison Journal* 80:379-390.

Struckman-Johnson, Cindy, David Struckman-Johnson, Lila Rucker, Kurt Bumby, and Stephen Donaldson. 1996. "Sexual Coercion Reported by Men and Women in Prison." *Journal of Sex Research* 33:67-76.

Sykes, Gresham. 1958. *The Society of Captives*. Princeton, NJ: Princeton University Press.

Toch, Hans. 1992. *Mosaic of Despair: Human Breakdowns in Prison*. Washington DC: American Psychological Association.

Useem, Burt and Anne M. Piehl. 2006. "Prison Buildup and Disorder." *Punishment & Society* 8: 87-115.

Walters, Glen D. 1998. "Time Series and Correlational Analysis of Inmate-Initiated Assaultive Incidents in a Large Correctional System." *International Journal of Offender Therapy and Comparative Criminology* 42:124-132.

Wells, James B., Kevin I. Minor, Earl Angel, L. Carter and M.Cox. 2002. *A Study of Gangs and Security Threat Groups in America's Adult Prisons and Jails.* Indianapolis, IN: National Major Gang Task Force.

Wener, Richard. 2006. "Effectiveness of the Direct Supervision System of Correctional Design and Management." *Criminal Justice and Behavior* 33: 392-410.

Wooldredge, John. 1991. "Correlates of Deviant Behavior among Inmates of U.S Correctional Facilities." *Journal of Crime and Justice* 14:1-25.

CHAPTER SEVEN

Addictions in Corrections

P. Ann Dirks-Linhorst

Correctional institutions in the United States serve an ever increasing number of men and women who committed crimes under the influence of drugs, or for drug-related purposes. The Bureau of Justice Statistics reported that at year-end 2005 some 2.3 million inmates were incarcerated, which amounts to an increase of 3.3 percent per year over the last ten year period (Harrison and Beck 2006). One-third of state prisoners and one-fifth of federal prisoners reported drug use at the time of their committing crime (Mumola 1999). Acquiring money to purchase drugs was identified as the criminal rationale for both federal and state prisoners, 16 and 19 percent respectively (Mumola 1999). Approximately four million individuals were on probation at year-end 2005 (Glaze and Bonczar 2006). Of that number, approximately 1,165,000 were sentenced for drug offenses (Glaze and Bonczar 2006). Also, drug crimes were the committing offenses for 290,230 parolees that same year, constituting the largest parolee population (Glaze and Bonczar 2006).

Jails also reported a population increase. Hence, in 2005 some 3,300 local jails housed nearly 750,000 inmates (Harrison and Beck 2006). The jail population at the close of 2005 represented a 76 percent increase from midyear 1990 and a 189 percent increase from midyear 1978 (Frase, 1998; Harrison and Beck 2006). Sixty-six percent of jail inmates regularly used alcohol and 69 percent regularly used drugs. Fifty-seven percent were unemployed, and 14 percent were homeless at least once in the year before incarceration (Lamb and Weinberger 1998). In 2002, there was either drug or alcohol usage for 85 percent of jail inmates who were convicted (Karberg and James 2005). Further, substance abuse has been consistently identified as a predictor of recidivism (Schroeder, Giordano and Cernkovich 2007).

The increase in the correctional population—coupled with the numbers of individuals who commit crimes while under the influence of legal or illicit substances—reflects an increasing need to consider what treatment or rehabilitation options should be in place for substance use at all levels of corrections. Support for such programming has come in the form of federal and state funding opportunities as well as technical assistance. Support from the federal government, for example, was provided in the Violent Crime Control and Law Enforcement Act of 1994. That act created a funding source for states that provided substance abuse treatment approaches for offenders (Patenaude 2005).

A number of agencies have responded to the need for addictions programs in correctional settings. For example, the Federal Bureau of Prisons provides guidance and suggestions for substance abuse screening, referral, education, and both residential and non-residential treatment via the National Institute of Corrections (Arcidiacono and Saum 1995). The American Correctional Association (2002), by contrast, developed performance based standards for general health care within correctional settings, including the management of chemical dependency. Also, the National Commission on Correctional Health Care provides comprehensive standards for juvenile and adult corrections addiction programs. Further support has come from the Substance Abuse and Mental Health Services Administration (SAMSHA) and the Center for Substance Abuse Treatment (CSAT), which among other efforts, have both been working toward the development of a National Treatment Plan to promote evidence-based substance abuse treatment in a variety of settings, including criminal justice systems (Clark 2002). Another resource is the U. S. Department of Justice's Corrections Program Office, which provides lists of federal resources that can assist states with substance abuse treatment programs.

These forms of assistance come with the underlying assumption that if treatment programs result in reduced recidivism, public safety will benefit. This support is also based upon a growing body of empirical studies that report positive treatment outcomes for offenders who participate in these interventions (Knight, Hiller and Simpson 1999).

There is increasing emphasis on evidence-based practices—correctional programs that have demonstrated their effectiveness (MacKenzie 2005), in part to offset the "nothing works" mindset (Tims and Leukefeld 1992; Wexler 2003). This chapter identifies the challenges of operating substance abuse programs in correctional settings. These issues include funding, admission criteria, the methods of interventions, referral source, as well as program capacity, duration, and staffing. The importance of community reintegration and program evaluation are also examined. Last, this chapter highlights interventions that have demonstrated to be effective in correctional settings.

Implementation Challenges – Substance Abuse Programs

The primary function of correctional institutions is to incapacitate individuals who are accused or convicted of criminal offenses. While fulfilling this goal, however, prisons and jails have the potential to serve identify individuals with medical, mental health, or social problems and then refer them to the appropriate services or in some cases providing services to them (Bowker 2002; Mullen et al. 2003; Peters and Matthews 2002). Peters and Matthews outline a rationale for assuming this secondary function. "This changing mission has been influenced by the recognition that jails serve as the repository for growing numbers of disadvantaged individuals who have been displaced from traditional 'safety nets', ... and by the fact that without meaningful interventions, these individuals often cycle repeatedly through the courts, jails, and prisons" (2002:187). This revolving-door pattern of admissions and discharges, coupled with ongoing substance abuse, has an impact upon public health. That impact is seen in HIV and hepatitis related cases requiring costly medical care both in correctional settings and in the community after these inmates are released (Allen et al. 2003).

Despite the substance abuse service needs of prison and jail inmates, and the existence of some model programs, developing and implementing rehabilitative programs in correctional settings is also posed with severe challenges (Farabee et al. 1999; Gendreau, Goggin and Smith 1999; Linhorst et al. 2001; Mullen et al. 2003; Taxman and Bouffard 2002). Chief among these challenges for jails is that most are small, poorly financed, or lack the expertise to operate such programs (Frase 1998). Also, a majority of inmates stay a relatively short time - as arrestees generally make bail in a day or two. As a result, sheriffs have been reluctant to invest in educational, vocational or treatment programs.

The lack of services is particularly notable in the area of substance abuse treatment (Springer, McNeece and Arnold 2003). Compared to prisons, jails have been slow to develop these services, and we are missing an opportunity for treatment and to reduce future criminal activity (Harrison and Martin 2003; Hughey and Klemke 1996). The most recent national survey of substance abuse treatment in jails finds that only 43 percent provide professional treatment to at least a segment of the jail population (Wilson 2000).

In contrast to these statistics, Mumola (1999) found that 94 percent of federal prisons and 56 percent of state prisons offered substance abuse treatment. That investigator also reported that approximately 24 percent of federal and state prisoners participated in substance abuse treatment programs. When correctional substance abuse treatment programs, including those in jails, are properly designed and implemented they can decrease criminal activity and substance use (Pearson and Lipton 1999; Springer et al. 2003). Despite this need, there are a number of challenges to implementing substance abuse treatment programs, some of which are outlined in the following pages.

Funding

Despite the fact that local, state, and federal correctional spending exceeded $60.8 billion dollars in 2003 (Hughes 2006), cost remains a major obstacle to offering substance abuse treatment. Adequate and stable funding of correctional substance abuse treatment programs is critical to their long-term success (Leukefeld and Tims 1993). This, however, is difficult to achieve in jail and prison settings, and funding is especially scarce in small or rural jails (Ruddell and Mays 2007). A survey of jail-based substance abuse treatment programs identified inadequate funding as the most frequent barrier to program implementation (Peters and Matthews 2002). Programs have a wide range of funding sources but the most frequent are county sheriff's budgets. These budgets often are supplemented by federal, state, or local grants. Peters and Matthews (2002) also found that some sheriffs use state liquor excise taxes, inmate funds, and inmate employment contracts to fund rehabilitative programs.

To counter the financial barriers to program implementation and maintenance, funding opportunities for correctional institutions can often be found through a variety of federal sources —including SAMHSA, the U. S. Department of Justice, the National Institute of Corrections, and the Council of State Governments. No matter the funding source, whether the agency is delivering an effective and cost-efficient service is a critical matter given the scarcity of resources. Research has demonstrated the cost-effectiveness of corrections-based substance abuse treatment, yet this issue requires additional studies, especially as they relate to long-term treatment outcomes.

Admission Criteria

A key issue affecting treatment deals with who should be admitted to correctional treatment programs. Since prisons hold inmates for extended periods of time, this matter presents a variety of treatment challenges: such as, when to initiate treatment, how to best maintain a prisoner's motivation, and how to best reintegrate them into the community. Due to the nature of their populations, jail administrators have somewhat different challenges to consider. Jail-based substance abuse treatment programs have a unique admission dilemma: whether to accept pretrial inmates. The primary disadvantage of treating pretrial clients is that they may not complete the treatment, as many are granted bail or resolve their criminal charges (Peters 1993). As a result, limiting treatment to sentenced jail inmates may be a better use of scarce resources. The percentage of clients completing substance abuse treatment programs varies widely, and largely is determined by the percentage of pretrial clients who participate. In a study of six Virginia jails that accepted pretrial clients, program completion rates ranged from nine to 20 percent (Taxman and Bouffard 2000). In a study of jails in California and New York, rates of program completion ranged from 10 to 68 percent, which again fluctuated due to the participation of pretrial clients. By contrast, jail-based substance abuse programs in Arizona, Florida, and New York, that served only sentenced inmates, reported program completion rates of 88 to 96 percent (Glider et al. 1997; Peters et al. 1993; Turley et al. 2004).

Given the low completion rates of pretrial clients, Krebs, Brady and Laird recommend that jails serve only sentenced inmates, arguing, "Targeting inmates who have already been sentenced represents a more practical policy implication, since doing so would likely conserve valuable resources and produce measurably better outcomes" (2003:1251). Consistent with this argument, many programs now serve only sentenced inmates (Glider et al. 1997). Others, however, argue that jail-based substance abuse treatment programs should serve pretrial clients. Peters (1992) contends that serving pretrial defendants greatly increases the number of inmates who can benefit from treatment, while Field (1998) believes that even brief programming with pretrial clients introduces treatment concepts and forms the basis of community referrals to treatment. A second argument against serving pretrial defendants is that some are eventually sentenced to prison and any gains made in jail-based treatment decrease over time. In one program serving pretrial inmates, for example, 50 percent were sentenced to prison (Swartz and Lurigio 1999).

A second admission decision is whether to accept alcohol or drug-addicted inmates with a co-occurring mental illness (also known as 'dual diagnosis'). Failure to address either challenge can result in decreased program success (Springer et al. 2003). A study of inmates participating in substance abuse treatment in five jails found that having a history of mental illness increased the odds of non-completion by almost three times (Brady, Krebs and Laird 2004). Program completion may especially be difficult for inmates experiencing psychiatric symptoms (Peters 1992). Because of their size and ability to provide specialized interventions, larger jails can often provide a separate program for inmates with co-occurring disorders that integrates mental health and substance abuse treatment (Burgess, Swanson and Fallon 1999).

A number of states and the federal prison system have developed co-occurring treatment units (Springer et al. 2003). Typically these programs feature a separate living unit within a prison, with specific referral and eligibility criteria (Katz 1999). SAMHSA has also recognized the need for integrated dual diagnosis treatment programs. In 2004, SAMHSA created the Co-Occurring Center for Excellence (COCE). One of COCE's goals is to collect and disseminate information on best practices for this disadvantaged population (Mental Health Weekly 2004).

Treatment programs may have other admission requirements. One jail, for example, requires potential participants to admit they have a substance abuse problem (Peters 1992). Another requires them to participate in community substance abuse treatment upon release, thus highlighting the issue of mandated or coerced treatment as a key ethical consideration (Farabee and Leukefeld 2001). Subsequently, it raises several key questions: Should costly treatment be given to inmates who are not committed to sobriety? In addition, can we afford to exclude inmates from treatment if public safety is the ultimate goal of the correctional intervention?

Referrals

Referrals to prison and jail-based substance abuse treatment programs come from a number of sources. These include booking officers (staff who conduct the initial admission of inmates as they enter prisons or jails), mental health and medical staff, correctional officers, judges, defense attorneys, other inmates, and self-referrals (Peters 1992). Referral sources are likely to vary across programs. In one substance abuse treatment program in a Texas jail, for example, 65 percent of clients were self-referred, about one-fifth were referred by medical staff, and 14 percent were sentenced to participate by the courts (von Sternberg and Carbonari 2000). By contrast, in one Maryland jail, courts referred 80 percent of all participants (Peters 1992). Many referrals for institutionally based programs originate from both the initial intake and assessment, and case reviews as the inmate approaches their release date (Knight et al. 1999).

Referrals from classification officers deserve special attention. Classification is the process of assessing the risks and needs of inmates as they enter a correctional facility. From this assessment, the facility staff makes housing assignments, determines the level of supervision, and identifies inmate service needs (Bowker 2002). Van Voorhis (2004) describes a model classification system that includes risk, needs, and responsivity assessments. Risk assessment involves the collection of information about past institutional violence, severity of current offenses and prior convictions, escape history, stability factors—such as age, education, and employment status—and time to release. A needs assessment, on the other hand, gathers information on physical and mental health, intellectual ability, alcohol and drug abuse, and educational or vocational status. Responsivity assessments gather information about the inmate's intelligence, maturity, personality, and other personal factors useful for determining an inmates' ability to function in the jail.

As a result of the scope of the information collected, the classification process is an excellent opportunity to identify an inmate's service needs. For this opportunity to be realized, however, classification officers must gather the appropriate information, and make appropriate referrals. Assessment of need is critical to ensure that inmates are matched with appropriate substance abuse services. A wide variety of screening instruments, such as the Alcohol Dependence Scale and the Simple Screening Instrument for Substance Abuse, are recommended by CSAT (2005). Assessment and screening is the focus of the CJ-DATS research initiative (Fletcher and Wexler 2005) and are important because treatment interventions rely upon appropriate assessments, accurate screening, and timely referrals.

Program Capacity

The number of inmates that can be served in prison and jail substance abuse treatment programs is another programmatic consideration. Program capacity varies widely across jail-based substance abuse treatment programs, determined in large part by jail size and funding. New York's Rikers Island jail—one of the largest in the country—developed four separate specialized substance abuse treatment programs ranging in bed capacity from 50 to 324 beds, with a total substance abuse treatment capacity of 648 beds (Burgess et al. 1999). Because urban jails serve a large population, they generally have little difficulty in placing inmates in specialized treatment units. Smaller jails, by contrast, have different challenges. There are some 1775 jails with less than 100 beds in the United States (Ruddell and Mays 2007). Subsequently, it is difficult to develop appropriate substance abuse treatment programs for small numbers of residents (Persinger 1999).

Mumola (1999) reports that approximately one-third of state prison inmates and one-fourth of federal inmates took part in substance abuse treatment since their prison admissions. Comparing these numbers to the prevalence of persons who committed their offenses under the influence of drugs or alcohol highlights the "capacity gap." One of the dilemmas of sentencing and corrections is that although judges are sentencing hundreds of thousands of inmates to jails and prisons for drug offenses—or crimes committed under the influence of drugs or alcohol—correctional systems provide few opportunities for drug and alcohol treatment for these prisoners.

Program Duration

The length of the treatment program is another key consideration for substance abuse interventions. Prisons can often provide longer duration treatment. Examples include: Delaware's Key Therapeutic Community (one year), Texas' Kyle New Vision Program's (nine months), and New York's Stay 'N Out program (nine to 12 months) (Ichiho et al. 1990; Knight et al. 1999). In addition to formal treatment programs, state and federal prisoners may be able to take advantage of "in-house" Alcoholics Anonymous and Narcotics Anonymous groups. Despite the fact prisoners serve longer sentences and they can participate for a longer amount of time, a critical question is if they can sustain the motivation to "remain clean and sober" over the duration of their sentences.

Program duration varies widely for jail-based substance abuse treatment programs. The shortest reported programs range from three to six weeks (Peters 1992; Peters et al. 1993; Peyrot, Yen and Baldassano, 1994). Longer interventions range from 90 to 120 days (Nichols 1990; Turley et al. 2004); and, while some programs run from six to 12 months, the mean length of attendance is much shorter (Taxman and Bouffard 2000; von Sternberg and Carbonari 2000). In a study of program length and community outcomes, Swartz, Lurigio and Slomka (1996) concluded that optimal length of jail-based treatment is three to five months. Harrison and Martin (2003) argue, however, that shorter programs—those with durations of six to eight weeks—can provide inmates with the necessary skills needed to begin the recovery process. Although all correctional substance abuse treatment programs should link clients with community treatment, this is especially important for programs with shorter durations (Field 1998).

Not only is program length important, but the amount of time an inmate spends within substance abuse treatment also matters. In a study of jail-based substance abuse programs, weekly treatment time was 26 hours (Peters and Matthews 2002). In a national sample of jails, however, average weekly time in treatment was five hours across all programs, although this ranged from an average of 3.4 hours in jails with less than 50 beds to 13.4 hours in jails with more than 2,000 beds (Peters et al. 1992). One seldom considered factor in correctional studies is the disconnect between an agency's claims to that which actually occurs. As a result, it is plausible hypothesis that many programs actually deliver fewer hours of treatment than "advertised."

Program Components

Corrections-based substance abuse treatment may include many different components. An American Jail Association (1991) report identified basic models of jail-based substance abuse treatment including, the self-help model (such as Alcoholics Anonymous and other 12-step or peer-run activities). Other classroom-based interventions are more formal than the self-help groups, and include the educational model led by an instructor covering a specific curriculum about alcohol, drugs, and recovery. In addition, some jails employ an outpatient model that requires trained counselors to deliver individual and group treatment. Another type is the residential model, in which everybody in a living unit participates in treatment. Last, some programs incorporate a case management approach that emphasizes assessment, treatment, and referrals to meet the inmate's needs.

In his review of program components for jail-based substance abuse treatment, Peters (1993) lists detoxification, drug testing, assessment, drug education, AIDS education and prevention, life skills training, educational and vocational training, interpersonal skills training, counseling (individual, group, and family), psychiatric services, confronting criminal thinking errors, relapse prevention, self-help groups, case management, transition planning, and aftercare services. Such key components are also recommended for prison-based substance abuse programs (Springer et al. 2003).

Given the wide range of treatment options, intervention approaches within jails and prisons vary widely. A survey of 3,172 jails found that of the one-third of jails that provided substance abuse programs, 64 percent offered assessment of treatment needs, 60 percent afforded self-help groups, 43 percent offered alcohol and drug education and awareness activities, 42 percent conducted drug testing, and 28 percent provided detoxification services (Office of Applied Studies 2000). Similarly, the study of jail-based substance abuse treatment services undertaken by Peters and Matthews (2002) found that most included HIV education and prevention (100%), individual counseling (100%), relapse prevention (100%), education and GED courses (94%), parenting skills (94%),

12-step groups (94%), modifying criminal thinking (82%), domestic violence treatment (77%), vocational and job training services (65%), and services for inmates with co-occurring disorders (47%). The existence of a centralized substance abuse intake unit has had promising results, and the Target Cities Project used this approach to improve and coordinate treatment outcomes (Barron, McFarland and McCamant 2002).

Many of the program components described above form the foundation of prison-based substance abuse programs. One successful approach to substance abuse treatment is the therapeutic community (TC) model. First created for non-correctional settings, the concept of building a community environment has since been adopted in prison living units (Hooper 2003). Substance abuse treatment programs based on the TC model cannot be implemented effectively unless participants reside in the same living unit (Inciardi et al. 1992). While counselors are part of the treatment structure, the inmates form the community, and are instrumental in facilitating changing behaviors (Hooper 2003). The use of peer counselors is an integral component of the TC approach (De Leon 1995). Given the positive outcomes for prison-based TC programs, grants were made available from the U.S. Department of Justice for states to develop these models (Wexler 2003). The Therapeutic Communities of America have published standards from implementation to operation of TCs, which are available on the White House Drug Policy website.

Programs should also be tailored to special needs populations. Women are one example of a special needs group (Field 1998; Taxman and Bouffard 2000). Since 1995, the female population in state and federal institutions has increased 57 percent (Harrison and Beck 2006). Approximately seven percent of all state and federal prisoners and about 13 percent of jail inmates are women (Harrison and Beck 2006). Given these changes, some jail-based programs, for example, have augmented their substance abuse programs for women by addressing self-esteem, family violence, and goal fulfillment. Other important issues for female prisoners include child care, health issues (including counseling and testing for sexually transmitted diseases), and employment (Field 1998). Baletka and Shearer (2005) summarized the development of gender specific correctional programming and highlighted 17 specific treatment issues for women, including self and relationships.

Another special needs correctional population is minority substance abusers. Limited research exists regarding which treatment approaches are most effective with African-American and Hispanic substance abusers (Arroyo, Westerverg and Tonigan 1998; Rounds-Bryant, Motivans and Pelissier 2003). A study of the Federal Bureau of Prisons residential drug treatment programs, however, found that providing culturally competent treatment improves outcomes (Rounds-Bryant et al. 2003). In a correctional context, cultural competence implies that the service providers have knowledge of the culture (including forms of interaction, norms, and beliefs) of the minority groups that they work with, factors that are very important to ensure that interventions are effective.

A recent addition to the substance abuse treatment philosophy is the harm reduction model. This approach differs from a traditional abstinence only philosophy of rehabilitation in that the desired outcome may be a reduction in the amount of use, but not complete abstinence. Harm reduction has been linked to the goal of improving overall health, rather than focusing on the sanctions for specific drug offenses (Springer et al. 2003). Although this model may produce positive outcomes, this method is not without its critics. Regardless, other countries (notably England) for example, are finding that the harm reduction model is a successful treatment strategy within prison settings (Hughes 2003).

Program Location Within the Institution

The location of the treatment program within the correctional institution has been the subject of much debate. It is highly recommended that inmates participating in corrections-based substance abuse treatment programs be housed separately from the general population (Leukefeld and Tims 1993). Housing program participants together allows them to develop a supportive community (Taxman and Bouffard 2000). This concept of community is critical when the correctional institution initiates a TC program (De Leon 2001). In addition, by design, it reduces the number of correctional officers needed to be trained to understand the treatment program and approach.

In some cases, large jail systems have the ability and capacity to dedicate a separate building for substance abuse treatment programs. For example, a 320 bed medium security building that is part of the Chicago Cook County jail is reserved for participants in the substance abuse treatment program (Swartz and Lurigio 1999). Other jails dedicate entire floors to substance abuse treatment (von Sternberg and Carbonari 2000) or pods (e.g., separate living units) within a floor (Glider et al. 1997; Taxman and Bouffard 2000). Still, in other programs, usually smaller jails, program participants are dispersed throughout the jail (Hughey and Klemke 1996).

Despite the desirability of housing program participants separately from other inmates, a survey of over 1,700 jail-based programs found that only 12 percent of jails housed program participants in separate housing units (although this statistic ranged from four percent of programs in jails with 50 to 250 beds to 90 percent of programs in jails with 2000 or more beds) (Peters et al. 1992). A 1997 survey of over 3,000 jails reported similar findings, with approximately two-thirds of jails providing treatment only to inmates in the general population, 18 percent housing program participants in units separate from the general population, and 10 percent housing some participants in separate units and others in the general population (Office of Applied Studies 2000). Maintaining separate units can be challenging. Some jails housed female substance abusers in the general population because their numbers were too small to fill a living unit (Glider et al. 1997; Peters 1992; Peters et al. 1993). When overcrowding occurs, even jails with separate treatment units may assign inmates without addictions problems to vacant beds in treatment units (Swartz and Lurigio 1999; Tunis et al. 1996).

Staffing

Another program component, which poses a significant cost for correctional operations, is staffing and training. Maintaining a qualified, well-trained program staff, including counselors and correctional officers, is essential for effective substance abuse interventions. This can be challenging because in correctional facilities addictions counselors traditionally received low pay and suffered from high turnover rates (Farabee et al. 1999). In order to deliver the best substance abuse treatment with limited resources, a number of different approaches have been used.

For example, one choice correctional administrators must make is how to secure counselors. For instance, they can hire counselors as employees, contract with private agencies to provide substance abuse services, or use a combination of both approaches. A survey of jail-based treatment programs found that most relied upon "in house" employees (Peters and Matthews 2002).

Little has been written about the positive and negative aspects of in-house versus contract staff delivering substance abuse treatment programs. One study of contract staff in a prison substance abuse treatment program identified challenges to writing, bidding, and overseeing treatment contracts (Linhorst et al. 2001). Positive examples exist of staff employed by the jail (Peters et al. 1993), of contract staff only (Swartz and Lurigio 1999), and of mixed models (Glider et al. 1997). Taxman and Bouffard (2000) outlined some negative aspects of using contract staff. In their evaluation of six Virginia jails, they reported that contract counselors had a high turnover rate and did not meet expectations for developing formal relationships with community agencies.

A second staffing consideration is deciding whether to require substance abuse counselors to be licensed professionals, or setting other educational requirements for these staff. Peters and Matthews' (2002) survey found that 83 percent of counselors were licensed professionals, although they did not collect information about educational standing. One large jail required that all clinicians in the substance abuse treatment program hold a master's degree and be certified or licensed in substance abuse counseling, social work, or psychology (Burgess et al. 1999). Recruiting counselors with advanced degrees and with licensure or certification to work in jails can be a significant challenge, especially in rural areas (Farabee et al. 1999). While prison systems can typically afford to pay higher wages, the austere environment, professional isolation, and the workload demands of prisons often make it difficult to recruit and retain qualified professionals.

A third staffing dilemma is whether or not to hire ex-offenders or people who are in substance abuse recovery. Many substance abuse counselors are in recovery, and as ex-offenders, they can be highly effective as counselors. Peters and Matthews' (2002) found that about one-half of counselors were former substance abusers. Many correctional facilities do not permit ex-offenders or people in recovery to serve as counselors (Harrison and Martin 2003). Some critics view this as a major obstacle to developing effective jail-based programs (see von Sternberg and Carbonari 2000). One prison program, for example, was highly committed to hiring people in recovery and ex-offenders, but a state law prevented them from working in prisons as state employees. To circumvent this obstacle, the prisons contracted with treatment services because state law does not restrict a contract agency from hiring ex-offenders as counselors (Inciardi et al. 1992).

The last staffing decision is how to incorporate correctional officers into the substance abuse treatment program. Some officers are interested in assisting with treatment in addition to fulfilling their custodial roles (Stohr, Lovrich and Mays 1997). Their level of involvement in the program depends in part on the treatment model that is used. Residential program models, particularly therapeutic communities, require that correctional officers receive extensive training so they can effectively intervene with clients in ways that support the program (Burgess et al. 1999; De Leon 2001). Even in other program models in which correctional officers are not as directly involved, it remains important that officers support inmates in the recovery process and communicate with substance abuse counselors. In practice, however, this rarely is the case.

Peters and Matthews' (2002) survey of jail-based addictions programs found that poor communication between correctional officers and counselors was a factor in 38 percent of programs, and was cited as the second most frequent barrier to effective program implementation, after inadequate funding. In their evaluation of six Virginia jails, Taxman and Bouffard (2000) recorded instances when correctional officers undermined treatment efforts and were disrespectful to program clients and staff. One way to address this issue is to cross-train correctional officers and substance abuse counselors so that each understands the duties of the other (Farabee et al. 1999; Peters 1993; Tunis et al. 1996). Farabee and colleagues (1999) also recommend offering certification and financial incentives to correctional officers who volunteer to participate in classroom and on-the-job training in the substance abuse treatment program.

Community Reintegration

Aftercare, or community reintegration, is a critical component for successful release from correctional settings (Pelissier, Jones and Cadigan 2007) and should be included as part of the treatment plan from the initial assessment and classification (Osher, Steadman and Barr 2003). Research has consistently found that the positive outcomes of prison and jail-based substance abuse treatment quickly diminish when inmates do not continue treatment in the community following release from custody (Inciardi et al. 2002; Wexler, De Leon et al. 1999; Wexler, Melnick et al. 1999). As such, staff in corrections-based substance abuse treatment programs have an obligation to facilitate their clients' access to community treatment (Martin et al. 1999; Tims and Leukefeld 1992). When participants are in a short-term jail-based program, staff should make referrals to community services (Burgess et al. 1999; Field 1998). Despite its importance, a survey of over 1,700 jail-based substance abuse treatment programs found that only 44 percent of jails provided transition planning, although 84 percent made referrals to community treatment (Peters et al. 1992). A survey of moderate to large jails found that all provided services to facilitate access to community treatment. Such services include assessing community treatment needs, planning discharge, and actively linking clients with community services (Peters and Matthews 2002). Despite this need, however, aftercare programs that provide transitional help are not always delivered (Tunis et al. 1996).

Some barriers to linking clients with community substance abuse treatment include the following: the fact that many community agencies do not want to work with ex-offenders (Farabee et al. 1999); limited availability of substance abuse treatment in the community, especially residential and intensive outpatient services (Farabee et al. 1999; Harrison and Martin 2003; Peters and Kearns 1992; Peters and Matthews 2002); unstable housing and homelessness (Peters and Matthews 2002); poor coordination with probation and parole officers (Taxman and Bouffard 2000); and courts not requiring inmates to participate in substance abuse treatment as conditions of release or probation (Field 1998; Peters et al. 1993; Peters and Matthews 2002). A review of these factors suggests poor integration between courts, correctional facilities, and community resources.

Differences exist in aftercare planning for programs serving offenders with short jail stays and those sentenced to long-term imprisonment (Osher et al. 2003). Cooperation between all service delivery providers—such as substance abuse providers and mental health providers (if co-occurring diagnoses are relevant), and correctional authorities—is critical to the success of community aftercare programs. The reason being is that such cooperation can also reduce costs, and improve program implementation (Osher et al. 2003). Planning for the offender's community reintegration should account for individual needs, housing, medication and medical care, income supports (to support the individual's basic needs of food, clothing and transportation), and child care (Osher et al. 2003). Given this range of services, collaboration is an important dimension of effective aftercare. If offenders do not participate in aftercare, treatment gains are typically lost (Melnick et al. 2001). Thus, not only must coordinated services be available, but encouragement, possibly in the form of coerced participation through conditions of release or parole, may also be necessary to increase compliance.

A number of strategies have been successful at increasing participation in aftercare. These interventions include: working with courts to offer early release or suspended sentences if offenders participate in treatment (Farabee et al. 1999; Peters 1992); advocating that probation (or parole) officers include community treatment as a condition of release from custody (Peters 1992; Peters et al. 1993; Peters and Matthews 2002); creating specialized probation and parole officer positions who work exclusively with inmates who have completed jail-based substance abuse treatment (Taxman and Bouffard 2000); funding counselor positions within treatment programs dedicated exclusively to aftercare planning (Peters 1992; Taxman and Bouffard 2000); enabling community agencies to make presentations to offenders and referring them to community services prior to their release (Field 1998); and funding aftercare services for three to six months so that the probationers or parolees can participate in community treatment (Field 1998; Peters and Matthews 2002; Taxman and Bouffard 2000). Ultimately, these studies revealed that completing a period of aftercare upon release from either jail or prison leads to less recidivism (Knight et al. 1999) and greater public safety.

The need for this aftercare planning for aftercare was recognized in the Brad H. v. City of New York (Barr 2003) lawsuit. Attorneys in this class action litigation argued that a lack of aftercare services for inmates discharged from New York City jails was unconstitutional, and the court agreed. Subsequently, the Court held that the jail system had an obligation to provide discharge planning (Barr 2003). In the future, it is likely that this decision will also stimulate more effective discharge planning for offenders with substance abuse treatment needs, as well as those with co-occurring disorders.

Program Evaluation and Evidence Based Corrections

Increasing attention is being placed on evaluating correctional programs to determine if they are effective (Friedmann, Taxman and Henderson 2007). For example, Pearson and Lipton (1999) conducted a meta-analysis to evaluate the effects of substance abuse treatment on recidivism. They discovered that boot camps and group counseling did not decrease recidivism, therapeutic communities had a small positive effect, and that methadone maintenance, substance abuse education, 12-step programs, and cognitive-behavioral programs were promising. Hiller and colleagues (2002) summarized a number of evaluations finding support for long-term substance abuse treatment programs in prisons, including therapeutic communities.

Measuring the success of these endeavors is problematic as programs often have different goals, and jurisdictions sometimes measure recidivism in different ways. Beyong merely collecting "yes/no" data about recidivism, Prendergast, Hall and Wexler (2003) suggest that agencies evaluate multiple outcome variables. Should a technical violation of parole or probation (such as a failed urine test), for example, be considered as treatment failure? Heinrich and Lynn (2002) suggest a variety of policy, program, and participant-level variables need to be included in any analysis in order to properly explain treatment outcomes. In addition to including funding and offender characteristics, these studies should also measure political climate, organizational mission, leadership as well as management style and capacity (Heinrich and Lynn 2002).

The issue of what constitutes "effective treatment" is key to any discussion about program evaluation. An attempt to define effective treatment was undertaken by the Office of National Drug Control Policy.

It included the following goals: "reduced primary drug use; improved employment functioning; improvements in educational status and interpersonal relationships; improved health and mental health status; improved legal status; and improved noncriminal public safety factors" (Springer et al. 2003:182). Program evaluation should be identified as a high priority, to properly evaluate the costs and benefits of an intervention, and also to serve as a step towards evidence-based corrections policies (De Leon 2001; Tims and Leukefeld 1992; Wexler 1996).

In addition to adding to the literature on evidence-based corrections, Field (1998) argues that program evaluation can also increase our understanding of costs, determining program outcomes, improving program implementation, assisting with policy making, obtaining funding, and promoting program expansion. Publicizing information about successful interventions is also helpful to other correctional programs (Wexler 1996). Yet, meaningful program evaluations require sound data (Leukefeld and Tims, 1993). Field (1998) contends that program evaluators should be involved in program development to assist with the creation of databases. Key evaluation questions include: What data should be collected? And, who will collect, analyze and disseminate the data? Peters (1993) recommends comprehensive information be collected from each program participant; and Patenaude (2005) suggests that correctional staff must also provide feedback about program effectiveness.

Conclusion

The high numbers of men and women convicted of drug-related offenses highlights the importance of offering substance abuse treatment programs in jails and prisons. Correctional administrators have responded to this need by implementing a number of substance abuse interventions that can be described as "best practices." Such programs cannot exist in isolation though: Often these interventions bridge the correctional facility and community. There is a growing acknowledgement that supporting an inmate's transition to the community is of key importance. In support of these programs, there has been an expansion in the amount of federal, state, and local funding. Resources, including technical assistance and, to some extent, funding opportunities, are increasingly contingent on implementing evidence-based practices.

A growing body of research has emphasized the need for evidence-based correctional interventions (Friedmann et al. 2007; MacKenzie 2005). There are several implementation issue that correctional administrators must address. Consistent terms and measures for outcome evaluation are necessary to allow meaningful comparisons among programs.

As outlined in this chapter, issues such as funding, staffing, program duration, capacity, as well as program admission criteria are of key importance. In addition, collaboration between the criminal justice system and community treatment providers is an absolute priority. Through improved addictions treatment, public safety and public health may both be increased.

References

Allen, Scott A., Josiah D. Rich, Beth Schwartzapfel and Peter D. Friedmann. 2003. "Hepatitis C Among Offenders – Correctional Challenge and Public Health Opportunity." *Federal Probation* 67:22-26.

American Correctional Association. 2002. "Performance-Based Standards for Correctional Health Care in Adult Correctional Institutions." Lanham, MD.

American Jail Association. 1991. *Design and Implementation Issues for Drug Treatment in the Jail Setting* (NCJ 152360). Washington, DC: U. S. Department of Justice, Office of Justice Programs, Bureau of Justice Assistance.

Arcidiacono, Anita and Christine A. Saum. 1995. "Substance Abuse Treatment Options: A Federal Initiative." *Journal of Psychoactive Drugs* 27:105-107.

Arroyo, Judith A., Verner S. Westerberg and J. Scott Tonigan. 1998. "Comparison of Treatment Utilization and Outcome for Hispanics and Non-Hispanic Whites." *Journal of Studies on Alcohol* 53:286-291.

Baletka, Dawn Marie and Robert A. Shearer. 2005. "Assessing Program Needs of Female Offenders Who Abuse Substances." Pp. 227-242 in *Substance Abuse Treatment with Correctional Clients*, edited by B. Sims. New York: The Haworth Press.

Barr, Heather. 2003. "Transinstitutionalization in the Courts: Brad H. v. City of New York, and the Fight for Discharge Planning for People with Psychiatric Disabilities Leaving Rikers Island." *Crime & Delinquency* 49:97-123.

Barron, Nancy, Bentson H. McFarland and Lynn McCamant. 2002. "Varieties of Centralized Intake: The Portland Target Cities Project Experience." *Journal of Psychoactive Drugs* 34:75-86.

Bowker, Gary M. 2002. *Jail Resource Issues: What Every Funding Authority Needs to Know* (NIC 017372). Washington, DC: U. S. Department of Justice, National Institute of Corrections.

Brady, Thomas. M., Christopher P. Krebs and Glen Laird. 2004. "Psychiatric Comorbidity and Not Completing Jail-Based Substance Abuse Treatment." *American Journal on Addictions* 13:83-101.

Broner, Nahama, Huy Nguyen, Anne Swern and Stephen Goldfinger. 2003. "Adapting a Substance Abuse Court Diversion Model for Felony Offenders with Co-Occurring Disorders: Initial Implementation." *Psychiatric Quarterly* 74:361-385.

Burgess, John D., Arthur J. Swanson and Bryan Fallon. 1999. "Therapeutic Community Services: A Jail-Based Substance Abuse Treatment Program at Rikers Island." *American Jails* 3:25-30.

Center for Substance Abuse Treatment. 2005. *Substance Abuse Treatment for Adults in Criminal Justice System: Treatment Improvement Protocol (TIP)* Series 44. Rockville, MD: U. S. Department of Health and Human Services, Substance Abuse and Mental Health Services Administration.

Center for Substance Abuse Treatment. 2002. *Treatment Drug Courts: Integrating Substance Abuse Treatment with Legal Case Processing: Treatment Improvement Protocol* (TIP) Series 23. Rockville, MD: U. S. Department of Health and Human Services, Substance Abuse and Mental Health Services Administration.

Clark, H. Westley. 2002. "Bridging the Gap Between Substance Abuse Practice and Research: The National Treatment Plan Initiative." *Journal of Drug Issues* 32:757-768.

Cunningham, Debbie S. and William E. Stone. 2005. "Effects of a Drug Diversion Court on Client Recidivism." Pp. 135-149 in *Substance Abuse Treatment with Correctional Clients,* edited by B. Sims. New York: The Haworth Press.

De Leon, George. 2001. "Therapeutic Communities for Substance Abuse: Developments in North America." Pp. 79-104 in *Therapeutic Communities for the Treatment of Drug Users,* edited by B. Rawlings and R. Yates. Philadelphia PA: Jessica Kingsley Publishers.

De Leon, George. 1995. "Residential Therapeutic Communities in the Mainstream: Diversity and Issues." *Journal of Psychoactive Drugs* 27:3-15.

Dynia, Paul and Hung-En Sung. 2000. "The Safety and Effectiveness of Diverting Felony Drug Offenders to Residential Treatment as Measured by Recidivism." *Criminal Justice Policy Review* 11:299-311.

Farabee, David and Carl G. Leukefeld. 2001. "Recovery and the Criminal Justice System." Pp. 40-59 in *Relapse and Recovery in Addictions,* edited by F. M. Tims, C. G. Leukefeld and J. J. Platt. New Haven, CT: Yale University Press.

Farabee, David. Michael Prendergast, Jerome Cartier, Harry Wexler, Kevin Knight and M. Douglas Anglin. 1999. "Barriers to Implementing Effective Correctional Drug Treatment Programs." *The Prison Journal* 79:150-162.

Field, Gary. 1998. *Continuity of Offender Treatment for Substance Use Disorders from Institution to Community*. Rockville, MD: U. S. Department of Health and Human Services, Substance Abuse and Mental Health Services Administration, Center for Substance Abuse Treatment.

Fletcher, Bennett W. and Harry K. Wexler. 2005. "National Criminal Justice Drug Abuse Treatment Studies (CJ-DATS): Update and Progress." *Justice Research and Statistics Association: The Forum* 23:1-7.

Frase, Richard S. 1998. "Jails." Pp. 474-506 in *The Handbook of Crime and Punishment,* edited by M. Tonry. New York: Oxford University Press.

Friedmann, Peter D., Faye S. Taxman and Craig E. Henderson. 2007. "Evidence-Based Treatment Practices for Drug-Involved Adults in the Criminal Justice System." *Journal of Substance Abuse Treatment* 32: 267-277.

Gendreau, Paul, Claire Goggin and Paula Smith. 1999. "The Forgotten Issue in Effective Correctional Treatment: Program Implementation." *International Journal of Offender Therapy and Comparative Criminology* 43:180-187.

Glaze, Lauren E. and Thomas P. Bonczar. 2006. *Probation and Parole in the United States, 2005* (NCJ210676). Washington, DC: U. S. Department of Justice, Office of Justice Programs, Bureau of Justice Statistics.

Glider, Peggy, Rod Mullen, Dianne Herbst, Catherine Davis and Bette Fleishman. 1997. "Substance Abuse Treatment in a Jail Setting: A Therapeutic Community

Model." Pp. 97-112 in *Community as Method: Therapeutic Communities for Special Populations and Special Settings,* edited by George De Leon. Westport, CT: Praeger.

Harrison, Lana D. and Steven S. Martin. 2003. *Residential Treatment Abuse Treatment for State Prisoners: Implementation Lessons Learned* (NCJ 195738). U. S. Department of Justice Programs, Office of Justice Programs, National Institute of Justice.

Harrison, Paige M. and Allen J. Beck. 2006. *Prisoners in 2005* (NCJ210677). Washington, DC: U. S. Department of Justice, Office of Justice Programs, Bureau of Justice Statistics.

Harrison, Paige M. and Allen J. Beck. 2006b. *Prison and Jail Inmates at Midyear 2005* (NCJ208801). Washington, DC: U. S. Department of Justice, Office of Justice Programs, Bureau of Justice Statistics.

Heinrich, Carolyn J. and Laurence E. Lynn Jr. 2002. "Improving the Organization, Management, and Outcomes of Substance Abuse Treatment Programs." *The American Journal of Drug and Alcohol Abuse* 28:601-622.

Hiller, Matthew L., Kevin Knight, Sandhya R. Rao and D. Dwayne Simpson. 2002. "Assessing and Evaluating Mandated Correctional Substance-Abuse Treatment." Pp. 41-68 in *Treatment of Drug Offenders: Policies and Issues,* edited by C. G. Leukefeld, F. Tims and D. Farabee. New York, NY: Springer.

Hooper, Robert M. 2003. "Something Works – Therapeutic Communities in the Treatment of Substance Abuse". Pp. 12-2-12-17 in *Correctional Psychology: Practice, Programming, and Administration,* edited by B. K. Schwartz. Kingston, NJ: Civic Research Institute.

Hughes, Kristen A. 2006. *Justice Expenditure and Employment in the United States,* 2003 Washington, DC: U. S. Department of Justice, Office of Justice Programs, Bureau of Justice Statistics.

Hughes, Rhidian. 2003. "Drugs, Prisons and Harm Reduction." *Journal of Health and Social Policy* 18:43-54.

Hughey, Ray and Lloyd W. Klemke. 1996. "Evaluation of a Jail-Based Substance Abuse Treatment Program." *Federal Probation* 60:40-44.

Ichiho, Henry, Gerard DeLisio, Theodore Sakai and Sandra Moritsugu. 1990. "The Hawaii State Department of Corrections Substance Abuse Strategy." *Hawaii Medical Journal* 49:196-208.

Inciardi, James A., Steven S. Martin, Dorothy Lockwood, Robert M. Hooper and Bruce M. Wald. 1992. "Obstacles to the Implementation and Evaluation of Drug Treatment Programs in Correctional Settings: Reviewing the Delaware KEY Experience." Pp. 176-191 in *Drug Abuse Treatment in Prisons and Jails,* edited by C. G. Leukefeld and F. M. Tims. Rockville, MD: U. S. Department of Health and Human Services.

Inciardi, James A., Hilary L. Surratt, Steven S. Martin and Robert M. Hooper. 2002. "The Importance of Aftercare in a Corrections-Based Treatment Continuum." Pp. 204-216 in *Treatment of Drug Offenders: Policies and Issues,* edited by C. G. Leukefeld, F. M. Tims and D. Farabee. New York: Springer.

Jessup, Mary. 2001. "Therapeutic Jurisprudence: Judicial and Corrections Panel." *Journal of Psychoactive Drugs* 33:355-367.

Karberg, Jennifer C. and Doris J. James. 2005. *Substance Dependence, Abuse, and Treatment of Jail Inmates, 2002.* NCJ209588. Washington, DC: U. S. Department of Justice, Office of Justice Programs, Bureau of Justice Statistics.

Katz, Randall I. 1999. "The Addiction Treatment Unit: A Dual Diagnosis Program at the California Medical Facility-A Descriptive Study." *Journal of Psychoactive Drugs* 31:41-46.

Knight, Kevin, Matthew L. Hiller and D. Dwayne Simpson. 1999. "Evaluating Corrections-Based Treatment for the Drug-Abusing Criminal Offender." *Journal of Psychoactive Drugs* 31:299-304.

Krebs, Christopher P., Thomas Brady and Glen Laird. 2003. "Jail-Based Substance User Treatment: An Analysis of Retention." *Substance Use and Misuse* 38:1227-1258.

Lamb, H. Richard and Linda E. Weinberger. 1998. "Persons with Severe Mental Illness in Jails and Prisons: A Review." *Psychiatric Services* 49:483-492.

Leukefeld, Carl G. and Frank M. Tims. 1993. "Drug Abuse Treatment in Prisons and Jails." *Journal of Substance Abuse Treatment* 10:77-84.

Linhorst, Donald M., Kevin Knight, J. Scott Johnston and Myrna Trickey. 2001. "Situational Influences on the Implementation of a Prison-Based Therapeutic Community." *The Prison Journal* 81:436-453.

Lo, Celia C. and Richard C. Stephens. 2002. "Arrestees' Perceived Needs for Substance-Specific Treatment: Exploring Urban-Rural Differences." *The American Journal of Drug and Alcohol Abuse* 28:623-642.

MacKenzie, Doris Layton. 2005. "The Importance of Using Scientific Evidence to Make Decisions About Correctional Programming." *Criminology & Public Policy* 4:249-257.

Martin, Steven S., Clifford A. Butzin, Christine A. Saum and James A. Inciardi. 1999. "Three-Year Outcomes of Therapeutic Community Treatment for Drug-Involved Offenders in Delaware: From Prison to Work Release to Aftercare." *The Prison Journal* 79:294-320.

Melnick, Gerald, George De Leon, George Thomas, David Kressel, and Harry K. Wexler. 2001. "Treatment Process in Prison Therapeutic Communities: Motivation, Participation, and Outcome." *American Journal of Drug Alcohol Abuse* 27:633-650.

Mental Health Weekly. 2004. "SAMHSA Creates Assistance Center for Co-Occurring Disorders." 14:6.

Mullen, Patricia D., A. Gaye Cummins, Mary M. Velasquez, Kirk von Sternberg and Raul Carvajal. 2003. "Jails as Important but Constrained Venues for Addressing Women's Health." *Family and Community Health* 26:157-168.

Mumola, Christopher J. 1999. *Substance Abuse and Treatment, State and Federal Prisoners, 1997* (NCJ172871). Washington, DC: U. S. Department of Justice, Office of Justice Programs, Bureau of Justice Statistics.

Mumola, Christopher J. 1998. *Substance Abuse and Treatment of Adults on Probation, 1995* (NCJ166611). Washington, DC: U. S. Department of Justice, Office of Justice Programs, Bureau of Justice Statistics.

Nichols, Jennifer. 1990. "Facing Society with Sobriety: Virginia Jail Helps Offenders Get Out from Under the Influence." *Corrections Today*, 108-110.

Office of Applied Studies. 2000. *Substance Abuse Treatment in Adult and Juvenile Correctional Facilities: Findings from the Uniform Facility Data Set 1997 Survey of Correctional Facilities.* Rockville, MD: U. S. Department of Health and Human Services, Substance Abuse and Mental Health Services Administration, Office

of Applied Studies.
Osher, Fred, Henry J. Steadman and Heather Barr. 2003. "A Best Practice Approach to Community Reentry from Jails for Inmates with Co-Occurring Disorders: The APIC Model." *Crime and Delinquency* 49:79-96.
Patenaude, Allan L. 2005. "A Qualitative Exploration into a Prison Substance Abuse Treatment Program: "I Tell Them What They Want to Hear"." Pp. 73-93 in *Substance Abuse Treatment with Correctional Clients*, edited by B. Sims. New York: The Haworth Press.
Pearson, Frank S. and Douglas S. Lipton. 1999. "A Meta-Analytic Review of the Effectiveness of Corrections-Based Treatments for Drug Abuse." *Prison Journal* 79:384-410.
Pelissier, Bernadette, Nichole Jones and Timothy Cadigan. 2007. "Drug Treatment Aftercare in the Criminal Justice System: A Systematic Review." *Journal of Substance Abuse Treatment* 32: 311-320.
Persinger, Bill D., Jr. 1999. "Local Agencies Cooperate to Deliver Substance Abuse Counseling in Rural Jails: A Program Report from the Field." *American Jails* 3:31-34.
Peters, Roger H. 1993. "Drug Treatment in Jails and Detention Settings." Pp. 44-80 in *Drug Treatment and Criminal Justice*, edited by James A. Inciardi. Newbury Park, CA: Sage.
------. 1992. "Referral and Screening for Substance Abuse Treatment in Jails." *Journal of Mental Health Administration* 19:53-75.
Peters, Roger H. and William D. Kearns. 1992. "Drug Abuse History and Treatment Needs of Jail Inmates." *American Journal of Drug and Alcohol Abuse* 18:355-366.
Peters, Roger H., William D. Kearns, Mary R. Murrin, Addis S. Dolente and Robert L. May, II. 1993. "Examining the Effectiveness of In-Jail Substance Abuse Treatment." *Journal of Offender Rehabilitation* 19:1-39.
Peters, Roger H. and Charles O. Matthews. 2002. "Jail Treatment for Drug Offenders." Pp. 186-203 in *Treatment of Drug Offenders: Policies and Issues,* edited by C. G. Leukefeld, F. M. Tims, and D. Farabee. New York: Springer.
Peters, Roger H., Robert L. May, II and William D. Kearns. 1992. "Drug Treatment in Jails: Results of a Nationwide Survey." *Journal of Criminal Justice* 20:283-295.
Peyrot, Mark, Sherman Yen and Carole A. Baldassano. 1994. "Short-Term Substance Abuse Prevention in Jail: A Cognitive Behavioral Approach." *Journal of Drug Education* 24:33-47.
Prendergast, Michael L., Elizabeth A. Hall and Harry K. Wexler. 2003. "Multiple Measures of Outcome in Assessing a Prison-Based Drug Treatment Program." Pp. 65-94 in *Treating Substance Abusers in Correctional Contexts: New Understandings, New Modalities,* edited by N. J. Pallone. New York, NY: The Haworth Press.
Rounds-Bryant, Jennifer L., Mark A. Motivans and Bernadette Pelissier. 2003. "Comparison of Background Characteristics and Behaviors of African-American, Hispanic, and White Substance Abusers Treated in Federal Prison: Results from the TRIAD Study." *Journal of Psychoactive Drugs* 35:333-341.
Ruddell, Rick and G. Larry Mays. 2007. "Rural Jails: Problematic Inmates, Overcrowded Cells, and Cash-Strapped Counties." *Journal of Criminal Justice* 35: 251-260.
Schroeder, Ryan D., Peggy C. Giordano and Stephen A. Cernkovich. 2007. "Drug

Use and Desistance Process." *Criminology* 45: 191-222.
Springer, David W., C. Aaron McNeece and Elizabeth M.Arnold. 2003. *Substance Abuse Treatment for Criminal Offenders: An Evidence-Based Guide for Practitioners.* Washington, DC: American Psychological Association.
Stephan, James J. 2004. *State Prison Expenditures, 2001.* NCJ202949. Washington, DC: U. S. Department of Justice, Office of Justice Programs, Bureau of Justice Statistics.
Stohr, Mary K., Craig Hemmens, Brian Shapiro, Brian Chambers and Laura Kelley. "Comparing Inmate Perceptions of Two Residential Substance Abuse Treatment Programs." *International Journal of Offender Therapy and Comparative Criminology* 46:699-714.
Stohr, Mary K., Nicholas P. Lovrich and G. Larry Mays. 1997. "Service v. Security Focus in Training Assessments: Testing Gender Differences Among Women's Jail Correctional Officers." *Women and Criminal Justice* 9:65-85.
Swartz, James A. and Arthur J. Lurigio. 1999. "Final Thoughts on IMPACT: A Federally Funded, Jail-Based, Drug-User-Treatment Program." *Substance Use and Misuse* 34:887-906.
Swartz, James A., Arthur J. Lurigio and Scott Slomka. 1996. "The Impact of IMPACT: An Assessment of the Effectiveness of a Jail-Based Treatment Program." *Crime and Delinquency* 42:553-573.
Taxman, Faye S. and Jeffrey A. Bouffard. 2000. *Residential Substance Abuse Treatment (RSAT) in Jail: Comparison of Six Sites in Virginia* (NCJ 182858).U. S. Department of Justice, National Institute of Justice.
Taxman, Faye S. and Jeffrey A. Bouffard. 2002. "Assessing Therapeutic Integrity in Modified Therapeutic Communities for Drug-Involved Offenders." *Prison Journal* 82:189-212.
Tims, Frank M. and Carl G. Leukefeld. 1992. "The Challenge of Drug Abuse Treatment in Prisons and Jails." *National Institute on Drug Abuse Research Monograph Series: Drug Abuse Treatment in Prisons and Jails.* Rockville, MD: U.S. Department of Health and Human Services, Public Health Service, National Institute of Health.
Tunis, Sandra, James Austin, Mark Morris, Patricia Hardyman, and Melissa Bolyard. 1996. *Evaluation of Drug Treatment in Local Corrections.* Washington, DC: U.S. Department of Justice, Office of Justice Programs, National Institute of Justice.
Turley, Alan, Tim Thornton, Craig Johnson and Sue Azzolino. 2004. "Jail Drug and Alcohol Treatment Program Reduces Recidivism in Nonviolent Offenders: A Longitudinal Study of Monroe County, New York's, Jail Treatment Drug and Alcohol Program." *International Journal of Offender Therapy and Comparative Criminology* 48:721-728.
Van Voorhis, Patricia. 2004. "An Overview of Offender Classification Systems." Pp 133 -160 in *Correctional Counseling and Rehabilitation* 5th ed., edited by P. Van Voorhis, M. Braswell, and D. Lester. Washington, DC: Anderson.
von Sternberg, Kirk and Joseph P. Carbonari. 2000. An Evaluation of the "New Choices" *Substance Abuse Treatment Program in the Harris County Jail, Houston, Texas – PROJECT CARE Final Report.* Houston, TX: University of Houston, Change Assessment Research.
Walker, Robert and Carl G. Leukefeld. 2002. "Employment Rehabilitation." Pp. 69-

79 in *Treatment of Drug Offenders: Policies and Issues*, edited by C. G. Leukefeld, F. Tims and D. Farrabee. New York, NY: Springer Publishing Company.
Wexler, Harry K. 2003. "The Promise of Prison-Based Treatment for Dually Diagnosed Inmates." *Journal of Substance Abuse Treatment* 25:223-231.
------. 1996. "Evaluation of Prison Substance Abuse Treatment Programs: Outcome Studies and Methodology." Pp. 109-131 in *Drug Treatment Behind Bars: Prison-Based Strategies for Change*, edited by K. E. Early. Westport, CT: Praeger.
Wexler, Harry K., George De Leon, George Thomas, David Kressel and Jean Peters. 1999. "The Amity Prison TC Evaluation: Reincarceration Outcomes." *Criminal Justice and Behavior* 26:147-167.
Wexler, Harry K., Gerald Melnick, Lois Lowe and Jean Peters. 1999. "Three Year Reincarceration Outcomes for Amity In-Prison Therapeutic Community and Aftercare in California." *The Prison Journal* 79:321-336.
Wilson, Doris J. 2000. *Drug Use, Testing, and Treatment in Jails* (NCJ 179999). Washington, DC: U.S. Department of Justice, Office of Justice Programs, Bureau of Justice Statistics.

CHAPTER EIGHT

Saving Lives Through Suicide Prevention

Christine Tartaro and David Lester

Prisons and jails typically house people who have an elevated risk for suicide due to their mental health status, substance abuse, and their understandably high levels of anxiety due to uncertainty about the future. An inmate's stress and discomfort levels are often exacerbated by the prison or jail environment. In this chapter, we examine the scope of problems related to suicide in correctional facilities and the role that the correctional system plays in influencing inmate behavior.

Who Commits Suicide in Custody?

One consistent finding in suicide research, whether inside a correctional facility or in a community, is that male suicides outnumber female suicides (for studies of the prevalence of prison and jail suicides see; Daniel and Fleming 2006; Fruehwald, Frottier, Matschnig, Koenig, and Eher 2003; Home Office 1999; United States Bureau of Justice Statistics 2005). For correctional settings, this should come as little surprise, since men far outnumber women within the incarcerated population. When discussing rates of suicides as opposed to raw numbers, findings have been mixed with regard to whether women are more likely than men to commit suicide while incarcerated. For instance, Liebling (1994) reported that the suicide rates for males and females in correctional facilities are similar, and Loucks (1997), Tatarelli and colleagues (1999) and Mackenzie, Oram and Borill (2003) reported that the self-inflicted death rates for Scottish, Italian and British female inmates, respectively, were higher than for male inmates. In contrast, Crighton and Towl (1997) reported that the rate of suicide for men in British facilities was higher than for women. Casale (1995) also researched suicides among those incarcerated in England and Wales. He found that the male suicide rate was 2.5 times higher than women's, but he also cautioned that these statistics could be misleading. For example, Casale cited Liebling's

(1999) research that reported that incarcerated women's suicides are more likely to be officially labeled a misadventure or unknown cause of death. Dooley (1990) found similar results in coroner's findings of cause of death for female suicide cases. The United States Bureau of Justice Statistics (2005) reported that male inmates in the United States are 56 percent more likely than females in jails to commit suicide.

Compared to males, female inmates tend to be at a higher risk for attempted suicide. This gender difference is similar in the general population. Researchers suggest that a possible explanation for this can be linked to histories of physical and sexual abuse (Liebling 1994; Loucks 1997). Darby and colleagues (1998), and Liebling (1992, 1994), found that while a history of abuse distinguished juvenile male suicide attempters from non-attempters, prior abuse was more prevalent among incarcerated females. Another possible contributing factor that most incarcerated women must face is separation from their children. Three quarters of female inmates in the United States are mothers. Unlike most male inmates, many of these women were the primary care-givers for their children prior to incarceration (Liebling 1994). As a result, Liebling (1994) observed that women tended to report separation from the family as one of the toughest aspects of incarceration.

Race

Another consistent finding across research on suicide is that whites tend to commit suicide more frequently than African-Americans or Hispanics. The Bureau of Justice Statistics (2005) reported that white males in United States jails are six times more likely than African-American inmates, and three times more likely than Hispanics, to commit suicide. This difference in racial groups is not exclusive to the United States. Researchers from Great Britain, Canada, and Australia have also reported that whites tend to be over-represented among prison suicides (British Home Office 1999; Serin, Motiuk and Wichmann 2002). The racial differences in suicide and attempted suicides are also present across gender (Mackenzie et al. 2003). In some settings, racial and ethnic minorities do have higher suicide rates. For example, Native Americans in the United States and Australian Aborigines have been found to have higher suicide rates in prison than other groups (Lester 1997; Biles, MacDonald and Fleming 1990; Serin et al. 2002).

Age

Juveniles who are incarcerated appear to be at a disproportionate risk for suicide. The United States Bureau of Justice Statistics (2005) reported that inmates under the age of 18 years of age have much higher suicide rates (101 per 100,000 inmates) than prisoners in the 18 to 24 year range (38 per 100,000 inmates). In a study of suicide among English and Welsh prisoners, researchers also found that juveniles between the ages of 15 and 17 years were over-represented among suicides (Towl and Crighton 1997). It is possible, however, that the high suicide rates in the American and British institutions can be at least partially explained by the higher turnover of the juveniles, since this group tends to receive shorter sentences than adults. On the other hand, juvenile inmates may find it more difficult than adults to deal with the stress of incarceration (see Toch's [1992] work on 'self-destructive breakdown' in custody). Hales, Davison, Misch and Taylor (2003) surveyed young men in a juvenile facility in London and found that approximately 20 percent had attempted suicide or harmed themselves at some point in their lives. Liebling (1999, 1992) emphasizes the importance of coping skills, or lack thereof, among incarcerated juveniles. A deficiency in coping skills might make incarcerated life more difficult and ultimately contribute to a suicide attempt. This population is also at-risk for being victimized by bullies. As a result, Liebling suggests that this group might be particularly dependent on violence-reduction and suicide prevention programs within the prison and frequent contact with family and staff.

Mental Illness

The United States Bureau of Justice Statistics (BJS) reported that, "at midyear 2005 more than half of all prison and jail inmates had a mental health problem, including 705,600 inmates in State prisons, 78,800 in Federal prisons, and 479,900 in local jails" (2006:1). While a smaller percentage of this population had a severe mental illness, these statistics illustrate the potential risk for suicide as mentally-ill inmates are over-represented among the suicides in correctional facilities.[1] Liebling (1993) compared incarcerated juveniles who had attempted suicide while in custody to those who had not. Subsequently she found that attempters were more likely to have received prior psychiatric treatment, and to have intentionally injured themselves in the past. Kovasznay, Miraglia, Beer and Way (2004) reviewed psychological autopsies of a sample of completed suicides occurring within the New York prison system between 1993 and 2001. They found that 70 percent of these victims had mental health treatment prior to their most recent incarcerations, and that over half had a history of at least one prior suicide attempt. Also, nearly two-thirds had been seen by a mental health professional in the prison system in the two weeks prior to their suicide.

Alcohol and Drug Use

Since suicidal behavior is much more common among drug users and abusers than others who refrain from such activities (Lester 2000), having a higher proportion of drug users in custody is expected to lead to higher rates of suicidal behavior. In 1998, the BJS (2000) reports that 70 percent of the inmates in American jails (about 417,000 individuals) had committed drug offenses or used drugs regularly, and that over half of all jail and prison inmates (about 56 percent) reported using drugs in the month prior to their offense. Moreover, one-third of state and one-fifth of federal prisoners reported using drugs at the time they committed their offense (BJS 1999b). Also, approximately half of female state prison inmates had been under the influence of drugs and/or alcohol at the time of their offenses (BJS 1999a).

Hayes (1989) found that over 60 percent of suicides in the National Center for Institutions and Alternatives (NCIA) national study were under the influence of drugs, alcohol, or both at the time of arrest. In addition, 44 percent were reported to be intoxicated at the time of the suicide. Marcus and Alcabes (1993) reported that all of the suicidal inmates in their study used excessive amounts of alcohol and drugs prior to incarceration. Over 40 percent of the cases in Davis and Muscat's (1993) study had in the past been arrested for alcohol-related offenses. Researchers speculate that the depressive effects of alcohol exacerbate the despair felt by inmates immediately upon incarceration.

The role of alcohol and drugs must be considered whenever anyone discusses suicide in correctional facilities. Jail officers have an added burden of dealing with arrestees who come from the streets while still under the influence of drugs or alcohol. Those in this condition are likely feeling less inhibited and, as a result, are more prone to attempt suicide. After these individuals "sober-up," they are faced with the challenges of withdrawal, as well as the reality of their current situation, and the fact that their next intoxicant will be difficult to obtain. The awareness of their current troubles, combined with the physical and psychological aspects of withdrawal, can bring about stress and feelings of hopelessness.

Offense Type

Information regarding the charges or conviction for the "typical" suicidal offender has been inconsistent. Whereas some researchers have found the typical prison suicides to be committed by violent offenders (Kovsaznay et al. 2004; Salive, Smith and Brewer 1989), others found that the typical offender who committed suicide was involved in non-violent crimes (Tatarelli, Mancinelli, Taggi and Polidori 1999; Topp 1979). Regarding jail suicides, Hayes (1989) and Jordan and colleagues (1987) reported that inmates were more often than not being held for non-violent offenses. The Bureau of Justice Statistics (2005), Kennedy and Homant (1984) and Copeland (1989) report that suicides tend to involve people being held for violent offenses. The lack of consistency, even within similar types of facilities, should serve as a caution to any corrections staff member interested in drafting a profile of the typical suicidal inmate based on offense characteristics.

Profiles of Suicidal Inmates

Thus far, we have provided information about who tends to commit suicide in prisons and jails. Some readers may believe that if white male inmates, and those who have substance abuse problems, make up the typical correctional suicide, then correctional employees would benefit from paying special attention to these inmates. After Lindsey Hayes of the National Center of Institutions and Alternatives published the profile of the typical suicide victim, he became concerned about institutional over-reliance on inmate profiles (Hayes 1989). In fact, not every inmate who attempts or commits suicide is white, and many female inmates attempt suicide. Over-reliance on demographic and offense information for suicide prevention policies may likely result in the overlooking of suicidal inmates who do not fit pre-selected profiles (false-negatives); while non-suicidal inmates who do fit are subject to extra supervision (false-positives) (Liebling 1992).

As a consequence, Liebling's (1999) work illustrates the importance of moving away from profiles that rely too heavily on demographic and offense characteristics. Referencing data from prisons in England and Wales from 1987 to 1993, Liebling identified three groups of inmates with specific treatment needs. The first group consists of inmates who are either serving life or long sentences, which includes pretrial inmates facing lengthy sentences if convicted. These inmates are usually older and tend to be serving time for violent offenses. They are likely to take their lives much later into their sentences than others. The second set of inmates consists of ones with mental illnesses. These individuals tend to commit suicide earlier in their stays and are generally over-represented in jails. The last group is the "poor copers," who tend to share similar demographic characteristics to the general inmate population. They are distinguished from other inmates by their vulnerability. This is the largest of the three groups mentioned. Staff members who use the profile of the "typical" victim would likely miss the distinctions between these groups. Correctional staff would also have a very difficult time identifying the poor copers using only demographic or offense data. In most cases, corrections personnel will be better equipped to meet the needs of inmates if they focus less on profiles and more on the behavioral cues of inmates, as well as situational factors that might increase stress or depression.

When Suicides Occur

Prisons hold inmates who serve years in those facilities, whereas jails house inmates who stay anywhere between a few hours to over a year. In terms of raw numbers, jails will experience more suicides than prisons. For example, slightly over 300 suicides were reported in local jails in the United States in 2002, contrasted to 168 suicides in state prisons. Comparing suicide rates between jails and prisons can be somewhat misleading because jails do not count the large numbers of inmates passing through these facilities each year (instead reporting the average daily population). Despite these differences, each type of facility has its own challenges in suicide prevention.

Research has revealed rather consistent findings about the point at which most jail inmates attempt suicide. According to the National Center on Institutions and Alternatives (Hayes 1989), over half of the inmates who commit suicide in jail do so within the first 24 hours of incarceration. The BJS reports that 48 percent of jail suicides in the United States, from 2000 to 2002, occurred in the inmates' first week of incarceration, and 29 percent of these suicides occurred during the first three hours. Other researchers report similar results (Frottier et al. 2002; Ingram et al. 1997).

The first few hours of a person's incarceration is not the only high-risk period. In their study of suicide victims in a New York jail, for instance, Marcus and Alcabes (1993) found that half of these suicides also occurred within three days of a court appearance. The National Commission on Correctional Health Care's (NCCHC) standards has (cited in Hayes, 1996) identified the following high risk periods for jail inmates: immediately after admission to the facility, immediately after adjudication, following an inmate's return to the facility from court, following the receipt of bad news, and after suffering humiliation or rejection.

Findings have been mixed about the times of greatest risk for prison inmates. The Victoria Department of Justice Correctional Service Task Force (1998) reports that the time suicidal Australian prison inmates spend in custody has no relation to when a suicide attempt occurs. Schlosar and Carlson (1997), however, reported that Canadian inmates were more likely to commit suicide during either the first six months or the last six months of their sentences. Eyland, Corben and Barton (1997) believe that the first two weeks after an inmate has been transferred to a new facility should be considered as an elevated risk period. Daniel and Fleming's (2006) study of prison inmates within one state found that transfers were also a risk factor for suicide. The BJS (2005), however, reports that only seven percent of prison suicides in the United States occur within the first month of incarceration. By contrast, sixty-five percent of suicides, occur after the first year. While these results appear to be contradictory, state or regional differences within the U.S. statistics, along with variation within inmate groups enhance the complex nature of these matters.

Where Suicides Occur

Isolation is used to protect inmates who may be at-risk of being victimized. It is also frequently used when inmates are determined to be at-risk for harming themselves. While isolation is a reliable way of preventing inmate-on-inmate violence, it also increases the opportunity for self-inflicted violence to occur. Inmates who are alone and who are not under constant supervision have the time to plan and execute a suicide attempt. The presence of someone else, even another inmate, will likely interrupt or prevent the suicide attempt.

Researchers find that the majority of inmates who succeed in killing themselves do so when they are housed alone (Eyland, Corben and Barton 1997; Hayes 1989; Way, Sawyer, Barboza and Nash 2007). Inch and colleagues (1995) noted that while isolating inmates "for their own protection" may prevent them from being assaulted, this isolation might increase and inmates' sense of despair, thus providing extra motivation for suicide. Placement in isolation may also increase the inmates' chances of a successful attempt, since detection and intervention might not occur until it is too late. Hayes (1989:20) has been particularly critical of the use of isolation as a response to suicidal inmates, stating, "In most instances, the use of isolation is for the convenience of the staff, and usually to the detriment of the inmate because it unconsciously causes reduced staff supervision/observation."

Methods Used to Commit Suicide

Nearly every piece of academic and practitioner research finds that the most common way to commit suicide in prison or jail is through hanging. The term hanging does not always refer to suspension of the person off the ground. While hanging can involve suspension of the entire body, it can also be accomplished in a sitting or kneeling position. In the correctional setting the term hanging can also be used to describe suffocation, self-suspension, and/or strangulation (Ingram et al. 1997).

There is a rather simple explanation for the frequent use of this method of self-harm: hanging is one of the few conventional methods of suicide available to inmates in most parts of the facility. Firearms are clearly not available, nor do inmates have access to carbon monoxide or other deadly gasses. Overdosing on drugs is rare as it is difficult to gain access to a lethal amount. Suicide by drowning or automobile crash is not possible either. Jumping from a high place is rarely possible, since multi-tier cell blocks tend to have "people-catchers" (e.g., netting) to prevent suicide and murders.

Cutting (also called 'slashing') is another option for inmates. Prisoners are generally permitted to possess more belongings than jail inmates, so it is easier for them to obtain sharp items. Researchers have found that cutting is a popular method of self-harm (Eyland et al. 1997; Liebling 1992; Serin et al. 2002).

The most common form of completed suicide, however, is strangulation or hanging (Borrill 2002; Crighton and Towl 1997; Eyland et al. 1997; Joukamaa 1997; Serin et al. 2002; Victoria Department of Justice Correctional Services Task Force 1998). There are two possible explanations for this. One is that the behavior of cutters is more of an attention-seeking act than an actual attempt to die. The second is that hanging is a more dangerous method as the victim loses consciousness faster than does a cutter. Jail inmates who attempt suicide typically resort to hanging. This is likely due to the lack of availability of cutting tools. They do, however, have clothing and a blanket that can be used to make a noose.

Implications for Suicide Prevention

Let's review what we have discussed thus far. While it is true that incarcerated males commit suicide more often than females, Whites more often than African-Americans and Hispanics, and the very young more often than adults, suicide prevention plans that rely primarily on demographic characteristics of an offender are risky and therefore not recommended. Such interventions will place unnecessary attention on inmates who are not in danger of suicide while missing those who are truly at-risk. Not all inmates who are mentally ill will commit suicide, nor will all of those who are intoxicated, but these two groups need to be watched carefully. State and federal courts have ruled that corrections officials' knowledge of a serious mental illness or high levels of intoxication warrant extra supervision of these inmates due to their elevated risk of self-harm (Kapeler, Vaughn and del Carmen 1991). Correctional officers and facility staff should be trained to monitor how each inmate appears to be coping with incarceration (see Liebling 1992, 1993).

Information about when these incidents occur as well as the methods of self-harm used by inmates is important to consider when developing suicide prevention programs. While studies of prison suicides revealed no consistent high-risk periods, jail research proves to be very informative about periods of elevated risk for those inmates. Jail inmates are at high risk during their initial admission and the periods immediately before and after a court appearance. For both prison and jail inmates the period following receipt of bad news from home or a serious rejection or humiliation might bring about a suicidal crisis.

The popularity of hanging for suicide in prison and jail stems from the lack of access to other methods. This fact has been widely recognized by practitioners. Many suicide prevention plans in prisons and jails focus on restricting the inmate's ability to make a noose and attach it to something in their cells. These strict opportunity reduction measures, however, have been criticized for ignoring the root-causes of inmate problems. For example, suicidal inmates are typically stripped of all personal belongings. Their clothes are removed – they are likely given a gown that is either tear-proof or made of paper. And they are placed alone in an empty isolation cell. The inmate is kept in these conditions until the person who is responsible for releasing them from suicide watch (often a psychologist or other mental health professional) approves his or her return to the general population. Wortley (1998; 2002) cautions that prevention techniques that are too heavy-handed might actually encourage the same behaviors it is intended to prevent. Placing an inmate into a bare cell alone and without any belongings or personal clothing might increase that person's sense of despair. The remainder of the chapter will focus on prevention strategies that avoid the use of isolation and strip cells.

Prevention Strategies

In the 1960s, during the development of suicide prevention centers in the United States and other countries, it was posited that suicidal individuals could be identified by using psychological inventories and tests, and that suicide could be predicted and, therefore, prevented. This proved to be impossible. In actuality, psychological tests were found to be of little use (Lester, 1970), and the simple screening devices devised for crisis counselors were used primarily for triage rather than prediction: Given two clients calling a telephone crisis line, for instance, which one should be put on hold?

These screening devices focused on five areas (Lester 1989). The first is concerned with race, age and gender. The second focused on the type and severity of psychiatric disturbance. Suicide risk is greater in inmates who are psychotics, substance abusers, and the severely depressed. These guidelines are probably valid for all populations. The third area refers to recent stressors in the person's life: losses of significant others, jobs, money, prestige and status, illnesses, accidents, criminal involvement and changes in residence. The greater the recent stress, the greater the risk. The fourth section of the instrument is concerned with suicidal behavior, and whether the person has recently attempted suicide (especially using a method of high lethality), if they have a specific plan for committing suicide, and whether the tools to commit suicide are readily available. The fifth and final section of the scale inquires about the availability of resources and support for the person and whether these people are able and willing to provide encouragement and assistance. For example, are the significant others hostile or sympathetic?

The usefulness of such screening devices in correctional settings is limited. The population is quite homogenous in terms of simple demographic characteristics (race, age and sex) as compared to the general population. There are also a large proportion of inmates with psychiatric disorders, recent stressors, current and prior suicidality, and limited resources. Thus, using such a scale without the aide of clinical judgment would likely result in unmanageable numbers of false positives, that is, inmates judged to be potential suicides but who did not harm themselves.

In recent years, there has been a change in focus from identification and prediction to assessment of suicidal individuals (Maris et al. 1992). This has occurred partly because of the failure of simple screening devices, but also as a result of the litigation brought by the families and significant others of suicides who have sued psychotherapists, psychiatric institutions, and correctional facilities for negligence or malpractice. It has become important to document the psychological and psychiatric state of patients and inmates. Assessment is also useful if there is to be a treatment plan for the potentially suicidal individual, for the assessment will help in the formulation of treatment goals.

For example, if an inmate appears to be depressed, it is useful to administer a self-report questionnaire to assess the level of depression (There are several standardized scales for the assessment of depression). Beck and his colleagues (1974) found that one particular component of the set of depressive symptoms is very strongly associated with prior, current, and future suicidality: the feeling of hopelessness. Therefore, it is important to assess hopelessness as well as depression in potentially suicidal inmates.

Similarly, there are several scales that assess the magnitude of recent stressors (Sarason et al. 1978). These can provide an objective and accurate measure of overall stress. However, these scales have not been tailored for correctional inmates. It would be useful if such scales could be devised for use in prisons and jails.

There are also standardized scales for measuring the extent of suicidal intention, based on interviews with those who are contemplating suicide (Beck et al. 1979) and detailed accounts from previous suicidal attempts (Beck et al. 1976). Reynolds (1988, 1990) has developed both a scale and a semi-structured interview to assess the extent of suicidal ideation in adolescents, and the results of which may be useful for unsophisticated inmates.

Jobes (2006) has recently published a manual for assessing suicidality and his Collaborative Assessment and Management of Suicidality (CAMS) has been field tested in many populations, including the military. This approach is characterized by a blend of assessment and a therapist-based intervention, and CAMS may prove to be a useful approach in correctional settings.

Some correctional staff members are concerned with distinguishing genuine suicidal behavior from manipulative behavior in inmates. For example, Correia (2000) argued that a simple depression self-report instrument is susceptible to malingering. He noted that a cursory interview should be used to identify those inmates pretending to be suicidal to get attention or to amuse themselves. If no evidence of a genuine psychiatric illness or withdrawal from substance abuse is present, malingering should be assumed.

If an inmate reports suicidal ideation, Correia (2000) believes that the presence of clear risk factors (such as a significant impairment or disorder, a clear triggering stressor, or withdrawal from alcohol and drugs) were necessary to decide that suicide risk was present. Correia contends that even suicide attempts should not always be viewed as "true" suicide attempts rather as "suicidal gestures." He was also concerned with distinguishing self-mutilation from suicidal behavior. It is likely that such a skeptical position, without any clear guidelines for making these distinctions, will lead to potential suicides being missed during screening. Some researchers have suggested that acts of self-harm can lead to suicide, so these incidents should be taken seriously (see Dexter and Towl 1995; Liebling 1999).

Estimates of the proportion of persons who use suicide to manipulate others range from 28 to 50 percent (Dear, Thomson and Hills 2000). In a sample of Australian inmates, Dear and colleagues showed that about 24 percent of their sample of attempted suicides reported motives that were coded as manipulative, 43 percent as seeking psychological relief and 32 percent as escape. Only about 20 percent of the attempts posed a risk to life. However, suicidal intent (objectively measured with a suicidal intent scale) was only weakly associated with the medical seriousness of the suicide attempt, and there was no association between the motive for the suicide attempt and its medical seriousness. Thus, correctional staff should not use the medical seriousness of a suicide attempt as a guide to the motive (manipulative or not) of the suicide attempt or to the suicidal intent.

With suicide, perhaps the best approach is similar to that which a physician might use for detecting the possibility of cancer in a patient. It is better to err on the side of caution. Therefore, if, in the self-reports of inmates, there appear to be indications of an increased risk of suicide, then the inmate should be considered as potentially suicidal and be assessed in a one-on-one interview with a mental health professional who has been trained and skilled in evaluating suicidality. It is better to assume "suicidal" inmates are a real danger to themselves than to dismiss them as "malingerers." Malingering should be easy to detect after an in-depth interview and close monitoring.

It is important to note that inmate screening is only helpful in preventing suicide if the information is shared with the appropriate staff members. Administrators may decide to adopt a screening instrument, and intake staff might do a superb job screening inmates. This means nothing, however, if the information is not passed on to the mental health and medical staff or the corrections officers, a problem identified by Hayes (2007). The information also needs to be passed on to all shifts. While this seems like a simple task, inmates and staff are often shuffled between units, and the hundreds of requests and staff-inmate interactions in a single shift might result in an inmate's risk going unreported.

Housing and Supervision

Screening inmates is an important task, but it will not uncover all suicidal inmates. Researchers have found that some inmates will deny their having suicidal ideation (thoughts of suicide), when asked by correctional staff members (Marcus and Alcabes 1993). Reasons for this denial range from cultural explanations to fear of being perceived as weak by other inmates.[2] Admission of a previous suicide attempt or current suicidal ideation can result in the inmate being placed in special clothing, placement in isolation, restricted privileges and ostracism from the other inmates. As noted earlier, placement in an isolation cell or area tends to result in the removal of most or all privileges, plus, it gives inmates ample opportunity for an inmate to initiate and complete a suicide attempt.

Unit Management and the Direct Supervision Design

Facilities operating under unit management or the direct supervision approach offer some hope of providing a correctional environment that is more receptive to the needs of vulnerable inmates. The Federal Bureau of Prisons developed unit management strategies in response to not only suicide, violence, vandalism, escapes and other threats to order, as well as the need for services to be delivered to inmates in the most efficient way determined possible. Prisons and jails operating using the unit management approach are divided into several semi-autonomous units. Each wing, unit, or pod is run by a supervisor and is staffed with its own counseling staff. The purpose of this approach is to allow for the same custody and treatment staff to work consistently with a particular group of inmates. In this setting, staff members are able to get to know this small group of inmates and understand their needs. The goal of this program is to offer services faster and better than in the antiquated linear-management institution that is characterized by inmates living in cells arranged along corridors (Levinson 1999).

During the 1970s, architects contracted by the Federal Bureau of Prisons developed a new correctional design and management strategy called the podular direct supervision model. Also known as the "new generation jail," the direct supervision model begins with unit management; so all pods (or units) are semi-autonomous. Architecturally, these facilities are different from the traditional linear-style jail. In the linear jails, for example, the facility tends to have a rectangular design with corridors leading to either single or multiple occupancy cells (Nelson 1983). The corridors are typically arranged either at acute or right angles, and which, by design, makes it difficult for officers to directly supervise the inmates. As a result, officers conduct intermittent supervision, which means that they periodically walk through the corridors and observe the inmates within their cells. The problem is that the supervision is not constant. Subsequently, hanging, the most popular form of suicide while in custody, can be done quickly and is highly lethal.

Podular jails, by contrast, have inmate cells arranged around a common dayroom, thus providing the officers better sight-lines to conduct surveillance. Consequently, one officer can typically observe the activities of all the inmates from a central location. Another difference between the direct supervision facilities and traditional jails is the use of non-institutional furnishings and fixtures. For example, traditional jails contain austere and "indestructible" furnishings for inmates made of metal, plastic or concrete, and which some researchers have suggested communicate negative expectations to inmates (Reser 1989). Non-institutional furnishings in the new generation jails, by contrast, are expected to provide inmates with more incentives to behave, since misbehavior is met with placement in a less desirable part of the jail.

Perhaps the most important feature of the new generation jail is the supervision strategy used by the officers. Correctional officers in traditional facilities typically have some type of physical barrier, usually bars or Plexiglas—between the staff and inmates. These architectural obstacles produce barriers to communication. In direct supervision facilities, officers and inmates share the same physical space. In this setting, officers mingle with the inmates, however, since this work is quite different from what is found in traditional correctional institutions, it is necessary for these officers to receive specialized training.

Direct supervision correctional officers receive communication skills and problem-solving training that teaches them how to work closely with inmates and diffuse conflicts before they escalate. The combination of the officers' proximity to the inmates and this proactive supervision technique has been credited with helping to create a more relaxed and safer environment in these jails. Evaluations of these facilities have indicated that, if the direct supervision model is implemented properly, these institutions are successful in reducing violence and suicides among inmates (Bayens, Williams and Smykla 1997a, 1997b; Jackson 1992; Sense 1997; Wener 2006). The more relaxed and safer environment in these facilities has the potential to reduce the stress and despair that could lead to a suicide attempt. A limitation to this approach, however, is the problem of partial implementation of this model. Tartaro (2002, 2003, 2006) has found that many jails that use this model are being referred to as direct supervision when in fact they are not providing the officers with the necessary training, nor are they making the appropriate changes to the physical environment.

Supervising Inmates Known to Be Suicidal

Hayes (1999) recommends that corrections staff avoid canceling privileges (such as telephone access, visits and recreation time) for inmates known to be suicidal. Eliminating privileges contributes to feelings of isolation, distress, or hopelessness. When at all possible, staff members should avoid placing inmates in isolation cells, especially offenders who are under the influence of intoxicants or experiencing psychological problems. Given the prevalence of suicide during the initial hours of jail incarceration, it may be better to refrain from placing newcomers in isolation during their first 48 hours, since this may allow the offender to adjust to the new setting, as well as to detoxify. However, in a situation where inmates are a danger to themselves and their roommates, isolation rooms may be used provided that the staff is able to maintain constant supervision (Hayes 1996).

The Mobile County Jail in Alabama developed a suicide prevention program in the early 1980s that successfully reduced the need to isolate inmates. The program involves a combination of training, constant supervision, and cooperation from the suicidal inmate (Manning 1989). All officers are trained to detect signs that the inmate is under the influence of drugs, since these inmates have been found to be at a high risk for suicide. In the event that a suicide attempt does occur, all officers are trained in cardiopulmonary resuscitation.

Suicide prevention begins at the time of admission (Manning 1989). At the Mobile County Jail, for example, inmates complete medical questionnaires that include questions about suicidality. Even if the inmate does not answer affirmatively to the suicide questions, the booking officer has the discretion to send a report to the nurse's station. It is at this point when the jail employees face a common problem with suicide prevention: the nursing staff works only during the day in most facilities.

The Mobile County jail administrators decided to deal with the absence of evening and late-night nursing staff by implementing the "buddy system" (Manning 1989). Buddies are trained trustee-inmates. They are told not to intervene in a suicide attempt nor give suicidal inmates any advice. The purpose of the buddy system is to avoid the use of strip cells and isolation. Under the program, inmates are placed in a cell with a buddy with all of their personal belongings, and they lose no privileges. Subsequently, the at-risk inmate maintains access to telephones and televisions. The buddy provides constant supervision of the at-risk inmate, and jail officers make rounds to check on the inmates every 15 minutes. If nurses are available, they will periodically check with the buddies to receive updates. To be released from the buddy system, the jail psychiatrist must interview the suicidal inmate and approve the release. Suicidal inmates are also required to sign a behavioral contract, which releases them from the buddy system. These contracts outline the following expectations: "I promise not to attempt suicide while at the Mobile County Jail. If I have these thoughts, I will contact a corrections officer or a nurse." Inmates who refuse to sign the contract remain on the buddy system until they feel ready to sign the document.

The Federal Bureau of Prisons also uses trained inmates to watch potentially suicidal inmates. The inmates are trained to summon staff if those being supervised attempt suicide, but they are also given instruction about suicidal behavior, listening skills, and general communication techniques. White and Schimmel (1995) report that 65 percent of federal institutions use inmate companions, and of the 75,363 hours of suicide watch in federal institutions in 1992, 72 percent of those hours were handled by inmates. Such peer suicide reduction programs have also been used in Canada. Research indicates that they seem to be an effective and inexpensive method for suicide prevention (Tripodi and Bender 2007).

Summary

Correctional suicide prevention programs range from the innovative to the counterproductive. Researchers and practitioners have observed that profiling inmates based on their demographic or offense characteristics is not an effective way to identify inmates who are at-risk. We have provided recommendations for screening instruments that might be helpful in a corrections setting. It is important to remember, however, that screening for risk is only one element in suicide prevention, and must be used in conjunction with trained professionals who can evaluate risk and develop appropriate interventions. Moreover, these activities are also dependent upon the quality of communication inside correctional facilities. Information about troubled inmates must be passed from shift to shift, and it must be shared with staff members who have contact with the individual—the security, educational (or other programming), and medical staff.

The housing characteristics in each facility play an important part in suicide prevention. We discussed a few ways in which housing can impact suicide prevention procedures. It is clear that suicidal inmates should not be housed alone in a cell unless there is constant supervision. Suicidal acts can be completed quickly, so even 15 minutes alone and unsupervised in a cell is dangerous. But, it is difficult and expensive, especially in understaffed or overcrowded facilities, to dedicate a staff member exclusively to the supervision of a single inmate. As a result, some prison and jail administrators have addressed the need for supervision by utilizing trained inmates to remain in constant sight-and-sound contact with at-risk inmates.

Some county governments are changing the design and management strategies within their jails, with the understanding that a dangerous and negative jail environment can contribute to an increase in the number of suicide attempts. Living areas in the direct supervision jails are made to look and feel as non-institutional as possible, and officers are trained to maintain order through use of their communication skills. This proactive approach to violence and disorder inside jails has great potential, but only if it is done properly.

Endnotes

1. Jails tend to house higher percentages of mentally ill inmates than prison (Liebling, 1999).
2. For a discussion about issues pertaining to screening Native Americans for suicidal ideation, see Lester (1997).

References

Bayens, Gerald J., Jimmy J. Williams and John O. Smykla. 1997a. "Jail Type Makes Difference: Evaluating the Transition from a Traditional to a Podular, Direct Supervision Jail Across Ten Years." *American Jails* 11(2):32-39.

------. 1997b. "Jail Type and Inmate Behavior: a Longitudinal Analysis." *Federal Probation* 61:54-62.

Beck, Aaron T., Maria Kovacs and Arlene Weissman. 1979. "Assessment of Suicide Intention." *Journal of Consulting and Clinical Psychology* 47:343-352.

Beck, Aaron T., Arlene Weissman, David Lester and Larry Trexler. 1974. "The Measurement of Pessimism." *Journal of Consulting and Clinical Psychology* 42:861-865.

Beck, Aaron T., Arlene Weissman, David Lester, and Larry Trexler. 1976. "Classification of Suicidal Behavior." *Archives of General Psychiatry* 33:835-837.

Biles, David, David McDonald and Jillian Fleming. 1990. "Aboriginal and Non-Aboriginal Deaths in Custody." *Australian and New Zealand Journal of Criminology* 23:5-23.

Casale, Silvia. 1995. "Suicide and Custody." *AIDS Care* 7:139-144.

Copeland, A. 1989. "Fatal Suicidal Hangings Among Prisoners in Jail." *Medicine, Science and the Law* 29:341-345.

Correia, Kevin M. 2000. "Suicide Assessment in a Prison Environment." *Criminal Justice and Behavior* 27:581-599.

Crighton, David and Graham Towl. 1997. "Self-inflicted Deaths in Prison in England and Wales." *Issues in Criminological and Legal Psychology* 28:12-20.

Daniel, Anasseril E. and Jennifer Fleming. 2006. "Suicides in a State Correctional System, 1992-2002: A Review." *Journal of Correctional Health Care* 12:24-35.

Darby, P. J., W. D. Allan, J. H. Kashani, K. L. Hartke, and J. C. Reid. 1998. "Analysis of 112 Juveniles Who Committed Homicide: Characteristics and a Closer Look at Family Abuse." *Journal of Family Violence* 13:365-375.

Davis, Mark S. and Joshua E. Muscat. 1993. "An Epidemiological Study of Alcohol and Suicide Risk in Ohio Jails and Lockups, 1975-1984" *Journal of Criminal Justice* 21:277-283.

Dear, Greg E., Donald M. Thomson and Adelma M. Hills. 2000. "Self-harm in Prison." *Criminal Justice and Behavior* 27:160-175.

Dexter, Polly and Graham Towl. 1995. "An Investigation into Suicidal Behaviours in Prison." *Issues in Criminological and Legal Psychology* 22:45-53.

Dooley, Enda. 1990. "Unnatural Deaths in Prison." *British Journal of Criminology* 30:229-234.

Eyland, Simon, Simon Corben and Jenny Barton. 1997. "Suicide Prevention in New South Wales Correctional Centres." *Crisis* 18:158-164.

Frottier, Patrick, Stefan Fruhwald, K. Ritter, Reinhard Eher, J. Schwalzler, and P. Bauer. 2002. "Jailhouse Blues Revisited." *Social Psychiatry and Psychiatric Epidemiology* 37:68-73.

Fruehwald, Stefan, Patrick Frottier, Teresa Matschnig, Franz Koenig, Stephan Lehr, and Reinhard Eher. 2003. "Do Monthly or Seasonal Variations Exist in Suicides in a High-risk Setting?" *Psychiatry Research* 121:263-269.

Hales, H., S. Davison, P. Misch and P. J. Taylor. 2003. "Young Male Prisoners in a Young Offenders' Institution: Their Contact with Suicidal Behaviour by Others." *Journal of Adolescence* 26:667–685.

Hayes, Lindsay M. 1989. "National Study of Jail Suicides: Seven Years Later." *Psychiatric Quarterly* 60:7-29.

------. 1996. "National and State Standards for Prison Suicide Prevention: A Report Card." *Journal of Correctional Health Care* 3:5-38.

------. 1999. "Suicide in Adult Correctional Facilities: Key Ingredients to Prevention and Overcoming the Obstacles." *Journal of Law, Medicine and Ethics* 27:260-269.

------. 2007. "Key Components of a Suicide Prevention Program." Retrieved April 15, 2007 (http://www.ncianet.org)

Home Office. 1999. Suicide is Everyone's Concern. London, England: Home Office.

Inch, H., P. Rowlands, and A. Soliman. 1995. "Deliberate Self-harm in a Young Offenders' Institution." *Journal of Forensic Psychiatry* 6:161-171.

Ingram, Alan, Graham Johnson and Ian Hayes. 1997. *Self Harm and Suicide by Detained Persons: A Study.* London: Home Office Police Research Group.

Jackson, P. G., 1992. *Detention in Transition: Sonoma County's New Generation Jail.* Rohnert Park, CA: Department of Criminal Justice Administration, Sonoma State University.

Jobes, David A. 2006. *The Collaborative Assessment and Management of Suicidality.* New York: Guilford.

Jordan, F. B., K. Schmeckpeper and M. Strope. 1987. "Jail Suicides by Hanging." *American Journal of Forensic Medicine and Pathology* 8:27-31.

Joukamaa, Matti. 1997. "Prison Suicide in Finland, 1969-1992." *Forensic Science International* 89:167-174.

Kappeler, Victor E., Michael S. Vaughn. and Rolando V. Del Carmen. 1991. "Death in Detention: An Analysis of Police Liability for Negligent Failure to Prevent Suicide." *Journal of Criminal Justice* 19:381-393.

Kennedy, Daniel B. and Robert J. Homant. 1984. "Predicting Custodial Suicides." *Justice Quarterly* 5:441-456.

Kovasznay, Beatrice, Richard Miraglia, Richard Beer, and Bruce Way. 2004. "Reducing Suicides in New York State Correctional Facilities." *Psychiatric Quar-*

terly 75:61-70.
Lester, David. 1970. "Attempts to Predict Suicidal Risk Using Psychological Tests." *Psychological Bulletin* 74:1-17.
------. 1989. *Can we Prevent Suicide?* New York: AMS.
------. 1997. *Suicide in American Indians*. Commack, NY: Nova Science.
------. 2000. "Alcoholism, Substance Abuse, and Suicide." Pp. 357-375. In *Comprehensive Textbook of Suicidology*, edited by R. W. Mars, A. L. Berman and M. M. Silverman. New York: Guilford.
Levinson, Robert B. 1999. *Unit Management in Prisons and Jails.* Lanham, MD: American Correctional Association.
Liebling, Alison. 1992. *Suicides in Prison*. New York: Routledge.
------. 1993. "Suicides in Young Prisoners: A Summary." *Death Studies* 17:381-409.
------. 1994. "Suicide Amongst Women Prisoners." *Howard Journal of Criminal Justice* 33:1-9.
------. 1999 "Prisoner Suicide and Prisoner Coping." Pp. 283-358. In *Crime and Justice,* edited by M. Tonry and J. Petersilia. Chicago, IL: University of Chicago Press.
Loucks, Nancy. 1997. *Research Into Drugs and Alcohol, Violence and Bullying, Suicides and Self-injury and Backgrounds of Abuse.* Edinburgh, Scotland: Scottish Prison Service.
Mackenzie, Nichola, Chris Oram, and Jo Borill. 2003. "Self-inflicted Deaths of Women in Custody." *The British Journal of Forensic Practice* 5:27-35.
Manning, R. 1989. "A Suicide Prevention Program that Really Works." *American Jails* 3:18-22.
Marcus, Paula and Phillip Alcabes. 1993. "Characteristics of Suicides by Inmates in an Urban Jail." *Hospital and Community Psychiatry* 44:256-261.
Maris, Ronald W., Alan L. Berman, John T. Maltsberge and Robert I.Yufit. 1992. *Assessment and Prediction of Suicide*. New York: Guilford.
Nelson, W. Ray. 1983. "New Generation Jails." *Corrections Today* 45:108-112.
Reynolds, William M. 1988. *Suicidal Ideation Questionnaire*. Odessa, FL: Psychological Assessment Resources.
------. 1990. "Development of a Semi-structured Clinical Interview for Suicidal Behavior in Adolescents." *Psychological Assessment* 2:382-390.
Reser, Joseph P. 1989. *The Design of Safe and Humane Police Cells.* Royal Commission into Aboriginal Deaths in Custody.
Salive, Marcel E., Gordon S. Smith and T. Fordham Brewer. 1989. "Suicide Mortality in the Maryland State Prison System, 1979 through 1987." *Journal of the American Medical Association* 262:365-369.
Sarason, Irwin G., James H. Johnson and Judith Siegel. 1978. "Assessing the Impact of Life Change." *Journal of Consulting and Clinical Psychology* 46:932-942.
Schlosar, Hilde and L. Wayne Carlson. 1997. "Befriending in Prisons." *Crisis* 18:148-151.
Senese, Jeffrey D. 1997. "Evaluating Jail Reform: A Comparative Analysis of Podular/direct and Linear Jail Inmate Infractions." *Journal of Criminal Justice* 25:61-73.
Serin, Ralph C., Larry Motiuk and Cherami Wichmann. 2002. "An Examination of Suicide Attempts Among Inmates." *Forum on Corrections Research* 14:40-42.
Tartaro, Christine. 2002. "Examining Implementation Issues with New Generation

Jails." *Criminal Justice Policy Review* 13:219-237.
------. 2003. "Suicide and the Jail Environment: An Evaluation of Three Types of Institutions." *Environment and Behavior* 35:605-620.
------. 2006. "Watered Down: Partial Implementation of the New Generation Jail Philosophy." *The Prison Journal* 84: 284-300.
Tatarelli, Roberto, Iginia Mancinelli, Franco Taggi and Gabriella Polidori. 1999. "Suicide in Italian Prisons in 1996 and 1997: A Descriptive Epidemiological Study." *International Journal of Offender Therapy and Comparative Criminology* 43:438-447.
Toch, Hans. 1992. *Mosaic of Despair: Human Breakdowns in Prison*. 2nd ed. Washington, DC: American Psychological Association.
Topp, D. 1979. "Suicide in Prison." *British Journal of Psychiatry* 134:24-27.
Towl, Graham J. and David A. Crighton. 1998. "Suicide in Prisons in England and Wales from 1988 to 1995." *Criminal Behavior and Mental Health* 8:184-192.
Tripodi, Stephen J. and Kimberly Bender. 2007. "Inmate suicide: Prevalence, Assessment, and Protocols." *Brief Treatment and Crisis Intervention* 7: 40-54.
United States Bureau of Justice Statistics. 1999 Women Offenders. Washington, DC: U.S. Department of Justice.
United States Bureau of Justice Statistics. 2000. Drug Use, Testing, and Treatment in Jails. Washington, DC: U. S. Department of Justice.
United States Bureau of Justice Statistics. 2005. *Suicide and Homicide in State Prisons and Local Jails*. Washington, DC: U. S. Department of Justice.
United States Bureau of Justice Statistics. 2006. *Mental Health Problems of Prison and Jail Inmates*. Washington, DC: U. S. Department of Justice.
Victoria Department of Justice Correctional Services Task Force. 1998. *Review of Suicides and Self Harm in Victorian Prisons*. Melbourne, Australia: Victorian Government Printer.
Way, Bruce B., Donald A Sawyer, Sharen Barboza and Robin Nash. 2007. "Inmate Suicide and Time Spent in Special Disciplinary Housing in New York State Prison." *Psychiatric Services* 58: 558-560.
Wener, Richard. 2006. "Effectiveness of the Direct Supervision System of Correctional Design and Management." *Criminal Justice and Behavior* 33: 392-410.
White, Thomas W. and Dennis J. Schimmel. 1995. "Suicide Prevention in Federal Prisons: A Successful Five-step Program." Pp. 48-59 in *Prison Suicide: An Overview and Guide to Prevention*, edited by L. M. Hayes. Washington, DC: U.S. Department of Justice.
Wortley, Richard. 1998. "A Two-stage Model of Situational Crime Prevention." *Studies in Crime and Crime Prevention* 7:173-188
------. 2002. Situational Prison Control. Cambridge: Cambridge University Press.

CHAPTER NINE

Correctional Mental Health: Problems, Prevalence, and Public Health

P. Ann Dirks-Linhorst

Over the last few decades, there has been increasing attention paid to the growing numbers of individuals with mental illness who find their way into American jails and prisons. Everyone seems in agreement that the marriage of criminal justice and mental health is not a good match, and the phenomenon is referred to as the criminalization of the mentally ill. Mentally ill prisoners serve sentences up to 15 months longer than inmates without mental illness (Ditton 1999). Life within a correctional facility is difficult for these inmates: prisoners with mental illness are more likely to fight with other inmates and are themselves at high risk of victimization (Aufderheide and Brown 2005; Gould 2003; Smiley 2001). Some inmates may only be able to deal with the stress of incarceration by exhibiting psychotic behavior (Gould 2003). Gannon (2005) reminds us that mentally ill individuals are not often able to comply with the rigid rules and regulations associated with correctional facilities, and therefore are prone to being singled out for punishment for behaviors beyond their control.

High numbers of mentally ill prisoners also have negative long-term consequences for public health and community medical systems. Individuals with mental illness are more likely to have co-occurring disorders (such as substance abuse, mental retardation or developmental disabilities) and these problems increase both the likelihood of recidivism and engaging in behaviors which place them at higher risk for HIV/AIDS infection and/or hepatitis C (de Montfort and Oss 2003). Individuals who are diagnosed with severe mental illnesses also tend to have poor health (Kane and Blank 2004). The MacArthur Violence Risk Assessment study found that persons with mental illness and a co-occurring substance abuse increased the odds of becoming violent, typically toward a family member, friend or acquaintance (Steadman et al. 1998). Mentally ill offenders are also more likely to be in prison for a violent offense than other prisoners, and are at higher risk for being homeless, unemployed, or physically or sexually abused prior to the current charge (Ditton 1999).

All these problems, if not identified and treated, can lead to a long-term strain on the public health system. Funding that has gone to community health initiatives in the past may be utilized instead to pay for incarceration (Freudenberg 2001). The lack of treatment for the mentally ill population in general is a growing public health concern (Wang, Demler and Kessler 2002). In fact, the President's New Freedom Commission on Mental Health (PNFCMH) found that the public mental health system was inadequate (PNFCMH 2003).

What factors led to the high numbers of mentally ill individuals in jails and prisons? Many point to the deinstitutionalization movement. Deinstitutionalization in the 1960s and 1970s transferred mentally ill individuals from large psychiatric institutions to community living and treatment. This was considered an innovative and a positive move, allowing patients to return to their home communities with better living conditions (Aufderheide and Brown 2005; Linhorst 2006). From the 1950s to 2000, the state-operated psychiatric hospital population dropped approximately 90 percent, from 550,000 to almost 55,000 persons, and has continued to decrease (Center for Mental Health Services 2003). For deinstitutionalization to accomplish any improvement in the lives of mentally ill people, however, adequately funded community psychiatric services were required, but this has not occurred (Linhorst 2006).

Instead, many of these individuals became homeless or came to the attention of law enforcement after committing a range of crimes from petty theft or other misdemeanors to serious violent crimes (Lamb and Weinberger 1998). For many years Riker's Island in New York and the Los Angeles County Jail have held the distinction of serving as de facto psychiatric hospitals, with higher populations of inmates with mental illness than traditional state-operated psychiatric facilities (Gordon and Chabot 2004; Weedon 2005). A number of researchers contend that deinstitutionalization was not solely responsible for the population shift from the mental health to correctional system (Banks et al. 2000). Instead they argued that there may be other causes for holding large numbers of mentally ill individuals in correctional systems, such as more restrictive civil commitment laws, or a lack of coordinated treatment services for persons with mentally illness and co-occurring disorders (Lamb and

Weinberger 1998; Lurigio 2000).

Regardless of the cause, mentally ill individuals are in prisons and jails in high numbers, and this is a serious criminal justice and public health issue. This chapter focuses on the prevalence of these individuals in correctional populations, the health-related problems associated with managing this population in correctional facilities, as well as identifying evidence-based interventions to divert these offenders from corrections, treating persons with mental illness within jails and prisons, and collaborating with community service providers to facilitate more successful reintegration after their release from jail or prison.

Prevalence of Persons with Mental Illness in Corrections

Does current information support the idea of high numbers of mentally ill individuals in jails and prisons? The Bureau of Justice Statistics reports that at year-end 2005 some 2.3 million inmates were held in some form of federal, state or local corrections (Harrison and Beck 2006). Typically, 16 percent of those in jails and state prisons, and seven percent of federal prisoners meet the diagnostic criteria for mental illness (Ditton 1999; Munetz, Grande and Chambers 2001), and a higher number suffers from less serious emotional disorders (see James and Glaze 2006).

The incarcerated population with severe mental health problems is estimated to be five times the number of patients currently in state psychiatric hospitals (Weedon 2005). In addition to mentally ill inmates in jails and prisons, over 600,000 probationers were diagnosed with some form of mental illness as of December 31, 2000 (de Montfort and Oss 2003).

Whether or not treatment is provided once these individuals are incarcerated is a significant concern for many health policy analysts. Beck and Maruschak (2001) reported that 89 percent of state prisons offer mental health treatment. These investigators also found that therapy or counseling is provided to approximately 12.5 percent of all prisoners, and ten percent of state prisoners received some type of psychotropic medication (Psychotropic medications are prescribed to alleviate symptoms of depression, psychosis, anxiety, or bi-polar disorders). About 1.8 percent of state prisoners received 24-hour mental health care (Beck and Maruschak 2001). Forty-five percent of federal prisoners had received counseling or therapy and almost half were provided with medication (Ditton 1999). While approximately one-third of mentally ill jail inmates were prescribed psychotropic medications, only 16 percent had received therapy or counseling (Ditton 1999). Given the high percentage of this population in corrections, a number of guidelines for practice have been established that outline the expectations for interventions in correctional facilities, and community-based alternatives to incarceration such as probation or parole.

Guidelines and Standards for Mental Health Care

Cost concerns, staff safety, and the legal obligation to provide treatment for correctional inmates are challenges for correctional administrators (Maue 2001). To address those broad concerns, the Criminal Justice/ Mental Health Consensus Project (hereafter Consensus Project) was initiated by the Council of State Governments. Their purpose was to identify gaps in service delivery and develop strategies for responding to these challenges. The major themes identified by this group included collaboration between systems, staff training, and making mental health services more accessible (Consensus Project 2002).

The Council of State Governments and the National Institute of Corrections (NIC) have worked together in order to implement the recommendations made by the Consensus Project (NIC 2006). The NIC provides technical assistance that addresses shortfalls in mental health service delivery, offenders with co-occurring disorders and substance abuse treatment in correctional settings. The NIC disseminates a number of free publications from its website, including a publication entitled, *Effective Prison Mental Health Services: Guidelines to Expand and Improve Treatment* (Hills, Siegfried and Ickowitz 2004). That guidebook sets forth standards for mental health and substance abuse evaluations, as well as recommendations for screening and assessment, treatment interventions, medication, treatment of women and other special-needs populations, and community reintegration (Hills et al. 2004).

Other types of assistance for correctional administrators exist in the form of standards and accreditation for mental health treatment programs in correctional settings. A number of organizations, including the American Correctional Association (ACA), the National Commission on Correctional Health Care (NCCHC), and the Joint Commission for the Accreditation of Healthcare Organizations (JCAHO) have established accreditation standards to ensure that inmates receive appropriate medical and mental health treatment while incarcerated. The ACA (2002), for example, has developed performance-based standards for correctional health care, including mental health care. The current ACA standards include mandatory mental health screening, staff training in crisis intervention, and provision of service to inmates with co-occurring mental illness and developmental disabilities. The NCCHC also provides *Standards for Health Services* that guide the delivery of correctional mental health care to inmates within juvenile facilities, as well as adult jails and prisons. These standards are similar to those developed by the ACA. The Joint Commission for the Accreditation of Healthcare Organizations (JCAHO) also provides accreditation for hospitals, mental health facilities, as well as juvenile and adult corrections.

All of these organizations offer voluntary accreditation for correctional mental health care programs. Accreditation involves on-site surveys of programs to ensure compliance with the national-level standards. Because accreditation standards are voluntary and it is costly to meet these standards, only a small percentage of all jails or prison systems subscribe to these services. As of 2003, for example, the Federal Bureau of Prisons achieved JCAHO accreditation for 99 percent of their health-care facilities (Department of Justice Report 2003). The NCCHC, by contrast, reports on its website that some 450 correctional organizations are accredited with that organization.

The American Psychiatric Association (APA) also provides standards for prison and jail-based psychiatric treatment (APA 2000). Separate guidelines are provided for prisons and jails, and include recommendations for such key services as referral and screening, assessment and evaluation, crisis intervention, treatment, and discharge planning. Other organizations have also established guidelines for the treatment of persons with mental illness in correctional settings, including the American Jail Association, the Council on Juvenile Correctional Administrators, and the National Juvenile Detention Association. Altogether there is a wealth of knowledge about correctional mental health care, although there is often a reluctance to adequately fund these services.

Recent federal legislation has acknowledged the large numbers of persons with mental illness in jails and prisons, including juveniles, and the challenges that this group has to overcome. The Mentally Ill Offender Treatment and Crime Reduction Act of 2004 (hereafter CRA) recognized that persons with mental illness can often benefit from treatment, and advocates for treatment services to be part of a collaborative approach to reduce recidivism. One of the key goals of this legislation was to encourage mental health systems at the federal, state, county or municipal level to improve services through better coordination.

There is a growing acknowledgment that "evidence-based" treatment—interventions that have demonstrated their effectiveness through empirical research—will form the cornerstone of future mental health treatment. A similar emphasis on evidence-based interventions in criminal justice systems has also recently emerged (MacKenzie 2005). There is an intuitive appeal to the notion that we should invest our scarce treatment resources in programs that have demonstrated their effectiveness. Consistent with that theme the Substance Abuse and Mental Health Services Administration (SAMHSA) is currently expanding its National Registry of Evidence-Based Programs and Practices. This Registry contains information about effective and promising programs that have been supported by evaluation research.

The remainder of this chapter provides examples of programs deemed effective in corrections-based mental health treatment and identifies key programmatic issues that must be addressed when implementing these interventions in correctional or community settings.

Diversion: Community-Based Alternatives to Incarceration

One approach to addressing the number of mentally ill individuals in the criminal justice system is to divert them from becoming an inmate in the first place. The discretion that local law enforcement uses to deal with mentally ill individuals is not a new topic. Teplin stated that law enforcement officials have three options when responding to a call for service and confronting a person with mental illness; "transport that person to a mental hospital, arrest the person, or resolve the matter informally" (2000:9). In recent times attention has increasingly focused on diversion programs with community-based treatment components, implementing police programs to respond to mentally ill individuals, and supporting legal innovations such as mental health courts (Hails and Borum 2003; Steadman, Cocozza and Veysey 1999).

There are a number of different approaches to diversion, including pre-booking and post-booking diversion. In pre-booking diversion some persons with mental illness are diverted from jail altogether—usually to receive some type of supportive community-based service. The alternative is post-booking diversion, and this involves the suspect being admitted to jail, and then later released to receive services from a community agency. Police officers typically have considerable discretion whether to take the arrestee to jail, but in some cases—if the person with mental illness is under the influence of drugs or alcohol, or requires a period of stabilization—post-booking diversion may be a better alternative. The following paragraphs outline a number of different approaches to diversion.

Police-Based Diversion

One of the most promising police interventions for responding to mentally ill individuals in conflict with the law is the Crisis Intervention Team (CIT), which is also known as the Memphis Tennessee Model

(Hails and Borum 2003; Steadman et al. 2001). This approach pairs specially trained police officers with community mental health service providers to divert persons with mental illness from formal legal sanctions (Hails and Borum 2003; Steadman et al. 2001). Steadman et al. (2001) also cited programs in Montgomery County, Pennsylvania, and Multnomah County, Oregon as examples of exemplary programs with excellent police training components and relationships with other community services. Dupont and Cochran (2000:338) stated that the CIT method is a "best practice" and this approach is supported by the National Alliance for Mentally Illness (NAMI), a national organization that advocates on the behalf of persons with mental illness.

NAMI also supports the specialized training of police officers to enhance their skills working with individuals with mental illness. In many locations NAMI offers 40-hour blocks of training to help police officers better understand mental illness (NAMI 2005). Hails and Borum (2003), among others, contend that training alone may not be as effective as pairing officers with community service providers. Even when these collaborations occur, however, working with the mentally ill can be a difficult proposition (Dupont and Cochran 2000; Gordon and Chabot 2004). Sellers and colleagues (2005) found that law enforcement agencies that do not have a specialized response team, but enter into cooperative agreements with local mental health providers, have more effective interactions with suspects and arrestees with mental illnesses.

SAMHSA has sponsored studies on the outcomes of jail diversion programs (Steadman et al. 1999; Theuma 2001). Steadman and colleagues (1999) identified three types of jail diversion programs, the first involves pre-booking (such as the CIT model), and the others are court-based and jail-based initiatives. Jail diversion programs in general have positive outcomes (Steadman, Cocozza and Veysey 1999). In order to be successful, however, collaboration between the stakeholder groups was deemed critically important (Draine and Solomon 1999; Steadman et al. 2000), as well as the ability to access community-based psychiatric programming (Grudzinskas et al. 2005; Richmond 2001; Steadman et al. 1999).

Mental Health Courts

Mental health courts are another alternative for persons with mental illness who have come into conflict with criminal justice systems. Ruddell observes that mental health courts are, "Intended primarily for non-violent misdemeanor defendants [and the]...courts are typically characterized by a specialized docket, one judge who hears all such matters, and a diversionary orientation" (2006:10). Many persons with mental illness have had unsuccessful relationships with community service providers, and mental health courts can use their coercive power to ensure that these offenders comply with both the court and treatment requirements.

Broward County, Florida, introduced the first mental health court in 1997 (Lerner-Wren 2002; Theuma 2001) and in December 2005, there were more than 113 mental health courts across the country (Survey of Mental Health Courts 2005). Mental health courts do not yet have evidence-based support, and a limited body of research currently exists. Preliminary studies of mental health court participants, however, indicated that while rates of arrest did not significantly vary between participants and non-participants, the mental health court cohort was arrested for less serious charges (Steadman, Redlich et al. 2005). Steadman, Redlich and colleagues (2005:224) study of seven mental health courts found that referrals were significantly "...more likely to be older, White and female...", an outcome also found an Ohio study (Munetz, Grande and Chambers 2001).

There are a number of studies currently underway that examine recidivism and other outcomes, and this initial research is providing encouraging results (see Moore and Hiday 2006). A consistent theme in the literature is that mental health courts seem to be more effective when supported by an array of community-based programs that support the efforts of these speciality courts. Because of the limited data about outcomes, however, correctional mental health practitioners will have to review the literature in the next several years to gauge the effectiveness of these interventions. A further challenge of reviewing these studies is that there is little uniformity in these courts and the different populations that are served and the goals of these courts make it difficult to make generalizations about the efficacy of these courts (Levin 2006).

Corrections-Based Mental Health Programs

Mental health programming provided in correctional settings should be grounded in evidence-based practices (Norton 2005). A number of standards and guidelines already exist that provide some blueprints for corrections-based mental health programs. These guidelines typically address a number of key issues in the assessment and treatment of persons with mentally illness, and include classification, screening, staffing, medication, institutional management, and cultural competence issues. Each of these issues are reviewed in the following pages.

Assessment and Classification

The Bureau of Justice Statistics found that nearly two-thirds of state prisons conduct some form of assessment, and a slightly higher percentage screen inmates for mental health needs upon admission to prison (Beck and Maruschak 2001). Prisons are able to undertake more comprehensive intake assessments as inmates are typically brought to a reception center and after comprehensive physical and mental health assessments are completed, are transferred to the facility that will become their home. In addition, to be admitted to a prison the inmate must be serving a sentence of more than one year, which makes it feasible to conduct more comprehensive assessments and classification.

Jails, on the other hand, are not particularly adept at recognizing mental health needs, in some measure due to the high volume of admissions (Sigurdson 2000). Another complicating issue is that arrestees admitted to these facilities are often under the influence of alcohol or drugs, are frequently depressed or otherwise agitated, making it difficult to distinguish between short-term distress and longer-term psychiatric problems.

The APA (2000) recommends screening jail admissions using a standardized assessment instrument. All guidelines indicate that assessment should have some observational components that consider demeanor and behaviors, as well as some clinical or conversational components (Fagan 2003; Roesch, Ogloff and Eaves 1995). The ACA (2002) standards include inquiring about suicidal thoughts or actions, prescriptions for psychotropic medications, as well as histories of psychiatric treatment or substance abuse. If the person is perceived to be at-risk of self harm or in need of psychiatric services, they should be referred to mental health professionals before being assigned to a living unit (Fagan and Ax 2003).

Neither the APA, ACA, nor the NIC recommend the use of a specific assessment or screening instrument. The Brief Jail Mental Health Screen, however, was developed for jail populations, and is available from the National Gains Center. This screening tool is recommended for use with male jail detainees —although it was not recommended for female detainees—in Steadman, Scott and colleagues (2005) evaluation of the instrument. Admissions screening of female arrestees or inmates is particularly relevant, as they tend to have higher rates of depression due to histories of physical, sexual, or substance abuse (Gunter 2004; NCCHC 2005).

Screening, assessment and evaluation by themselves do not ensure that inmates seek out or participate in treatment, so correctional administrators and professional staff should identify any roadblocks to accessing treatment (Steffan and Morgan 2005). The opposite can also occur.

Screening may result in placing an inmate in high security housing units which may be stressful and non-therapeutic. As a result, objective instruments have to be supported by clinical assessments, especially when the inmate has severe mental illness, or is expressing suicidal ideation. These inmates should also be re-assessed on a regular basis. These ongoing assessments are necessary to assure that the inmate receives appropriate interventions throughout their custody term (White and Gillespie 2005).

Screening for malingering in correctional settings is also recommended. Malingering occurs when inmates fake physical or psychiatric symptoms in order to receive some type of benefit or advantage (e.g., to minimize responsibility for their actions, seek attention, or to avoid an unpleasant assignment). Vitacco and Rogers (2005) recommend that malingering be evaluated during the inmate's initial assessment and screening. They outlined a number of screening instruments that can detect malingering, such as the Miller Forensic Assessment of Symptoms Test, the Structured Inventory of Malingered Symptomatology, the Structured Interview of Reported Symptoms, the Minnesota Multiphasic Personality Inventory, and the Personality Assessment Inventory (Vitacco and Rogers 2005). Using these instruments might not be practical for a jail inmate who might be bailed out in a few hours, but may be useful for long-term inmates who are suspected of manipulating staff.

Staffing Issues

Staffing is a critical issue in correctional facilities. Both security as well as staff members who provide specialized medical and mental health services play key roles in responding to inmates with mental illnesses. The ACA (2002) standards require that correctional administrators identify the types of staff necessary for the services delivered, to set job descriptions with minimum qualifications for qualified mental health professionals, to comply with new employee orientation and in-service training requirements, and to monitor staff turnover. Staffing considerations also include the training needs of correctional officers. Officers should be able to recognize symptoms of mental illness so that they can make appropriate referrals for evaluation and treatment (Hafemeister, Hall and Dvoskin 2001; Norton 2005; Tahir 2003). Training is also important for the mental health staff so that they understand the security requirements of the institution (Schwartz 2003).

Physical Plant

The physical plant refers to the structure and layout of a jail or prison, and this is an important consideration in the delivery of programs. The ACA (2002) has outlined a number of standards, including how much space must be provided for each inmate. Some institutions have a set number of beds to serve mentally ill inmates, and have had to increase that number in the last decade (Stahl and West 2001). One dilemma is how to estimate the number of beds that are necessary to accommodate every inmate with severe mental health problems versus the level of treatment effectiveness that can be maintained. Some correctional systems construct separate residential units for persons with mental illness. The Colorado Department of Corrections, for example, has developed a 500-bed mental health unit (Stahl and West 2001). Such units have successfully decreased problematic behaviors (Holton 2003).

Some facilities are too small to construct their own mental health unit. It is not feasible to construct a separate mental health unit in a jail with 50 beds, for instance, especially if there are only a few mentally ill inmates. One alternative approach is to utilize mobile teams who assess the mental health needs of inmates in the general population (Lovell and Rhodes 1997). A less desirable alternative is to place persons with mental illness in isolation. Inmates housed in segregation pose an entirely different set of treatment issues, and the NCCHC has developed standards for these inmates, including their mental health care (Hills et al. 2004). Because placing a person with mental illness in isolation is akin to punishment, and places the inmate at higher risk of suicide, this approach must be considered a "last resort."

Some correctional facilities have used technology to improve the delivery of mental health services. Innovations in technology, such as electronic medical records or the ability to complete assessments using a hand-held computer, lend themselves to data collection that can be used for evidence-based practice (Freedman 2003). Telemedicine (conducting interviews by way of a television or computer screen utilizing web-based technology) can also assist with the delivery of mental health care. This approach can be used in all units or facilities without disrupting staffing and reducing the risks and costs of transportation (Fitzgibbons and Gunter-Justice 2000; Holton 2003; Magaletta et al. 2005). The NIC provides technical assistance for jails or prisons that are considering incorporating telemedicine into their correctional health care services.

Medication

A primary treatment for mental illness is psychotropic medication. When used appropriately, these medications can decrease problematic behaviors within a facility (Tahir 2003). There are a number of concerns regarding medications, including ensuring that inmates comply with the physician's orders, storage, and cost control. Psychotropic medications are costly and diagnostic tools are critical to ensure that the proper type and dose of medications are given to achieve the best outcomes at reasonable costs (Taylor 2001). In order to manage costs the state of Texas has introduced algorithms (set guidelines or best practices) for medication and treatment although some stakeholders have been critical of this approach (Taylor 2001).

The NCCHC and other accrediting bodies have established standards for medication storage and use (Hills et al. 2004). Filling prescriptions and the delivery of medications becomes a very complex issue when providing medications to thousands of inmates in a large jail or prison system. A key question is whether inmates should have access to their medications, or whether they should take their medications supervised by correctional officers or medical staff. Some inmates may not take their prescribed medications because they do not like the side effects, while others sell or barter their medications to other inmates. While staff members can dispense these medications directly to prisoners, it doesn't give these individuals the skills to independently manage their medications once they are returned to the community.

Co-occurring Disorders: Substance Abuse

A second type of co-occurring disorder is mental illness and substance abuse. There are high numbers of inmates with this designation, which is not surprising given the size of the mentally ill population who are incarcerated, and the high percentage of inmates charged with some type of alcohol- or drug-related offense. When the need for mental health or substance abuse treatment is indicated during screening, referrals for service should be made. If the inmate has co-occurring disorders, each condition exacerbates the other, resulting in a complicated treatment dilemma (Woody 1996). Individuals with co-occurring diagnoses are also likely to engage in risky behaviors that lead to increased health problems (Hiller et al. 2005). This finding has implications for providing medical and psychiatric care in correctional settings, and arranging for medical care upon release, which in turn impacts the public health care system (Hiller et al. 2005).

Treatment for co-occurring disorders starts upon admission to a facility. Evaluation, assessment and screening should identify treatment needs (Abram and Teplin 1991). Treatment plans should be developed with discharge in mind, and the problems associated with community re-entry. Relapse to substance use, for instance, can be a predictive factor for violence or recidivism (Draine et al. 2005; Steadman et al. 1998). As a result, the involvement of both mental health and substance abuse services are necessary for effective community reintegration (Drake, Wallach and McGovern 2005).

The American Psychiatric Association (2000) has recommended that co-occurring disorders be treated together in an integrated approach. A number of states and the federal prison system have developed co-occurring treatment units for prison inmates (Springer, McNeece and Arnold 2003). Typically these programs involve a separate residential unit within a prison, with specific referral and eligibility criteria (Katz 1999). An example of a prison-based treatment model is New York's Psychiatric Center (CNYPC) that houses inmates from the state Department of Corrections (Smith, Sawyer and Way 2002). In order to integrate services, the CNYPC works in conjunction with the Department of Corrections to ensure continuity of services for inmates released to the community (Smith et al. 2002). Treatment interventions for substance abusing inmates known as therapeutic communities have, in Colorado, and other locations, been adapted to work with co-occurring populations (Sacks, Sacks and Stommel 2003).

Some larger jails can provide a separate program for inmates with co-occurring disorders that integrates mental health and substance abuse treatment (Burgess, Swanson and Fallon 1999). Beaver County, Pennsylvania, found that one-fifth of their jail inmates had co-occurring treatment needs, so they initiated a jail-based program that has decreased recidivism (Bell et al. 2005). SAMHSA and the National Gains Center have sponsored jail diversion programs for this population, and investigators have reported that offenders participating in these diversion initiatives spent more time in the community than those who did not participate (Steadman and Naples 2005). A jail diversion study of offenders with co-occurring needs, by contrast, found that individuals who were diverted were at no greater risk for rearrest than those who served their sentence (Broner et al. 2004). Sherman and colleagues (2004) found that the success of these programs depended on screening and assessment, as well as long-term stable funding.

SAMHSA (2005) has also recognized the need for integrated co-occurring interventions and in 2004 created the Co-Occurring Center for Excellence (COCE) (Mental Health Weekly 2004). COCE is currently disseminating information about the best practices for individuals with co-occurring disorders in special settings, such as prisons. Some of these best practices involve responding to special needs correctional populations, such as women. Prison and jail administrators should consider different approaches for women with co-occurring disorders (Dolan et al. 2003). Abram, Teplin and McClelland (2003) found, for instance, that eight percent of women in Chicago's Cook County Jail had co-occurring disorders. Maryland has developed interventions for female inmates with co-occurring disorders that include corrections-based treatment units, with corresponding treatment available in the community upon release (Gillece and Russell 2002).

Co-occurring Disorders: Developmental Disabilities

Correctional administrators must be aware of the treatment needs of inmates with co-occurring disorders. Individuals with mental illness and mental retardation or other developmental disabilities are over-represented in correctional institutions (Giamp and West 2003; NCCHC 1992). Such individuals may be at higher risk of victimization in correctional settings due to their decreased intellectual functioning, lack of patience, and impulsive or annoying behaviors (Hills et al. 2004). Similar to inmates with mental illness, those with developmental disabilities often stay in prison longer and may not always have access to appropriate care (Giamp and West 2003).

In order to respond to this special needs population, living units for developmentally disabled inmates have been developed in Colorado, New York, and Texas (Giamp and West 2003; Hills et al. 2004). These programs identify strategies to confront problematic inmate behaviors in an effort to decrease recidivism once they are returned to a community setting (Gardner, Graeber and Machkovitz 1998). Just as training is necessary for correctional officers to interact effectively with the mentally ill, training on symptom recognition and intervention strategies for this dually diagnosed population is essential for program success (Richardson 2003).

Cultural Competence

Racial and ethnic minorities are disproportionately represented in correctional institutions (Bonczar 2003). Given this fact, there is a need for cultural competency in the delivery of mental health services. Research indicates that, compared to whites, more drugs were prescribed for African-Americans with a schizophrenia diagnosis (Chung, Mahler and Kakuma 1995). Chung and colleagues (1995) outline how African-Americans are treated differently than their white counterparts (more drug screens ordered, shorter lengths of stay in community-based psychiatric hospitals, and less likely to be identified as requiring one-to-one observation). African-Americans and Latinos also have less access to mental health treatment, have less tolerance for some antipsychotic medication, receive a lower quality of care, and are more likely to be misdiagnosed (Lawson and Strickland 2004).

The NASMHPD (2004) has issued a report on cultural competence in state-funded psychiatric settings, recommending culturally appropriate services, linguistic services, services for the hard-of-hearing, and suggested that cultural competence be included in service contracts. The finding that members of minority groups have less access to mental services is a critical weakness in community reintegration efforts. One important goal is to increase community-based services in general, while ensuring that the special needs of minority populations are not forgotten. The National Center for Cultural Competence promotes these services, and information about cultural competency can be accessed on their website.

Community Reintegration

Two important dimensions of correctional treatment for persons with mental illness are meaningful discharge plans and the availability of a wide range of community services to support the offender's reintegration (Roesch et al. 1995). All of the major correctional accrediting bodies—the ACA, APA, and NCCHC—recommend continuity of care upon release. Since lack of services has been correlated with increased recidivism, it is appropriate to apply the public health framework where an individual's protective factors are increased to offset the known risks (Ax 2003). As a result, planning for an offender's community reintegration should include attention to individual needs, housing, medication and medical care, income supports, and food, clothing, transportation and child care if relevant (Osher, Steadman and Barr 2003). Acknowledging the importance of these needs, the federal government has been supportive of expanding services such as public aid, housing, assistance with educational plans, and vocational rehabilitation in order to reduce recidivism (Pogorzelski et al. 2005). In the past there has been a cut in funding for public health, and a corresponding increase in correctional spending (Freudenberg 2001). New federal initiatives, however, may return funding to providing better services for persons with mental illness who are returning to the community.

Given the importance of aftercare to successful community reintegration, the issue then becomes what evidence-based services will be given the highest priority. Essock and colleagues evaluated evidence-based practices for community mental health services and found that best practices are ". . .assertive community treatment, integrated dual disorders treatment, family psychoeducation, supported employment, illness self-management, and medication practices" (2003:932). This list identifies areas in which the criminal justice, mental health, substance abuse, and public health systems can best direct their scarce resources. Assertive Community Treatment programs (ACT) are model interventions because they incorporate medication, housing, employment, medical support, therapy or other needed services to assist with community reintegration (Honberg and Gruttadaro 2005).

One significant question is how to best monitor probationers or parolees with histories of mental health problems. Probation and parole officers must be included as part of the aftercare planning process, and they should receive training about mental health issues (Slate et al. 2003). In fact, some federal probation and parole officers are classified as "mental health specialists" (Slate et al. 2003:16), to better serve the 18 percent of federal probationers who have mental health treatment as a condition of their release. Local and state probation and parole officers who have specialized mental health caseloads may also support the re-entry of persons with mental illness returning to the community.

Systems Collaboration

Cooperation between service delivery providers and correctional authorities is critical to the long-term success of community aftercare programs. Such cooperation can reduce costs, provide improved program implementation (Osher et al. 2003), and enhance public safety. The President's New Freedom Commission (2003), however, found that the public mental health system was scattered and it was difficult for some people to access services. Therefore, a major focus of the Consensus Project is to improve collaboration and coordination between criminal justice agencies and the mental health and substance abuse treatment systems (Consensus Project 2002). One of the goals of the Consensus Project is to provide technical assistance to states to encourage such interactions (Buell 2004). It is hoped that such collaboration will eventually lead to reduction in service overlap, and standardized data collection and analyses (Anzaldi and Buell 2005).

In addition to providing technical assistance to a number of states, a number of local programs have been recognized by the Consensus Project as models of inter-agency collaboration including Franklin County, Ohio, San Bernandino, California, Jefferson County, Colorado, and Monroe County, New York (Buell 2004). Moreover, Project Link in New York supports collaboration between criminal justice, mental health and other service agencies for mentally ill offenders (Weisman, Lamberti and Price

2004). Community treatment teams (Kane and Blank 2004), and therapeutic communities have also been recognized as effective programs (Weisman et al. 2004).

The State of Arizona, with funding assistance from SAMHSA, developed the Arizona Integrated Treatment Initiative to work with individuals with co-occurring diagnoses (Franczak and Dye 2001). This is an example of an evidence-based community system design. A key goal of these integrated services is the understanding that the offender should also join in community activities, which in turn becomes part of their support system (Draine et al. 2005; Lurigio 2000). An important part of that support system is local law enforcement, and they must be included in any collaborative efforts (Wooten and Hoelter 1998). Law enforcement awareness of the service delivery system assists them as first responders at calls involving persons with mentally illness (Roskes 2001).

Conclusion

The prevalence of persons with mental health needs in the criminal justice system is coupled with a lack of accessible, well staffed, culturally competent, and integrated treatment programs. These are problems identified in diversion programs, institutional corrections, and in community-based probation and parole services. The public health model identifies risks and then works toward enhancing protective factors. The same approach may successfully increase mental health initiatives in prisons, jails, and in community re-integration efforts to serve as protective actions against the risk of recidivism.

Failing to treat individuals with mental illness during their incarceration, and then releasing them into the community without appropriate supports, adversely affects the entire community. Increasing the scope of community resources for offenders with mental illness can protect both the offender and the community. There has been an increasing awareness that the failure to provide appropriate services for this population has decreased our public safety. One encouraging development is that federal and state governments are increasingly interested in expanding services for offenders with histories of mental health problems. It is hoped that this interest will be translated into more funding for community-based services.

References

Abram, Karen A. and Linda A. Teplin. 1991. "Co-Occurring Disorders Among Mentally Ill Jail Detainees: Implications for Public Policy." *American Psycholo-*

gist 46:1036-1045.

Abram, Karen A., Linda A. Teplin and Gery M. McClelland. 2003. "Comorbidity of Severe Psychiatric Disorders and Substance Use Disorders Among Women in Jail." *American Journal of Psychiatry* 5:1007-1010.

American Correctional Association. 2006. "Notice of Open Hearing: The American Correctional Association and the Commission on Accreditation for Corrections." Retrieved January 11, 2006 (http://www.aca.org).

------. 2002. "Performance-Based Standards for Correctional Health Care in Adult Correctional Institutions." Lanham, MD: Author.

American Psychiatric Association. 2000. *Psychiatric Services in Jails and Prisons: A Task Force Report of the American Psychiatric Association*, Second Edition. Washington, DC: Author.

Anzaldi, Monica and Maureen Buell. 2005. "Building Collaboration Between Criminal Justice and Mental Health." *Behavioral Health Management* 25:22-24.

Aufderheide, Dean H. and Patrick H. Brown. 2005. "Crisis in Corrections: The Mentally Ill in America's Prisons." *Corrections Today* 67:30-33.

Ax, Robert K. 2003. "A Viable Future for Correctional Mental Health Care." Pp. 303-327 in *Correctional Mental Health Handbook*, edited by T. J. Fagan and R. K. Ax. Thousand Oaks, CA: Sage Publications.

Banks, Steven M., James L. Stone, John A. Pandiani, Judith F. Cox and Pamela C. Morschauser. 2000. "Utilization of Local Jails and General Hospitals by State Psychiatric Center Patients." *The Journal of Behavioral Health Services & Research* 27:454-459.

Barr, Heather. 2003. "Transinstitutionalization in the Courts: Brad H. v. City of New York, and the Fight for Discharge Planning for People with Psychiatric Disabilities Leaving Rikers Island." *Crime & Delinquency* 49:97-123.

Beck, Allen J. and Laura M. Maruschak. 2001. *Mental Health Treatment in State Prisons, 2000* (NCJ188215). Washington, DC: U. S. Department of Justice, Office of Justice Programs, Bureau of Justice Statistics.

Bell, Arlene, Nancy Jaquette, David Sanner, Carol Steele-Smith and Holly Wald. 2005. *Corrections Today* 67:86-90.

Broner, Nahama, Pamela K. Lattimore, Alexander J. Cowell and William E. Schlenger. "Effects of Diversion on Adults with Co-Occurring Mental Illness and Substance Use: Outcomes from a National Multi-Site Study." *Behavioral Sciences and the Law* 22:519-541.

Broner, Nahama, Huy Nguyen, Anne Swern and Stephen Goldfinger. 2003. "Adapting a Substance Abuse Court Diversion Model for Felony Offenders with Co-Occurring Disorders: Initial Implementation." *Psychiatric Quarterly* 74:361-385.

Buell, Maureen. 2004. "Bridging the Gap." *Corrections Today* 66:26-31.

Burgess, John D., Arthur J. Swanson and Bryan Fallon. 1999. "Therapeutic Community Services: A Jail-Based Substance Abuse Treatment Program at Rikers Island." *American Jails* 3:25-30.

Center for Mental Health Services. 2003. *State and County Psychiatric Hospitals, Inpatient Census, End of 2000.* U. S. Department of Health and Human Services, Substance Abuse and Mental Health Services Administration, National Mental Health Services Center, Center for Mental Health Services.

Chung, Henry, John C. Mahler and Tatsu Kakuma. 1995. "Racial Differences in

Treatment of Psychiatric Inpatients." *Psychiatric Services* 46:586-591.
Criminal Justice/Mental Health Consensus Project. 2002. Washington, DC: Council of State Governments.
de Montfort, Deborah and Monica E. Oss. 2003. "Examining the Intersection of the Behavioral Health and Corrections Systems: A Look at the Numbers Shows That Many People are Caught Between Both Systems." *Behavioral Health Management* 23:10-14.
DeCou, Kate. 2001. "Incarcerated Women and Self-Harm — Security or Sanity." Pp. 36-1-36-13 in *Forensic Mental Health: Working with Offenders with Mental Illness* edited by G. Landsberg and A. Smiley. Kingston, NJ: Civic Research Institute.
Department of Justice. 2003. *Performance and Accountability Report* FY 2003. Washington, DC: U. S. Government Printing Office.
Ditton, Paula M. 1999. *Mental Health and Treatment of Inmates and Probationers.* (NCJ174463). Washington, DC: U. S. Department of Justice, Office of Justice Programs, Bureau of Justice Statistics.
Dolan, Lisa, Ken Kolthoff, Mike Schreck, Patti Smilanich and Ross Todd. 2003. "Gender-Specific Treatment for Clients with Co-Occurring Disorders." *Corrections Today* 65:100-107.
Draine, Jeffrey, Amy Blank, Petra Kottsieper and Phyllis Solomon. 2005. "Contrasting Jail Diversion and In-Jail Services for Mental Illness and Substance Abuse: Do They Serve the Same Clients?" *Behavioral Sciences and the Law* 23:171-181.
Draine, Jeffrey and Phyllis Solomon. 1999. "Describing and Evaluating Jail Diversion Services for Persons with Serious Mental Illness." *Psychiatric Services* 50:56-61.
Draine, Jeffrey, Nancy Wolff, Joseph E. Jacoby, Stephanie Hartwell and Christine Duclos. 2005. "Understanding Community Re-Entry of Former Prisoners with Mental Illness: A Conceptual Model to Guide New Research." *Behavioral Sciences and the Law* 23:689-707.
Drake, Robert E., Michael A. Wallach and Mark P. McGovern. 2005. "Future Directions in Preventing Relapse to Substance Abuse Among Clients with Severe Mental Illnesses." *Psychiatric Services* 56:1297-1302.
Dupont, Randolph and Sam Cochran. 2000. "Police Response to Mental Health Emergencies-Barriers to Change." *The Journal of the American Academy of Psychiatry and the Law* 28:338-344.
Essock, Susan M., Howard H. Goldman, Laura Van Tosh, William A. Anthony, Charity R. Appell, Gary R. Bond, Lisa B. Dixon, Linda K. Dunakin, Vijay Ganju, Paul G. Gorman, Ruth O. Ralph, Charles A. Rapp, Gregory B. Teague and Robert E. Drake. 2003. "Evidence-Based Practices: Setting the Context and Responding to Concerns." *Psychiatric Clinics of North America* 26:919-938.
Fagan, Thomas J. 2003. "Mental Health in Corrections: A Model for Service Delivery." Pp. 3-19 in *Correctional Mental Health Handbook*, edited by T. J. Fagan and R. K. Ax. Thousand Oaks, CA: Sage Publications.
Fitzgibbons, Mark F. and Tracy Gunter-Justice. 2000. "Telemedicine and Mental Health In Jails: A New Tool for an Old Problem." *Corrections Today* 62:104-107.
Fletcher, Bennett W. and Harry K. Wexler. 2005. "National Criminal Justice Drug Abuse Treatment Studies (CJ-DATS): Update and Progress." *Justice Research and Statistics Association: The Forum* 23:1-7.
Franczak, Michael and Christina Dye. 2001. "Treating Offenders with Mental Disor-

ders And Co-Occurring Substance Abuse Disorders — The Arizona Integrated Treatment Initiative." Pp. 10-1-10-20 in *Forensic Mental Health: Working with Offenders with Mental Illness*, edited by G. Landsberg and A. Smiley. Kingston, NJ: Civic Research Institute.

Freedman, Joshua. 2003. "The Role of Information Technology in Evidence-Based Practices." *Psychiatric Clinics of North America* 26:833-850.

Freudenberg, Nicholas. 2001. "Jails, Prisons, and the Health of Urban Populations: A Review of the Impact of the Correctional System on Community Health." *Journal of Urban Health: Bulletin of the New York Academy of Medicine* 78:214-235.

Gannon, John. 2005. "Mental Health in Corrections: The Continuing Dilemma." *Corrections Today* 67:8-10.

Gardner, William I., Janice L. Graeber and Susan J. Machkovitz. 1998. "Treatment of Offenders with Mental Retardation." Pp. 329-362 in *Treatment of Offenders with Mental Disorders*, edited by R. M. Wettstein. New York: Guilford Press.

Geller, Jeffrey L. 2001. "Donut Shop Diversion Program." *Psychiatric Services* 52:1559.

Giamp, Jacqueline S. and Mary E. West. 2003. "Delivering Psychological Services to Incarcerated Men with Developmental Disabilities." Pp. 8-1-8-17 in *Correctional Psychology: Practice, Programming, and Administration*, edited by B. K. Schwartz. Kingston, NJ: Civic Research Institute.

Gillece, Joan and Betty G. Russell. 2002. "Maryland's Programs for Incarcerated Women with Mental Illness and Substance Abuse Disorders." Pp. 165-171 in *Serving Mentally Ill Offenders: Challenges and Opportunities for Mental Health Professionals*, edited by G. Landsberg, M. Rock, L. K. W. Berg and A. Smiley. New York: Springer Publishing.

Glaze, Lauren E. and Seri Palla. 2005. *Probation and Parole in the United States, 2004* (NCJ210676). Washington, DC: U. S. Department of Justice, Office of Justice Programs, Bureau of Justice Statistics.

Gordon, Christopher and Lisa Chabot. 2004. "Jail Diversion Programs Show Power of Teamwork." *Behavioral Healthcare Tomorrow* 13:31-35.

Gould, Mark A. 2003. "Issues of Power and Oppression." Pp. 1-1-1-28 in *Correctional Psychology: Practice, Programming, and Administration*, edited by B. K. Schwartz. Kingston, NJ: Civic Research Institute.

Grudzinskas, Albert J., Jonathan C. Clayfield, Kristen Roy-Bujnowski, William H. Fisher and Maurice H. Richardson. 2005. "Integrating the Criminal Justice System into Mental Health Service Delivery: The Worcester Diversion Experience." *Behavioral Sciences and the Law* 23:277-293.

Gunter, Tracy D. 2004. "Incarcerated Women and Depression: A Primer for the Primary Care Provider." *Journal of the American Medical Women's Association* 59:107-112.

Haddad, Jane E. 2001. "Implementing Effective In-Prison Outpatient Care for Inmates with Serious Mental Illness — The Ohio Experience." Pp. 19-1-19-11 in *Forensic Mental Health: Working with Offenders with Mental Illness*, edited by G. Landsberg and A. Smiley. Kingston, NJ: Civic Research Institute.

Hafemeister, Thomas L, Susan R. Hall and Joel A. Dvoskin. 2001. "Administrative Concerns Associated with the Treatment of Offenders with Mental Illness." Pp. 419-444 in *Treating Adult and Juvenile Offenders with Special Needs*, edited by J. B. Ashford, B. D. Sales and W. H. Reid. Washington, DC: American Psychological

Association.

Harrison, Paige M. and Allen J. Beck. 2005. *Prisoners in 2004.* (NCJ210677). Washington, DC: U. S. Department of Justice, Office of Justice Programs, Bureau of Justice Statistics.

Hails, Judy and Randy Borum. 2003. "Police Training and Specialized Approaches to Respond to People with Mental Illnesses." *Crime & Delinquency* 49:52-61.

Hiller, Matthew L., J. Matthew Webster, Thomas F. Garrity, Carl Leukefeld, Egle Narevic and Michele Staton. 2005. "Prisoners with Substance Abuse and Mental Health Problems: Use of Health and Health Services." *The American Journal of Drug and Alcohol Abuse* 1:1-20.

Hills, Holly, Christine Siegfried and Alan Ickowitz. 2004. *Effective Prison Mental Health Services: Guidelines to Expand and Improve Treatment.* Washington, DC: U. S. Department of Justice, National Institute of Corrections.

Holton, Shelia M. B. 2003. "Managing and Treating Mentally Disordered Offenders in Jails and Prisons." Pp. 101-122 in *Correctional Mental Health Handbook*, edited by T. J. Fagan and R. K. Ax. Thousand Oaks, CA: Sage Publications.

Honberg, Ron and Darcy Gruttadaro. 2005. "Flawed Mental Health Policies and the Tragedy of Criminalization." *Corrections Today* 67:22-27.

Hulnick, Marjory J. 2003. "Treating the Offender with Mental Illness." Pp. 7-1-7-42 in *Correctional Psychology: Practice, Programming, and Administration*, edited by B. K. Schwartz. Kingston, NJ: Civic Research Institute.

James, Doris J. and Lauren E. Glaze. 2006. *Mental Health Problems of Prison and Jail Inmates*. Washington, DC: Bureau of Justice Statistics.

Kane, Catherine F. and Michael B. Blank. 2004. "NPACT: Enhancing Programs of Assertive Community Treatment for the Seriously Mentally Ill." *Community Mental Health Journal* 40:549-559.

Katz, Randall I. 1999. "The Addiction Treatment Unit: A Dual Diagnosis Program at the California Medical Facility-A Descriptive Study." *Journal of Psychoactive Drugs* 31:41-46.

Lamb, H. Richard and Linda E. Weinberger. 1998. "Persons with Severe Mental Illness in Jails and Prisons: A Review." *Psychiatric Services* 49:483-492.

Lawson, William B. and Tony Strickland. 2004. "Racial and Ethnic Issues Affect Treatment for Bipolar Disorder." *Psychiatric Annals* 34:17-20.

Lerner-Wren, Ginger. 2002. "Broward's Mental Health Court: An Innovative Approach to the Mentally Disabled in the Criminal Justice System." Pp. 128-132 in *Serving Mentally Ill Offenders: Challenges and Opportunities for Mental Health Professionals,* edited by G. Landsberg, M. Rock, L. K. W. Berg and A. Smiley. New York: Springer Publishing.

Levin, Aaron. 2006. "MH Courts Garner Mostly Favorable Reviews." *Psychiatric News* 41: 32-36.

Linhorst, Donald M. 2006. *Empowering People with Severe Mental Illness: A Practical Guide.* New York: Oxford University Press.

Lovell, David and Lorna A. Rhodes. 1997. "Mobile Consultation: Crossing Correctional Boundaries to Cope with Disturbed Offenders." *Federal Probation* 61:40-45.

Lurigio, Arthur J. 2000. "Persons with Serious Mental Illness in the Criminal Justice System: Background, Prevalence, and Principles of Care." *Criminal Justice Policy Review* 11:312-328.

MacKenzie, Doris Layton. 2005. "The Importance of Using Scientific Evidence to Make Decisions About Correctional Programming." *Criminology & Public Policy* 4:249-257.

Magaletta, Phillip R., Robert K. Ax, Marc W. Patry and Erik F. Dietz. 2005. "Clinical Practice in Segregation: The Crucial Role of Psychologists." *Corrections Today* 67:34-36.

Maue, Frederick R. 2001. "An Overview of Correctional Mental Health Issues." *Corrections Today* 64:8.

Mental Health Weekly. 2004. "SAMHSA Creates Assistance Center for Co-Occurring Disorders." *Mental Health Weekly* 14:6.

Mentally Ill Offender Treatment and Crime Reduction Act of 2004. 42 United States Code 3711 et seq.

Moore, Marlee E. and Virginia Aldige Hiday. 2006. "Mental Health Court Outcomes: A Comparison of Re-Arrest and Re-Arrest Severity Between Mental Health Court and Traditional Court Participants." *Law and Human Behavior* 30: 659-674.

Morris, Suzanne M., Henry J. Steadman and Bonita M. Veysey. 1997. "Mental Health Services in United States Jails: A Survey of Innovative Practices." *Criminal Justice and Behavior* 24:3-19.

Mumola, Christopher J. 1999. *Substance Abuse and Treatment, State and Federal Prisoners, 1997* (NCJ172871). Washington, DC: U. S. Department of Justice, Office of Justice Programs, Bureau of Justice Statistics.

Munetz, Mark R., Thomas P. Grande and Margaret R. Chambers. 2001. "The Incarceration of Individuals with Severe Mental Disorders." *Community Mental Health Journal* 37:361-372.

National Alliance for Mentally Ill. 2005. "Crisis Intervention Team (CIT) Resource Center." (NAMI Alert). Retrieved January 20, 2006 (http://www.nami.org).

National Commission on Correctional Health Care. 2006. "Standards for Health Services And Other Assistance." Retrieved January 11, 2006 (http://www.ncchc.org).

------. 2005. "Women's Health Care in Correctional Settings: Position Statement." Retrieved January 11, 2006 (http://www.ncchc.org).

------. 2004. "Treatment of Schizophrenia in Correctional Institutions." Retrieved January 11, 2006 (http://www.ncchc.org).

------. 1997. "Use of Telemedicine Technology in Correctional Facilities: Position Statement." Retrieved January 11, 2006 (http://www.ncchc.org).

------. 1992. "Mental Health Services in Correctional Settings: Position Statement." Retrieved January 11, 2006 (http://www.ncchc.org).

National Institute of Corrections. 2006. "Offender Mental Health Services: Learn More About NIC Technical Assistance Related to Mental Health Services in Corrections." Retrieved January 17, 2006 (http://www.nicic.org).

National Technical Assistance Center for State Mental Health Planning. 2004. *Cultural Competency: Measurement as a Strategy for Moving Knowledge into Practice in State Mental Health Systems, Final Report.* Alexandria, VA: National Association of State Mental Health Program Directors.

National Institute of Corrections. *Offender Mental Health Services*. Retrieved January 17, 2006 (http://www.nicic.org)

Norton, Steven C. 2005. "Successfully Managing Mentally Ill Offenders: Thoughts

and Recommendations." *Corrections Today* 67:28-37.
Osher, Fred, Henry J. Steadman and Heather Barr. 2003. "A Best Practice Approach to Community Reentry from Jails for Inmates with Co-Occurring Disorders: The APIC Model." *Crime and Delinquency* 49:79-96.
Pogorzelski, Wendy, Nancy Wolff, Ko-Yu Pan and Cynthia L. Blitz. 2005. "Behavioral Health Problems, Ex-Offender Reentry Policies, and the "Second Chance Act." *American Journal of Public Health* 95:1718-1724.
President's New Freedom Commission on Mental Health. 2005. Subcommittee on Evidence-Based Practices: Background Paper. Rockville, MD: U. S. Department of Health and Human Services.
President's New Freedom Commission on Mental Health. 2003. *Achieving the Promise: Transforming Mental Health Care in America: Final Report.* Rockville, MD: U. S. Department of Health and Human Services.
Report to Congress on the Prevention and Treatment of Co-occurring Substance Abuse Disorders and Mental Disorders. 2003. Washington, DC: U. S. Department of Health and Human Services, Substance Abuse and Mental Health Services Administration.
Richardson, Linda. 2003. "Other Special Offender Populations." Pp. 199-216 in *Correctional Mental Health Handbook,* edited by T. J. Fagan and R. K. Ax. Thousand Oaks, CA: Sage Publications.
Richmond, Linda L. 2001. "Evaluation of a Case Management Model in a Jail Diversion Program." Pp. 6-1-6-7 in *Forensic Mental Health: Working with Offenders with Mental Illness,* edited by G. Landsberg and A. Smiley. Kingston, NJ: Civic Research Institute.
Roesch, Ronald, James R.P. Ogloff and Derek Eaves. 1995. "Mental Health Research in the Criminal Justice System: The Need for Common Approaches and International Perspectives." *International Journal of Law and Psychiatry* 18:1-14.
Roskes, Erik. 2001. "Professional Collaboration to Effectively Manage Offenders with Mental Illness in the Community." Pp. 9-1-9-7 in *Forensic Mental Health: Working with Offenders with Mental Illness,* edited by G. Landsberg and A. Smiley. Kingston, NJ: Civic Research Institute.
Ruddell, Rick. 2006. "Jail Interventions for Inmates with Mental Illnesses." *Journal of Correctional Health Care* 12: 1-14
Sacks, Stanley, JoAnn Y. Sacks and Joe Stommel. 2003. "Modified Therapeutic Community Program for Inmates with Mental Illness and Chemical Abuse Disorders." *Corrections Today* 65:90-99.
Schwartz, Barbara K. 2003. "Establishing a Mental Health Unit Within an Institution." Pp. 3-1-3-20 in *Correctional Psychology: Practice, Programming, and Administration,* edited by B. K. Schwartz. Kingston, NJ: Civic Research Institute.
Sellers, Courtenay L., Christopher J. Sullivan, Bonita M. Veysey and Jon M. Shane. 2005. "Responding to Persons with Mental Illnesses: Police Perspectives on Specialized and Traditional Practices." *Behavioral Sciences and the Law* 23:647-657.
Sherman, Richard K., Larry K. Irvin, Paul Yovanoff and Susan Sowards. 2004. "Federal Demonstration Funds at the Interface of Mental Health and Criminal Justice." *Administration and Policy in Mental Health* 32:17-29.
Sigurdson, Chris. 2000. "The Mad and the Bad and the Abandoned: The Mentally Ill in Prisons and Jails." *Corrections Today* 62:70-78.

Slate, Risdon N., Erik Roskes, Richard Feldman and Migdalia Baerga. 2003. "Doing Justice for Mental Illness and Society: Federal Probation and Pretrial Services Officers as Mental Health Specialists." *Federal Probation* 67:13-19.

Smiley, Amy. 2001. "Forensic Mental Health in the United States – An Overview." Pp. 1-1-1-15 in *Forensic Mental Health: Working with Offenders with Mental Illness*, edited by G. Landsberg and A. Smiley. Kingston, NJ: Civic Research Institute.

Smith, Hal, Donald A. Sawyer and Bruce B. Way. 2002. "Central New York Psychiatric Center: An Approach to the Treatment of Co-Occurring Disorders in the New York State Correctional Mental Health System." *Behavioral Sciences and the Law* 20:523-534.

Springer, David W., C. Aaron McNeece and Elizabeth M.Arnold. 2003. *Substance Abuse Treatment for Criminal Offenders: An Evidence-Based Guide for Practitioners.* Washington, DC: American Psychological Association.

Stahl, Earl and Mary West. 2001. "Growing Population of Mentally Ill Offenders Redefines Correctional Facility Design." *Corrections Today* 63:72-74.

Steadman, Henry, J., Joseph J. Cocozza and Bonita M. Veysey. 1999. "Comparing Outcomes for Diverted and Nondiverted Jail Detainees with Mental Illnesses." *Law and Human Behavior* 23:615-627.

Steadman, Henry J., Martha Williams Deane, Randy Borum and Joseph P. Morrissey. "Comparing Outcomes of Major Models of Police Responses to Mental Health Emergencies." *Psychiatric Services* 51:645-649.

Steadman, Henry J., Martha Williams Deane, Joseph P. Morrissey, Mary L. Westcott, Susan Salasin and Steven Shapiro. 1999. "A SAMHSA Research Initiative Assessing the Effectiveness of Jail Diversion Programs for Mentally Ill Persons." *Psychiatric Services* 50:1620-1623.

Steadman, Henry J., Edward P. Mulvey, John Monahan, Pamela Clark Robbins, Paul S. Appelbaum, Thomas Grisso, Loren H. Roth and Eric Silver. 1998. "Violence by People Discharged From Acute Psychiatric Inpatient Facilities and by Others in the Same Neighborhoods." *Archives of General Psychiatry* 55:393-401.

Steadman, Henry J. and Michelle Naples. 2005. "Assessing the Effectiveness of Jail Diversion Programs for Persons with Serious Mental Illness and Co-Occurring Substance Use Disorders." *Behavioral Sciences and the Law* 23:163-170.

Steadman, Henry J., Allison D. Redlich, Patricia Griffin, John Petrila and John Monahan. "From Referral to Disposition: Case Processing in Seven Mental Health Courts." *Behavioral Sciences and the Law* 23:215-226.

Steadman, Henry J., Jack E. Scott, Fred Osher, Tara K. Agnese and Pamela Clark Robbins. 2005. "Validation of the Brief Jail Mental Health Screen." *Psychiatric Services* 56:816-822.

Steadman, Henry J., Kristin A. Stainbrook, Patricia Griffin, Jeffrey Draine, Randy Dupont and Cathy Horey. 2001. "A Specialized Crisis Response Site as a Core Element of Police-Based Diversion Programs." *Psychiatric Services* 52:219-222.

Steffan, Jarrod S. and Robert D. Morgan. 2005. "Meeting the Needs of Mentally Ill Offenders: Inmate Service Utilization." *Corrections Today* 67:38-41.

Substance Abuse and Mental Health Services Administration. 2005. SAMHSA's National Registry of Evidence-Based Programs and Practices (NREPP). (NREPP Overview, August 26). Washington, DC: SAMHSA. Retrieved January 30, 2006 (http://www.modelprograms.samhsa.gov).

Survey of Mental Health Courts. 2005. NAMI, National GAINS Center for People with Co-Occurring Disorders in the Criminal Justice System, TAPA Center for Jail Diversion, and Criminal Justice/Mental Health Consensus Project. Retrieved January 30, 2006 (http://www.mentalhealthcourtsurvey.com).

Tahir, Laura. 2003. "Supervision of Special Needs Inmates by Custody Staff." *Corrections Today* 65:108-111.

Taylor, Eulon Ross. 2001. "Using Algorithms and Protocols in Diagnosing and Treating Offenders with Mental Health Disorders." *Corrections Today* 63:80-83.

Teplin, Linda A. 2000. "Keeping the Peace: Police Discretion and Mentally Ill Persons." *National Institute Justice Journal* 9-23.

Theuma, Christine. 2001. "Community Mental Health Services for Offenders with Mental Disorders – Recent Innovations in the United States." Pp. 3-1-3-9 in *Forensic Mental Health: Working with Offenders with Mental Illness*, edited by G. Landsberg and A. Smiley. Kingston, NJ: Civic Research Institute.

Vitacco, Michael J. and Richard Rogers. 2005. "Assessment of Malingering in Correctional Settings." Pp. 133-153 in *Handbook of Correctional Mental Health*, edited by C. L. Scott and J. B. Gerbasi. Washington, DC: American Psychiatric Publishing, Inc.

Wang, Philip, Olga Demler and Ronald C. Kessler. 2002. "Adequacy of Treatment for Serious Mental Illness in the United States." *American Journal of Public Health* 92:92-98.

Weedon, Joey R. 2005. "The Incarceration of the Mentally Ill." *Corrections Today* 67:16-20.

Weisman, Robert L., J. S. Lamberti and N. Price. 2004. "Integrating Criminal Justice, Community Healthcare, and Support Services for Adults with Severe Mental Disorders." *Psychiatric Quarterly* 75:71-85.

White House. 2004. "Statement on the Second Chance Act 2004." (White House Press Release, June 23). Washington, DC: White House. Retrieved January 20, 2006 (http://www.whitehouse.gov/news/releases/2004).

White, Thomas W. and Elizabeth Gillespie. 2005. "Mental Health Programs: Addressing the Unfunded Mandate." *Corrections Today 67:108-115.*

Woody, George. 1996. "The Challenge of Dual Diagnosis." *Alcohol Health and Research World* 20:76-80.

Wooten, Harold B. and Herbert J. Hoelter. 1998. "Operation Spotlight: The Community Probation-Community Police Team Process." *Federal Probation.*

CHAPTER TEN

Gray Matters: Elderly Jail and Prison Inmates

Robynn Kuhlmann

In 2006, the first wave of baby boomers reached 60 years of age, and this aging population will place an economic strain on America's social systems. Some challenges this group will have to confront are health-related and quality-of-life issues such as housing, the rising cost of prescription medication, failure to plan for retirement, and an ailing Social Security system. Just as this population is growing, there is also an increase in America's aging correctional population - and this has been a focus of concern for researchers and policy analysts. Those over the age of 50 years are projected to form a growing proportion of the prison population (Neeley and Addison 1997). There were approximately 26,860 prisoners aged 55 years or older in 1991 (Gillard and Beck 1998). This number increased to 63,500 by year-end 2005 (Harrison and Beck 2006), which is indicative of a trend that is expected to continue.

Increased populations of the aged create a budget strain on correctional systems due to their health care needs (Adams 1995). The Texas Department of Criminal Justice, for example, reported a rapid growth in the number of elderly offenders admitted to prison (Fabelo 1999). New prison admissions for offenders aged 55 years and over in Texas increased 48.6 percent between 1994 and 1998 (Fabelo 1999). Washington's Department of Corrections reported in 1993 that inmates 50 and older made up 6.7 percent of their inmate population, but by 2004, this number had grown to 10.6 percent (Washington State Department of Corrections 2004).

Jail administrators have also noted an increase in the number of aged inmates. As a result of this type of growth, both county jail and state or federal prison systems have been struggling to find ways to modify their correctional programs to better respond to the needs of elderly prisoners. A recent budget analysis from the Legislative Analyst's Office (2003) highlights the economic challenges of providing health care to a large population of aging California prison inmates. Such findings underscore the importance of better understanding the characteristics of this growing population, the challenges they pose, and their special needs.

Research on this population often focuses on the challenges in treating, supervising, and paying the expense of housing and caring for elderly inmates (Aday 2003; Jones, Connelly, and Wagner 2001). Some research on elderly prisoners highlights the special needs of aging prisoners including health care costs (Anno et. al., 2004; Falter 1999; Marquart, Merianos, and Doucet 2000), the challenges of providing health programs within correctional systems (Aday 1994b; Booth 1989), and the effects of environmental and interpersonal stressors on the health of older prison inmates (Aday 2006; Williams et al. 2006). These studies highlight how elderly health care in prison systems is in urgent need of attention. It is important to understand the boundaries of this issue, and the implications of growing populations of elderly prisoners for correctional systems.

In addition to the special needs and increased costs of housing the aged in prison, the environmental conditions in prison may also exacerbate health problems. Research points out that aged inmates are viewed as being more likely to be victimized than their younger counterparts (Booth 1998; Kuhlmann and Ruddell 2005), which can increase personal stress, and decrease their ability to recover from illness. Such findings suggest that correctional systems should implement programs or special housing units that segregate these inmates. Further, these special housing units may be beneficial in reducing the need for security staff, as these inmates typically pose little risk of escape or misconduct.

Responding to the needs of elderly inmates such as special diets, medications, accessibility, health care, and segregated housing, creates a corresponding increase in correctional costs. It is no wonder, then, that health care costs for an elderly inmate are estimated to be three times higher than their younger counterpart (Adams 1995). In 1976 the United States Supreme court ruled that government officials must provide appropriate medical care for incarcerated populations (See *Estelle v. Gamble*). As a result, providing substandard health care is not a legal nor ethical option. Despite these rulings, however, health care is still the number one source of prisoner litigation (Schlanger, 2003).

Numerous programs have been created to meet this requirement. Subsequently, correctional administrators are increasingly adopting more comprehensive medical care programs, including special programs for elderly offenders. Compassionate release programs, separate housing units, and preventative health care programs are some of the best practices that corrections officials have introduced. The following pages outline our knowledge about aging offenders in American correctional systems.

Understanding Change: Why the Rapid Growth?

There are a number of reasons for the rapid increase in the elderly population behind bars. One often cited reason is the baby boom effect. The first wave of baby boomers born in 1946 recently turned 60 years of age. Just as this demographic group challenged schools and other public services a half-century ago, the effects of the baby boomers are still being felt in jails and prisons today. Adding to this, an increase in life expectancy is making their presence felt even more. Those who are currently approaching age 65 are expected to live an additional six to 18 years longer than those who were of the same age in 1940. Between 2002 and 2030 one in five individuals will be 65 years of age and older (U. S. Department of Health and Human Services 2004).

Hanser (2007) observes three different types of elderly prison inmates: 1) Habitual offenders who have led a lifetime of crime, 2) Inmates who have grown old in prison, and 3) First-time offenders. Interestingly, each type of offender may have different health needs, especially in terms of coping with the normal pains of imprisonment. Habitual offenders and those who have grown old in prison, for instance, are typically well aware of the expectations of the prison, are familiar with the rules and routines, and know how to cope with the deprivations in correctional environments. Typically either of these offender groups will have a greater need for health care services than first-time elderly prisoners, either from years of risky behaviors in the community, or long-term deprivation in prison.

First-time elderly prison inmates, by contrast, have often been convicted of violent offenses (Aday 2003). Because these prisoners have no experience with incarceration, and typically do not regard themselves as criminals, they have a greater problem with adjusting to prison life. In many cases, their violent offenses were directed at family members, which may increase their social isolation, as their relatives may be less likely to visit. Hanser (2007) observes that many of these offenders were probably maladjusted in society, have a poor ability to cope with environmental change, are likely to have a volatile personality, irascible, and often suicidal. Such behaviors may put this group at comparatively higher risk for victimization.

It is also feasible that "tough on crime" policies may have entangled some older Americans in criminal justice systems (Aday 2003). Because of these policies, prison inmates are often serving longer terms and are growing old in the correctional system. Lengthy prison sentences are due to mandatory-minimum sentences, three-strikes legislation, or truth-in-sentencing schemes that require inmates to serve 85 percent of their sentence before they are eligible for parole (Anno et al. 2004; Kempker 2003). A Washington State Department of Corrections (2004) report highlights the problem of prison overcrowding stemming from "tough on crime policies." It was reported that in 1993, 3.8 percent of the older offender population had been sentenced to 20 years or more, but by 2004 this percentage increased to 13.4 percent. Further, under three-strikes legislation, some states require offenders to serve mandatory sentences of 25 years to life (Jones and Newburn 2006). Offenders receiving their third-strike in their middle-ages will be spending their golden years in prison.

Defining the Elderly in Correctional Systems

There is a saying about aging: "You know you're getting old when your back goes out more than you do." Sadly, there is truth behind this observation. As we undergo the natural process of aging, it is inevitable that health problems will arise. The extent to which a person ages depends on a number of lifestyle choices and conditions. This factor is what makes defining who is considered to be "elderly" in the correctional system problematic, because many of those who end up in prison are likely to have lived unhealthy lifestyles (Aday 2003; Mara 2002; Marquart et al. 2000; Shimkus 2004).

To illustrate this point, the term elderly has been used to describe inmates 40 years and older in correctional research (Morton 1992). However, most correctional agencies use the age of 50 years as a baseline to define older or elderly offenders (see Aday 2003; Kuhlmann and Ruddell 2005; Morton 1992). Other scholars, government analysts, and correctional administrators, by contrast, have defined the older prison population as beginning at the age of 55 or 60 years (see Jones et al. 2001). Elderly persons who are repeat offenders are likely to have aged less gracefully than their community counterparts (Aday 2003; Mara 2002; Marquart et al. 2000; Shimkus 2004). As a result, the term elderly, when associated with correctional populations, is somewhat younger than Census Bureau definitions for elders in community populations.

Although the baseline age for the elderly prisoner is younger than their counterparts in the community, concerns about the health status of older inmates are similar to the chronic health issues that everybody undergoes as they age. A comprehensive review of the health status of elderly inmates reveals a range of serious health problems such as dementia, cancer, stroke, incontinence, arthritis, ulcers, hypertension, chronic respiratory ailments, chronic gastrointestinal problems, prostate problems, heart disease, and deteriorating kidney functions (Aday 2003; Anno et al. 2004; Booth 1998; Falter 1999; Marquart et al. 2000; Shimkus 2004). Overall physical ability is also expected to decrease as this geriatric population ages (Guralnik and Simonsick 1993).

While community and correctional populations of the elderly have similar health problems, poor lifestyles are probably what set these two groups apart. Offender populations are more likely to have more chronic illnesses due to lifestyle choices. Such illnesses are brought on by smoking, drug and alcohol addictions, homelessness, poor dietary habits, and risky behaviors (Marquart et al. 2000; Shimkus 2004). Conditions such as poverty and access to health care are also likely to hasten the aging process. Grecco (2004), for instance, reports that in the New York prison system, elderly inmates have an average of three chronic illnesses that require care.

Special Needs and Environmental Stressors

Due to the health problems that can occur as we age, many elderly inmates have special needs. Special diets are a common requirement for those suffering from chronic health conditions such as diabetes or heart disease. Further, many chronic health problems require medication. The National Commission on Correctional Health Care (NCCHC) reports that many inmates who have chronic diseases such as hypertension, diabetes, seizure disorder, asthma, and HIV are commonly under diagnosed (see Anno et al. 2004). This is problematic for both the health of the prisoner and the correctional system. If jails or prisons fail to assess and respond to inmate health concerns, then older prisoners have the potential to experience unnecessary suffering. Further, poor identification of health problems in prisoners might cost corrections more in the long run. Health problems that might require simple care could turn into more serious conditions if untreated. Preventative health care and health education may be positive approaches to cutting health care costs over the long term (Aday 2006).

It has been noted that the stress of incarceration accelerates the physical and mental deterioration of the elderly (Booth 1998). The process of going through trial, awaiting court dates, the financial costs of mounting a defense, and being sentenced to prison are stressful events (Aday 1994a; 1994b; Booth 1998). Aday (2006) observed that many elderly inmates fear dying in prison. Researchers point out how this stress contributes to physical and psychological reactions such as anxiety, nervousness, and hypertension, and these factors can aggravate existing health problems (Seymour and Black 2002).

Being incarcerated is a stressful event in the lives of most inmates. Correctional facilities are typically overcrowded, noisy, and chaotic places. Threats of violence, verbal abuse, and volatile surroundings are prevalent in prisons and jails (Tartaro 2005), and these conditions increase tension (Vega and Silvermann 1988). Due to these uncertain conditions, elderly inmates often report feelings of insecurity (Edgar and O'Donnell 1998). Being victimized while incarcerated is also a concern of older prisoners and many believe that their age places them at a higher risk (Aday 1994a; Marquart et al. 2000). Further, older prisoners might be less inclined to report abuse by younger inmates (Marquart et al. 2000). As a result, even though older inmates often seem serene, such adaptations are made in order to avoid projecting weakness (Gallagher 1990; Silverman and Vega 1990; Vega and Silvermann 1988).

Aday (2003) notes that elderly offenders admitted into a correctional facility for the first time often experience a great deal of stress. Late-life incarceration can lead to a kind of identity crisis, especially if they have "lived a majority of their lives as model citizens with no prior arrests" (Aday 2003:115). Further, psychological problems can develop from experiencing guilt and depression due to being incarcerated. The shame of conviction or being "found out" by family members of a hidden life of crime can cause an enormous psychological burden.

Although hiding weakness might be easy for some inmates, it is difficult for those who are suffering from visible health ailments. For example, a reduction in mobility can cause tension by hindering the ability to undertake basic tasks such as going to the bathroom or showering (Guralnik and Simonsick 1993). Older inmates who use wheelchairs or walkers—or have other assistive devices or prosthetic limbs—will often have a difficult time engaging in activities of daily living (ADLs) such as eating, bathing, and toileting (Anno et al. 2004). Taking part in ADLs might prove difficult if proper facilities are not available.

Accommodating elderly inmates who have physical or cognitive disabilities is a requirement of the Americans with Disabilities Act (ADA). The ADA stipulates that accommodations must be made for assisting persons with disabilities living within correctional facilities. Thus, correctional systems have a legal obligation to ensure that architectural barriers are removed and assistance be provided to inmates with special needs (e.g., hearing aids for elderly inmates). Correctional officers must also receive training to be sensitive to the needs of this group, their responsibility to comply with the ADA, and the legal consequences of non-compliance (Rubin and McCampbell 1995).

Booming Costs for Incarcerated Boomers: Policy and Programmatic Responses

Elderly inmates experience stress due to the normal aging process, their increased likelihood of victimization, and the inability (or unwillingness) of some correctional institutions to accommodate their medical needs. Over time, these stressors and lack of medical attention may contribute to decreases in physical functioning that requires increased health care, a significant concern for correctional administrators. Rising health care costs for inmates is a cause for concern, and has prompted correctional officials and legislators to reconsider sentence lengths, parole policies for geriatric inmates, and the types of health-related programs that are offered in corrections. In reaction to rising correctional costs, Connecticut, Louisiana, Mississippi, and North Dakota have revised mandatory and truth-in-sentencing policies (e.g., sentencing schemes that mandate fixed sentences for certain crimes or that offenders serve 85 percent of their sentence before being released).

A number of states are trying to form proactive policies to address the growing populations of aging inmates. Policy analysts in California have recommended that geriatric prisoners be released prior to the end of their sentences in order to save money (Legislative Analyst's Office 2003). Compassionate and pre-release options are possible solutions to this challenge. One variation of early release is a commutation process where a prisoner's eligibility for release on humanitarian or compassionate grounds is reviewed by the state governor. Upon review of the prisoner's circumstances, it is determined whether they can be released based on an evaluation of their medical condition, history within correctional institutions, and perceived risk to the community (Kempker 2003). Another potential option for early release is after they are determined to be terminally ill (typically within six months of their death) or if they are "incapable of physically functioning in the correctional system" (Aday 2003: 210). In 1997, a National Institute of Corrections survey found that 23 states had compassionate release policies. By 2001, however, this number jumped to 43 states (Criminal Justice Institute 2001).

The Washington Department of Corrections has an Extraordinary Medical Placement (EMP) program that has the authority to release inmates prior to the end of their sentence. To be considered for this program, inmates must either be severely ill, require high-cost care, or be of low-risk to the public. Under the EMP program between 1999 and 2003, it is estimated that of the 180 inmates whose cases were reviewed, 20 percent were released (Anderson and Hillard 2005). Although the EMP program is an example of reducing correctional health care costs, it is doubtful whether these policies will have any meaningful impact on prison overcrowding, and in most cases they simply transfer the health care costs to the community.

Prisoner Housing

The increase in the number of elderly prisoners has led to the introduction of health-promotion programs and other interventions designed to increase well-being. Some correctional systems provide separate housing facilities for older prisoners (Aday 2003; Anno et al. 2004; Legislative Analyst's Office 2003; Shimkus 2004), while others mainstream (place them within the general population) their elderly inmates. Taking into consideration the problems the aged might have in mainstream housing units (such as trouble with ADLs and a greater number of environmental stressors) this approach may have more pitfalls than benefits.

Four levels of housing for the older prisoner have been identified (Anderson and Hillard 2005). One is Environmental Support Housing (ESH). This program places geriatric inmates who do not need extensive help in conducting their ADL's in the general population. In some cases, modifications of correctional facilities are required, such as "grab-bars, ramps, and handicapped-accessible toilets, sink and bathing facilities" (Anderson and Hillard 2005: 60). Such features undoubtedly relieve much of the stress that older inmates might have while living in mainstream housing.

Another level is referred to as Assisted Living Housing (ALH). ALH is identified for elderly inmates who can still engage in ADL's but require some assistance. Non-medical personnel or volunteers can aide these inmates since they require little medical knowledge.

Extended Care Housing, by contrast, is for inmates who require greater access to licensed medical staff due to their health-related problems. Examples of inmates who might live in these units are those who are "terminally ill or need ongoing care for chronic diseases, including Alzheimer's, or are in rehabilitation after a stroke or injury" (Anderson and Hillard 2005: 60). The highest level of housing is infirmary care, and is intended for inmates who require 24-hour medical care.

Specialized housing and better classification of older inmates are two ways to manage the special needs of this population. Building separate housing units can be expensive. Some state prison systems are too small to care for many elderly inmates. As a result, geriatric inmates who need special housing are chosen from a pool of their contemporaries and placed in low-risk settings (Kempker 2003). In South Carolina, for instance, the state prison system has modified several tuberculosis treatment centers into geriatric inmate facilities (Morton 1992; Aday 1994b; 2003). While some require placement in a nursing home (Anno et al. 2004) or a secondary level housing environment (Anderson and Hillard 2005), it is argued that others must be placed in specialized housing units due to their risk of victimization (Marquart et al. 2000; Edgar and O'Donnell 1998).

However, opposing views question the benefits of specialized housing for elderly inmates who appear to be in good health (Strupp and Willmott 2005). Hanser (2007) found that some correctional administrators advocate mixing elderly inmates with the general population because they have a calming effect on the other prisoners. Separating older inmates from the general population may cause some elderly inmates to experience feelings of social isolation, which can be detrimental to their psychological well-being (Marquart et al. 2000). As a result, correctional administrators in conjunction with medical staff should carefully consider the costs and benefits of both approaches to managing this special needs population.

In some states, correctional facilities or systems offer placement choices to elderly inmates. The Minnesota Department of Corrections (MDC), for example, gives inmates over the age of 55 years a choice as to whether they want to live in the general population or be placed with their contemporaries and younger inmates with disabilities (Anno et al. 2004). However, these inmates must be able to engage in ADLs, otherwise they are transferred to an infirmary unit. Those deemed elderly by administrators at MDC have their own dining and recreational areas. MDC also provides senior dormitories, where older offenders are assigned to a specialized housing unit.

Elderly Inmates in Jails: Issues and Health Services

While most correctional research has focused on the elderly population residing within prisons, local jails must also deal with the crisis of housing geriatric offenders. Because of the short-term nature of jail incarceration, however, research about elderly jail inmates has not been a priority, and this makes it difficult to assess the boundaries of this problem. Elderly jail inmates are perceived by jail administrators as vulnerable to the same individual and environmental stressors as their counterparts in prison (Kuhlmann and Ruddell 2005). Further, populations in jail tend to be transitory and these facilities tend to be more unpredictable and risky for inmates (see Tartaro, 2002).

Much of the health-related jail research that exists focuses on the subject of controlling infectious diseases and blood borne pathogens (CDC 2001; 2005; Potter and Rapposelli 2002; Roberts et al. 2003). The jail environment has a constant ebb and flow of inmates, and has a very short-term orientation (in California the average stay is approximately 20 days, but many inmates make bail after just a day or two) and as a result health issues are rarely a priority (Roberts et al. 2003). Thus older inmates who have suppressed immune systems or frail health may be more vulnerable to communicable diseases in this environment. Finding such problems has led to the introduction of jail-based health-promotion programs and other public health interventions (Potter and Ropposelli 2002). But providing separate housing facilities for older prisoners is not practical in small jails (Aday 2003; Anno et al. 2004), especially if they hold only two or three elderly inmates.

Some larger jails have hospital units that are able to provide specialized care for inmates with serious and chronic illnesses. For instance, most mid-sized jails have regular health care programs which provide inmates with regular access to physicians. Unfortunately, not all jails have such facilities. Few specialists will provide in-jail services, and transporting offenders to appointments in the community is expensive and places both the offender and officer at some risk. As a result, programs such as "telemedicine" enable physicians and other health care providers to treat inmates using videoconferencing (Fallon 2007; Jones et al. 2001). In other jails, health practitioners have counseled elderly inmates about chronic health conditions, such as diabetes and prevention of communicable diseases (National Institute of Corrections 2003).

Despite the fact that their average stay in many jurisdictions is two to three weeks, it is important to screen jail inmates for health ailments and communicable diseases. Prompt medical assessments deter outbreaks of communicable diseases, guide preventative health care measures, and help control correctional health care costs, especially given that these inmates are at higher risk than community populations (CDC 2005; Potter and Rapposelli 2002; Roberts et al. 2003). Since most jail inmates return to their communities, inadequate screening methods for communicable diseases are a public health challenge. Thus, it is a good strategy for jail administrators to work in conjunction with local public health care agencies.

Special Programs for the Elderly Prison Inmate

Recently, there has been increased interest in programs that provide psychological and emotional support for elderly prisoners. Such prison-based interventions include designating different meal-times for the elderly, as well as offering programs such as; enhanced library services, chess, art classes, senior social "rap" groups, reminiscent therapy, horticulture, and work programs (Anno et al. 2004; Grecco 2004; Mara 2003; National Institute of Corrections 1997). Aged inmates who are socially isolated, have interpersonal problems, or require transitional assistance because they are new to corrections gain the most benefits from their involvement in these special programs (Aday 2003; Loeb and Steffensmeier 2006).

The process of aging—whether in corrections or the community—can bring about feelings of low self-worth, an increased fear of dying, social isolation, and a creeping loss of independence (Aday 2006; Morton 1992). This is a common process that people all experience as they age (Fried et al. 2004). Thus, most elderly inmates can benefit from the interactive activities that these special programs can provide. Work programs can also help aging inmates maintain a sense of independence and self-worth. Since there is a natural decline in mobility (Guralnik and Simonsick 1993), work could help the elderly prisoner focus on activities they can perform.

Participation in supportive or reminiscing groups, recreational programs, and volunteer groups reduce depression and anxiety (Aday 2003; McGarland 2005; Neely and Addison 1997). Incarceration is a stressful experience and support groups enable inmates to express emotions that would not normally be addressed in the prison environment. Listening to guest speakers, engaging in writing therapy, and participating in supportive groups can alleviate health ailments exacerbated by the stress of imprisonment. Further, reminiscing groups that involve reviewing life events can bring about a sense of accomplishment for the elderly inmate. Reminiscing about past life experiences can jog a sense of self-worth that is often lost while living in corrections.

Some prisons provide elderly inmates with opportunities for volunteer work (Anno et al. 2004). Activities such as repairing toys for children reinforce a sense of self-worth, psychological well-being, and recognition of their special skills. Engaging in recreational activities also benefits physical and psychological well-being. Also, leisure activities such as ping-pong or shuffleboard, for example, can provide a positive outlet for stress, enhance self-esteem, and foster new interests (Carter and Russell 2005). Altogether, much can be gained by offering these low-cost interventions to elderly prisoners.

An Overview of Best Practices

Participation in supportive groups, recreational programs, and voluntary activities help reduce depression and increase both life satisfaction and self-esteem (Aday 2003; Anno et al. 2004; Carter and Russell 2005; McFarland 2005). The programs that show the most promise for health promotion are activities that intertwine segregated housing and specialized programs for elderly inmates.

The following programs illustrate the best use of health care practices for America's aging correctional population:

*Minnesota***.** The Minnesota correctional system (MDC) has both compassionate and early-release planning (Aday 2003; Anno et al. 2004). Those policies could help reduce overcrowding and correctional health care costs (Kempker 2003; Legislative Analyst's Office 2003). Minnesota also provides special housing for its elderly inmates. The MDC offers a Senior Dormitory that houses those aged 50 years and over. These residents are self-sufficient but if there is a need for special medical attention they are assigned to a special health care unit. This dormitory also allows its older inmates to go to meal-times before other inmates, which is an effective way to reduce stress (Morton 1992). Devices that help inmates engage in ADL's such as walkers, hearing aids, and eyeglasses are provided. Warmer clothing and extra blankets are also given to the older inmate. Further, older inmates receive enhanced health appraisals (Anno et al. 2004). MDC also provides special work assignments for the elderly (Aday 2003; Morton 1992), but does not offer recreational programs that are specially designed for their elderly (Anno et al. 2004).

North Carolina. North Carolina is considered a leader in developing integrative housing and special programs for elderly prisoners (Aday 2003; Kempker 2003). McCain Correctional Hospital, for example, serves minium-security inmates with special health care needs. Devices that help inmates engage in ADLs such as walkers, hearing aids, and eyeglasses are provided. Warmer clothing and extra blankets are also given to these prisoners. Twenty-four hour medical care is available as well as physical therapy, nursing care, a laboratory, and an x-ray machine for those who need prompt assessments. Providing these services "in house" lowers the cost (and risk) of transporting inmates to local hospitals. Further, at the McCain Correctional Hospital, reminiscent therapy, support groups, and recreational activities such as horseshoes, ceramics, a walking program, and gardening are also offered to elderly inmates.

Ohio. The Ohio Department of Aging provides support to the Correctional Training Academy to train staff in recognizing the needs of aging inmates. These measures are intended to assist with accommodating special needs, enhancing preventative health care, and assigning correctional officers who are more sensitive to the needs of these prisoners. Ohio prisoners undergo comprehensive annual health appraisals at the age of 40 years (Anno et al. 2004). The state correctional department also provides segregated housing for geriatric inmates in the medium-security Hocking Correctional Facility. Educational programs such as general equivalency diploma (GED) and college-level courses are offered in this facility (Aday 2003). Work programs such as the Blue Bird Project—whereby inmates construct bird houses—are other activities that promote the constructive use of time. Other Ohio prisons also offer recreational competitions based on age groups and include team sports (Aday 2003). Further, the state of Ohio also has a medical parole policy that allows releases of inmates with a life expectancy of six months or less (Anno et al. 2004).

Assessing the Aging Prisoner Crisis

Understanding how and to what extent America's correctional system has responded to the aging prison population is critical for policy makers and correctional administrators to create effective responses to these challenges. A range of health problems affect the elderly prisoner (Aday 2003; Anno et al. 2004; Booth 1998; Falter 1999; Gallahger 1990; Marquart et al. 2000; Shimkus 2004) and the NCCHC reports that many inmates who have chronic diseases are commonly under-diagnosed in correctional institutions (see Anno et al. 2004). As a result all correctional systems must adopt comprehensive medical evaluations for elderly prisoners. While this approach typically takes place in larger correctional systems, county jails have been slow to respond to this need.

If prisons and jails lack information systems that track inmate health, then older prisoners can experience undue suffering, as a result of "falling through the cracks." Poor identification of health problems, and inadequate responses in prison populations might have a significant long-term cost. Some health problems that might require simple treatment could, over time, turn into chronic conditions. Preventative health care should be a way to reduce medical costs for all inmates. The most significant challenges facing corrections system include: management and housing of inmates with special needs; special accommodations; updating or retrofitting antiquated facilities; offering programs for elderly inmates; a comprehensive plan to contain costs in providing for geriatric prisoners; liberal compassionate release policies; and training correctional staff to respond to the health needs of the aging correctional population (Anno et al 2004).

Implementation of a comprehensive correctional health policy towards elderly inmates should be holistic in nature, and include housing needs, special programs (such as recreation and support groups), programs that track prisoner health, as well as the acknowledgment that elderly inmates are vulnerable to victimization. Moreover, programs for the elderly should also acknowledge the special needs of female prisoners (see Williams et al. 2006). Last, Collins and Bird (2007) suggest that prison systems retain geriatricians to provide specialized input and coordinate services.

A recent report about the conditions many geriatric inmates face in California prisons provides information that is disconcerting (Strupp and Willmott 2005). For example, attention to simple details such as assigning the elderly inmate to a lower bunk bed is an important element of preventing injuries, but these factors are sometimes overlooked (Strupp and Willmott 2005). Crawley (2005) has called these oversights as "institutional thoughtlessness" in the care of the elderly prisoners. Administrators and correctional officers sometimes forget that these inmates are frail and less coordinated than their younger counterparts. For example, work programs that can be used to stave off depression are counterproductive if the geriatric inmate experiences physical duress. There are reports, for instance, that some elderly California prisoners have been assigned to work outdoors in hot weather (Strupp and Willmott 2005; see also Williams et al. 2006).

It is apparent that alternatives to prison and jail confinement for elderly inmates should also be considered whenever practical, and when it is consistent with public safety. Home detention programs—such as ones introduced in Illinois—decrease the housing costs of inmates. Moreover, early medical release programs are also viable alternatives to incarceration in some cases (Lundstrom 1994). Annual conferences of correctional health organizations, such as the NCCHC, the American Correctional Association, and American Correctional Health Services Association that specifically address the problems associated with aging prisoners are also effective ways to disseminate "best practices." Forum topics that involve the logistics, housing options, and special programs for elderly inmates can create an open line of communication between medical care administrators from different jurisdictions. Attendance at such meetings and reviews of current programs may be instrumental in maximizing the resources of correctional facilities and minimizing the problems that come along with the aging inmate population.

References

Adams, William E. 1995. "The Incarceration of Older Criminals: Balancing Safety, Cost, and Humanitarian Concerns." *Nova Law Review* 19:465-486.

Aday, Ronald H. 1994a. "Golden Years Behind Bars: Special Programs and Facilities for Elderly Inmates." *Federal Probation* 58:47-55.

------. 1994b. "Aging in Prison: A Case Study of New Elderly Offenders." *International Journal of Offender Therapy and Comparative Criminology* 38:79-91.

------. 2003. *Aging Prisoners: Crisis in American Corrections.* Praeger: Westport CT.

------. 2006. "Aging Prisoners' Concerns Toward Dying in Prison." *OMEGA* 52: 199-216.

Anderson Elizabeth and Theresa Hillard. 2005. "Managing Offenders with Special Health Needs: Highest and Best Use of Strategies." *Corrections Today* 67:50-61.

Anno, Jaye B., Camelia Graham, James E. Lawrence, and Ronald Shansky. 2004. *Correctional Health Care: Assessing the Needs of Elderly, Chronically Ill, and Terminally Ill Inmates.* Longmont, CO: National Institute of Corrections.

Beck, John A. 1999. "Compassionate Release from New York State Prisons: Why re so Few Getting Out?" *Journal of Law, Medicine, & Ethics* 27:216-233.

Booth, Dorothy E. 1989. "Health Status of the Incarcerated Elderly: Issues and Concerns." *Journal of Offender Counseling Services and Rehabilitation* 13:193-213.

Carter, Marcia J. and Kelly J. Russell. 2005. "What is the Perceived Worth of Recreation? Results from a County Jail Study." *Corrections Today* 67: 80-91.

Centers for Disease Control and Prevention. 2001. *Drug Use, HIV, and the Criminal Justice System.* Atlanta: Centers for Disease Control and Prevention.

------. 2005. The Status of TB Prevention and Control Measures in Large City and County Jails in the U.S. Atlanta: Centers for Disease Control and Prevention. Retrieved April 17, 2007 (http://www.cdc.gov).

Collins, D. Ronan and Rachael Bird. 2007. "The Penitentiary Visit – A New Role for Geriatricians?" *Age and Ageing* 36: 11-13.

Conklin, Thomas, Thomas Lincoln, Rachel Wilson, and Gail Gramarossa. 2002. *A Public Health Manual for Correctional Health Care.* Ludlow, MA: Hampden County Sheriff's Department.

Crawley, Elaine. 2005. "Institutional Thoughtlessness in Prisons and its Impact on the Day-to-Day Lives of Elderly Men." *Journal of Contemporary Criminal Justice* 21: 350-363.

Criminal Justice Institute. 2001. *Managing the Needs of Aging Inmates with Chronic and Terminal Illnesses.* Middletown, CT: Criminal Justice Institute.

Edgar, Kimmett and Ian O'Donnell. 1998. "Assault in Prison: The 'Victim's' Contribution." *The British Journal of Criminology,* 38:635-650.

Ditton, Paula M. and James Wilson. 1999. *Truth in Sentencing in State Prisons.* Washington, DC: Bureau of Justice Statistics.

Estelle V. Gamble, 429 US (97), 1976

Fabelo, Tony. 1999. *Elderly Offenders in Texas Prisons.* Austin, TX: Criminal Justice Policy Council.

Fallon, Paul V. 2007. "Introducing Telemedicine to English Prisons." *International Journal of Prisoner Health* 3: 77-78.

Falter, Robert G. 1999. "Selected Predictors of Health Services Needs of Inmates

Over Age 50." *Journal of Correctional Health Care* 6: 149-75.

Fried, Linda P., Luigi Ferrucci, Jonathan Darer, Jeff D. Williamson, and Gerard Anderson. 2004. "Untangling the Concepts of Disability, Frailty, and Comorbidity: Implications for Improved Targeting and Care." *Journal of Gerontology* 59:255-263.

Gallagher, Elaine M. 1990. "Emotional, Social, and Physical Health Characteristics of Older Men in Prison." *International Journal of Aging and Human Development* 31:251-265.

Gillard, Darrell K. and Allen J. Beck. 1998. Prisoners in 1997. Washington, DC: Bureau of Justice Statistics.

Grecco, Rozann. 2004. *The Future of Aging in New York States Brief: Older Prisoners. New York State Department of Correctional Services Project 2015:* New York. Retrieved November 21, 2005 (http://www.nysofaelderly.org).

Guralnik, Jack M. and Eleanor M. Simonsick. 1993. "Physical Disability in Older Americans." *The Journals of Gerontology* 48:3-10.

Hanser, Robert D. 2007. *Special Needs Offenders in the Community.* Upper Saddle River, NJ: Pearson.

Harrison, Paige M. and Allen J. Beck. 2006. *Prisoners in 2005.* Washington, DC: Bureau of Justice Statistics.

Jones, Greg, Michael Connelly, and Kate Wagner. 2001. *Aging Offenders and the Criminal Justice System.* Baltimore, MD: State Commission on Criminal Sentencing Policy, Maryland.

Jones, Trevor and Tim Newburn. 2006. "Three Strikes and You Are Out: Exploring Symbol and Substance in American and British Crime Control Policies." *British Journal of Criminology* 46: 781-802.

Kempker, Erica. 2003. "Graying of American Prisons: Addressing the Continued Increase in Geriatric Inmates." *Corrections Compendium* 28:22-26.

Kuhlmann, Robynn and Rick Ruddell. 2005. "Elderly Jail Inmates: Problems, Prevalence and Public Health." *Californian Journal of Health Promotion* 3(2):49-60.

Legislative Analyst's Office. 2003. Analysis of the 2003-04 Budget: Judiciary and Criminal Justice. Sacramento: Legislative Analyst's Office.

Loeb, Susan J. and Darrell Steffensmeier. 2006. "Older Male Prisoners: Health Status, Self-Efficacy Beliefs, and Health-Promoting Behaviors." *Journal of Correctional Health Care* 12: 269-278.

Long, Lydia M. 1992. "A Study of Arrests of Older Offenders: Trends and Patterns." *Journal of Crime and Justice* 15:157-175.

Lundstrom, Susan. 1994. "Dying to Get Out: A Study on the Necessity, Importance, and Effectiveness of Prison Early Release Programs for Elderly Inmates Suffering from HIV Disease and Other Terminal-centered Illnesses." *BYU Journal of Public Law* 8:155-189.

Mara, Cynthia M. 2002. "Expansion of Long-term Care in the Prison System: An Aging Inmate Population Poses Policy and Programmatic Questions." *Journal of Aging & Social Policy* 14:43-91.

Marquart, James. W., Dorothy E. Merianos and Geri Doucet. 2000. "The Health Related Concerns of Older Prisoners: Implications for Policy." *Aging and Society* 20:79-96.

McFarland, Kay. 2005. "Short Term Psychotherapy for Depression in Older Adults—A Review of Evidence-Based Studies Since 2000." *Annals of the Ameri-*

can Psychotherapy Association Winter: 20-27.

Morton, Joann B. 1992. *An Administrative Overview of the Older Inmate.* Washington, DC: US Department of Justice.

National Institute of Corrections. 1997. *Prison Medical Care: Special Needs Populations and Cost Control.* Longmont, CO. National Institute of Corrections.

------. 2003. *Corrections Agency Collaborations with Public Health.* Longmont, CO: National Institute of Corrections.

Neely, Connie L. and Laura Addison. 1997. "Addressing the Needs of Elderly Offenders." *Corrections Today* 59:120-124.

Potter, Roberto H. and Karina Krane Rapposelli. 2002. "Large Jails and Communicable Disease: An Update on Why Public Health Must Go to Jail." *Large Jail Network Exchange* 25-28.

Roberts, Cheryl A., Mark N. Lobato, Lauri B. Bazerman, and Theodore M. Hammett. 2003. The Status of Tuberculosis Prevention and Control Measures in Large Cityand County Jails in the United States. Division of Tuberculosis Elimination, National Center for HIV, STD, and TB Prevention.

Rubin, Paula N. and Susan W. McCampbell. 1995. *The Americans With Disabilities Act and Criminal Justice: Mental Disabilities and Corrections.* Washington, DC: National Institute of Justice.

Seymour, Deborah H. and Kristen Black. 2002. "Stress in Primary Care Patients." Pp. 65-87 in *Twenty Common Problems in Behavioral Health,* edited by F. V. deGruy III et al. New York: McGraw-Hill.

Shimkus, Jaime. 2004. "Corrections Copes With Care for the Aged." *Correct Care* 18:1-2.

Silverman, Mitchell and Manuel Vega. 1990. "Reactions of Prisoners to Stress as a Function of Personality and Demographic Variables." *International Journal of Offender Therapy and Comparative Criminology* 34:187-195.

Strupp, Heidi and Donna Willmott. 2005. *Dignity Denied: The Price of Imprisoning Older Women in California.* Legal Services for Prisoners with Children: San Francisco.

Tartaro, Christine. 2002. "The Impact of Density on Jail Violence." *Journal of Criminal Justice* 30:499-510.

------. 2005. Suicide in Jails and Prisons. Pp. 72-85 in *Key Correctional Issues,* edited by R. Muraskin. Upper Saddle River, NJ: Pearson.

Vega, Manuel and Mitchell Silvermann. 1988. "Stress and the Elderly Convict." *International Journal of Offender Therapy and Comparative Criminology* 32:153-161.

Walsh, Eamon C. 1992. "Aging Inmate Offenders: Another Perspective." *Correctional Theory and Practice.* Chicago, IL: Nelson-Hall.

Washington State Department of Corrections. 2004. *Older Offender Briefing Paper.* Retrieved April 17, 2007 (http://www.doc.wa.gov/budget/).

Williams, Brie A., Karla Lindquist, Rebecca L. Sudore, Heide M. Strupp, Donna J. Wilmott and Louise C. Walter. 2006. "Being Old and Doing Time: Functional Impairment and Adverse Experiences of Geriatric Female Prisoners." *Journal of the American Geriatrics Society* 54: 702-707.

CHAPTER ELEVEN

Hospice and Palliative Care Behind Bars

John F. Linder

Despite the fact that the United States has the highest rate of imprisonment in the world, jail and prison populations continue to grow. There are now some 2.3 million incarcerated Americans (Harrison and Beck 2006). The unprecedented growth in correctional populations has created a number of compelling long-term health related challenges: the average inmate age is increasing, there are a large number of prisoners who are terminally ill or suffer from chronic diseases, and 3,138 state prisoners died behind bars in 2004 (Mumola 2007).

Aging inmates experience health concerns typical of the community population. Conversely, inmates have higher incidence of health complications associated with their risk behaviors, impoverished lifestyles, and a lack of community health care or access to it. Life in prison also poses challenges including prison violence, incarceration-related constraints on exercise, poor diets, and health care that is often found to be lacking. Inmates are more likely to have a history of alcohol or drug abuse or addiction and sex industry work. Risk-behavior conditions include HIV/AIDS, hepatitis B and C, liver disease, tuberculosis, endocarditis and cardiomyopathy. Other prisoners have chronic care conditions such as diabetes that have to be managed throughout the inmate's term of imprisonment, and are associated with a decreased life expectancy.

Although prison inmates have not traditionally elicited much public sympathy, during the 1980s and early 1990s, increasing numbers of deaths from AIDS attracted intense public scrutiny. Spotlighting deficiencies in end-of-life care for incarcerated populations, legal decisions have repeatedly affirmed prisoners' right to quality health care by explicitly prohibiting deliberate indifference while mandating "a medical care system that meets minimal standards of adequacy." This has been generally defined as care equal to community standards. Litigation over the delivery of health care, for instance, is the number one source of lawsuits in large jails and prisons (Schlanger, 2003).

Due in large part to the introduction of new medications, AIDS deaths have declined sharply since 1996 in both the free population and within correctional facilities. Mumola (2007) outlines how AIDS-related deaths within prison spiked in 1995, and have decreased since then.

The overall rate of deaths from natural causes during incarceration is steadily rising, however, and will continue to do so for the next 20-25 years given the increasing aging population. This chapter examines how jails and prison systems can best respond to the reality of deaths from natural causes in prisons.

Hospice is increasingly the preferred response to the health and care needs of terminally-ill prison inmates. Perhaps the best definition is that hospice is a philosophy and sometimes a physical place where care is delivered in a manner that increases the patient's ability to die with increased levels of support, care, compassion and dignity. The goal of medical care in these settings is palliation. Palliative health care strives to reduce the symptoms and suffering of terminal illness rather than providing a cure or delivering disease-directed therapy. According to Anno et al. (2004:36) such care involves:

> Keeping the patient comfortable and pain free, and also helping the inmate adjust to imminent death. Because terminally ill individuals may experience increased anger and depression and are at increased risk of suicide, the involvement of clergy, mental health professionals, and others who can offer supportive counseling is essential.

Implementing palliative care in a correctional setting has some unique challenges in addition to those inherent in hospice work.

Background and Extent of the Problem

State and federal prison systems are experiencing significant, sustained growth. Concurrently, the number of inmate deaths per year, the percentage of deaths from natural causes excluding AIDS, and the average prisoner age on entry into prison all show long-term increases. These demographic trends suggest that the prison population is "graying." The health concerns of older adults, including coping with chronic, degenerative or terminal illnesses, are also a source of growing concern for departments of corrections and public safety nationwide.

At year-end 2005, for instance, there were over 253,000 inmates aged 45 years and above (Harrison and Beck 2005) and many of these prisoners are serving lengthy sentences. Sentencing legislation such as "three strikes" has made longer sentences for repeat offenders more common. Approximately 22 percent of all prison inmates were serving sentences of 20 years or more (including life sentences) between 1989 and 1999 (see Bureau of Justice Statistics 2000). Extrapolating this to the entire U.S. prison population in 2004 would suggest that there are some 294,000 inmates serving these lengthy sentences. In addition, there are some 3,254 prisoners sentenced to death at year-end, and many will die on death row before their sentence is carried out (Snell 2006).

The average age of inmates at the time of admission to prison has grown in six of the eight year-to-year periods between 1990 and 1998. During that time, the average age at admission grew from 29.9 to 31.5 years (Bureau of Justice Statistics 2000). Moreover, the average age of jail inmates seems to parallel the prison population (Kuhlmann and Ruddell 2005). Along with an aging correctional population, the total number of deaths in prison is also on the rise. In 1987, for instance, 1,407 inmates died in U. S. prisons. By 2004, that number had risen to 3,138 for state prisoners alone, an increase of more than 100 percent. During that period, the high water mark for deaths per year occurred in 1995, when 3,345 inmates died in custody. The introduction of new antiretroviral medications in 1996 temporarily adjusted deaths per year downward. However, the steady year-over-year increases from non-HIV causes have continued uninterrupted.

Cause of death is an important consideration when examining these numbers. Aging by itself brings an increased incidence of death, in prison and in the general population. Reduction in prison mortality can result from successful violence reduction interventions and suicide prevention. However, a number of other risk factors increase the likelihood of death from natural causes in inmate populations.

A significant overlap exists between the populations at greatest risk of long-term incarceration and many groups at elevated risk of HIV infection, tuberculosis, hepatitis B and C and other liver diseases, as well as other chronic or life-threatening conditions. AIDS and hepatitis B, and C, disproportionately affect persons with substance-abuse histories, particularly injection drug users. One third of state and federal inmates participate in drug-treatment programs; a considerably larger number report substance use or abuse (Smyer, Gragert, and LaMere 1997). Sex-industry workers of both genders are more likely to be incarcerated and are at elevated risk of HIV seropositivity; many also have a history of substance abuse. Men who have sex with men are at elevated risk, whether that risk behavior is a result of sexual preference or environmental circumstance. Prison rape, for instance, not only has long-term physical and psychological effects, but has also been associated with the transmission of HIV/AIDS (McGuire 2005). Finally, women and men of color are disproportionately over-represented in the incarcerated population and the HIV population (Hightow-Weidman and Smith 2007; Jacob Arriola, Braithwaite and Newkirk 2006). Some populations of men and women of color are also at elevated risk of diabetes and hypertension when compared to the general population.

Improvements in AIDS treatment have significantly slowed both disease progression and mortality in community and correctional populations. However, AIDS remains an incurable, life-limiting health condition. AIDS treatment is costly, adherence (inside and outside the prisons) is problematic and the outcome of even the most successful treatment regimens remains uncertain. Clearly the new therapies, and particularly the introduction of the protease inhibitor class of antiretrovirals has had an effect nationwide. Their use in combination with other antiretroviral agents in HAART (Highly Active AntiRetroviral Therapy) has sharply reduced AIDS deaths in the free community and in prisons as well (Marushak 2006; Mumula 2007).

Prison deaths from other "natural causes" (excluding AIDS, suicide, homicide and execution) are also on the rise. A recent study by the U.S. Bureau of Justice Statistics revealed that deaths from natural causes dropped significantly in jails, but actually increased in prisons between 1980 and 2002 (Mumola 2005). It is with these inmate deaths that the provision of palliative or hospice care can have a significant impact on prison health services.

Prisoner Rights and Penal Health Care

Society's sentiment notwithstanding, the right of prisoners to quality health care has been addressed and affirmed repeatedly by the courts (Kay 1999). Two court rulings which have spoken clearly on this issue have held that incarceration—separation from family, community, and society—is the punishment, not poor health care. In *Estelle v. Gamble*, the U.S. Supreme Court found that the Eighth Amendment "establishes the government's obligation to provide medical care for those whom it is punishing by incarceration..." The Court concluded that "deliberate indifference to serious medical needs of prisoners constitutes the 'unnecessary and wanton infliction of pain'...proscribed by the Eighth Amendment."

In *Wellman v. Faulkner*, the Court concluded that a prison or jail must provide "a medical care system that meets minimal standards of adequacy." Though this term is not further defined, in general, correctional institutions have established the policy of measuring adequacy by requiring that correctional health care be equal to community standards. As Murphy (2005) observed, poor correctional health care due to indifference, apathy, inconvenience or claims of insufficient funds should not turn a period of incarceration into a death sentence.

"Community standards" have not been clearly defined by the courts, however, with respect to end-of-life or palliative care, the concept of community standards may not be the best measure to use, as decades of research suggest that the medical community does a less-than-adequate job of providing care to the dying (Byock 1997; Freeborne 2000). The Supreme Court did not intend to give correctional facilities license to perpetuate inadequate care by replicating substandard community practice. Anecdotal accounts suggest that many prisoners fear dying in prison chained to a bed and surrounded by indifferent correctional officers (Aday 2006). While prison inmates have committed crimes against their communities, they still deserve the opportunity to die with as much dignity as the state can provide. As Dostoevsky once observed, "The degree of civilization in a society can be judged by entering its prisons." Perhaps American corrections can also be evaluated by the treatment of our dying prisoners.

While ad hoc end-of-life care is not reliably of high quality, an established model of good end-of-life care does exist: the hospice movement. Issues addressed in this chapter are an examination of the types of hospice care that are delivered, and the characteristics of good community programs. Further, it is important to examine how prison systems have imported hospice and palliative care into their health care services, and the challenges of creating such units. Are there, for instance, jail or prison hospice programs that deliver quality care that do not compromise the safety and security of the facility or the community, and that are delivered in a cost-effective manner? In addition, are compassionate release programs an effective way to support dying inmates and their families? Perhaps these "best practices" might be imported into jail or prison systems to provide effective "end of life" treatment.

Hospice as the Standard of Care for the Terminally Ill

For more than three decades, hospice programs in the United States have provided services that constitute the best standard against which to measure the quality of care provided to the dying, in or out of prison. In 1979 Medicare initiated a number of hospice pilot projects nationwide. Incorporation of hospice into the Medicare entitlement structure through adoption of the "Hospice Medicare Benefit" in 1982 further cemented hospice's position as the standard. Medicare's "conditions of participation" delineate the required components of care for a certified hospice program. State practice guidelines and licensure standards, modeled closely on Medicare's conditions of participation, contribute to a high degree of uniformity of services in hospice programs nationwide. Guidelines and standards of care publicized by organizations like the National Hospice and Palliative Care Organization have set forth and refined the structure of hospice. The requirements necessary to qualify for reimbursement from federal and state funding agencies also drives greater homogeneity of services. Very few hospices remain in the United States that are financially independent. Codes and standards of professional organizations also lend support to the practice of hospice care (National Association of Social Workers 2007).

The hospice movement, as a modern incarnation, has been around for just under forty years. Dame Cecily Saunders is considered the founder of the modern hospice movement. Under her tutelage, St. Christopher's hospice, the first facility of its kind, opened its doors in Great Britain in 1967 (St. Christopher's Hospice 2006). The first hospice in the United States opened its doors seven years later in New Haven/Branford, CT. (Continuum Care Hospice 2006). In 2004, the latest year for which data are available, 3,650 hospice programs provided care to one million and sixty thousand patients in the United States (National Hospice and Palliative Care Organization 2006). In the United States, nearly 96 percent of all care is provided to persons in their homes. This is different than the British model, where most care is still provided in hospice residences.

The hospice model in the United States provides services to patients and caregivers in their home. The services provided are spelled out in Medicare's conditions of participation: hospices must provide nursing, social work, chaplaincy, bereavement and volunteer services to the home, using a broadly-defined concept of "family" as the unit of care. Hospice also provides prescription medications related to the terminal condition and necessary durable medical equipment like hospital beds, bedside commodes and oxygen. Many hospices also provide some level of bath or attendant care services, various therapies (primarily speech and physical therapy) and certain palliative interventions, for example palliative radiation; more commonly treatments like radiation are associated with curative treatment goals. The focus of all these professionals and interventions is patient comfort and the achievement and maintenance of the highest possible quality of life.

In the past decade, definitions of "home" used by US hospices have changed substantially. It now includes nursing homes, skilled facilities and other step-down units, assisted living and graduated care environments. Prison hospice most closely resembles hospice care as delivered in a skilled nursing environment, though programs nationwide vary considerably. Some programs have a dedicated hospice unit, wing or ward; some integrate hospice services into the general medical population, in some instances inmates stay in their cells and services come to them.

By definition, people who are admitted to a hospice must be certified as having a prognosis of six months or less to live. These patients are consciously electing to forego further curative therapy and must be recertified at frequent intervals as to their continued appropriateness for hospice services. Patients who improve significantly and who no longer have a prognosis of six months or less to live are graduated off hospice until their condition again meets the criteria.

Hospice in Prisons

Federal and state prisons are faced with a growing and aging prison population, an increasing number of deaths, older inmates serving long sentences and concerns about the conditions in which inmates in state and federal prisons die. Since the mid 1980s, a number of departments of corrections have developed hospice programs within jail or prison environments. While jails typically house short-term inmates, some larger facilities, such as the Broward County Sheriff's Office, have developed hospice programs (Schwartz and Bauersmith 2000). Most of the hospice programs within the United States, however, are located in state or federal prisons.

Hospice programs in corrections are a fairly new intervention. The U.S. Federal Bureau of Prisons, for instance, introduced its first hospice program in 1987. Mara, McKenna and Sims (2000) reported that eleven state prison systems had hospice programs, and another 25 hospice programs were in the planning or development stage. Anno and colleagues (2004:13) report that slightly more than one-half of the correctional agencies that they surveyed had hospice programs, and that "Five agencies (20%) offer hospice services in a separate unit; 22 (88%) operate the hospice as part of their infirmary; 4 (16%) operate the hospice as part of a housing unit; and 8 (32%) operate a hospice as part of an outpatient program." Clearly there is a wide variety of hospice programs that are offered, and the extent of these programs depends on the size of the correctional agency among other factors.

At the National Commission on Correctional Health Care Conference (NCCHC) in November, 1998, several presentations on hospice care in correctional settings were featured. Representatives from several of these programs met with representatives of the National Prison Hospice Association (NPHA) and the National Hospice Organization, now the National Hospice and Palliative Care Organization (NHPCO). These organizations outlined the challenges of providing hospice care within corrections settings, and a series of descriptive articles relating to corrections hospices was produced (Bauersmith 2002; Boyle 2002; Evans 2002; Linder 2002a; Linder, 2002b).

Hospice for inmates is comprised of the same core services as hospice in the free community: an interdisciplinary team with physician-supervised care, routine nursing and social work intervention, spiritual and bereavement care, volunteers and allied professionals. Additionally, custody, classifications and administration are integral to prison hospice programs; winning institutional supporters within the ranks of these groups is essential to establishing and sustaining a prison hospice program. In prisons, the role of the hospice volunteer and the decision of who will fulfill that role vary widely. Some programs utilize inmates as volunteers or assigned workers in hospice. Strong prohibitions exist against inmates having authority over one another, so the duties inmate volunteers can perform are often carefully circumscribed.

Inmate volunteers often sit vigil with the dying, assuaging the fear of dying alone voiced by many inmates. In some settings, inmate volunteers can assist professional staff with some direct patient care, for example helping patients dress, bathe, eat and ambulate. One issue that programs utilizing inmate volunteers often must contend with is inconsistencies in the duties these volunteers can perform based on the variable interpretation of individual medical and custody staff. Staffing levels and the relative shortage or surplus of paid staff, and changes in an institution's operational status, for instance lockdowns, can also cause variability in the availability of volunteer service delivery.

Inmate volunteers are very carefully screened and trained by those institutions that make use of them. These volunteers take the commitment to the dying seriously, particularly when sitting vigil with someone whose death is imminent. Disruptions in their ability to be there for fellow inmates are very distressing, yet their place at the bottom of the prison hierarchy necessitates that they be able to adapt to the changing environment in which they serve, an environment that is mostly beyond their influence or control. Having an institutional liaison who understands these various emotions and forces promotes sustaining a quality hospice inmate volunteer program.

Some of these differences are substantive and others are more stylistic. Some of the variations relating to patient and care issues include:

- Programs must decide whether to integrate hospice patients with general medicine patients.
- Some medications, particularly opioids (such as morphine pills or liquid, and synthetic morphine patches), may be dispensed with restrictions in prisons, and some may not be available at all.
- The problem of patients coming into hospice and subsequently needing to be discharged due to improved prognosis is problematic in prisons as hospice may include benefits unavailable to the general prison population.
- The hospice team includes additional stakeholders: custody and security, inmate classifications, Medical Technical Assistants (a hybrid of patient care and security/custody) and others.
- Programs must make decisions about what role, if any, other inmates will play
- Are the patient's close inmate friends to be included as "family", and if so, with what rights and privileges?
- Should inmates be used to deliver health care services within the hospice, and if so, which services?
- What effect does an institution-based hospice program have on the compassionate discharge process in those states that release terminally ill patients to be cared for in the community or by their family?

The implementation of hospice in prisons is one strategy which begins to address the issue of prisoners "graying in place" and helps provide inmates with a dignified death free of unnecessary pain and suffering.

One of the challenges of correctional health care is to balance the need to provide a safe and secure environment for both inmates and staff with the medical and psychological needs of the inmates who are terminally ill. As mentioned above, some medications (such as narcotics) might not be dispensed in a correctional setting due to the possibility that other inmates might attempt to steal these medications. Another important consideration is whether all family members can visit the inmate in a hospice. In some cases, family members might have criminal records and not all prisons might allow them to visit someone receiving palliative care. A further question is whether prison officials will allow visits between siblings who are incarcerated in other state prisons, or even other units within the same prison?

Palliative Medicine

During the last 15 years, the field of palliative care has taken a quantum leap in importance. Palliative medicine is the broader category of interventions geared toward comfort goals, and includes hospice as the largest and most clearly articulated of palliative programs, but also including inpatient services, consult services and specialty outpatient clinics seeing a broad array of patients with palliative care needs, not just those terminally ill patients with a prognosis of six months or less to live. Palliative care as outlined by the World Health Organization (2000) includes the following key characteristics:

- provides relief from pain and other distressing symptoms;
- affirms life and regards dying as a normal process;
- intends neither to hasten nor postpone death;
- integrates the psychological and spiritual aspects of patient care;
- offers a support system to help patients live as actively as possible until death;
- offers a support system to help the family cope during the patients illness and in their own bereavement;
- uses a team approach to address the needs of patients and their families, including bereavement counseling, if indicated;
- will enhance quality of life, and may also positively influence the course of illness;
- is applicable early in the course of illness, in conjunction with other therapies that are intended to prolong life, such as chemotherapy or radiation therapy (in the case of cancer), and includes those investigations needed to better understand and manage distressing clinical complications.

Even as the prison hospice movement has been implemented or is in development in a number of federal and state prisons and local jail settings, the introduction of palliative care is serving to further diversify the care options available to inmates with chronic conditions or degenerative or progressive disease as well as with terminal conditions, and extend the availability of comfort-focused care beyond designated hospice environments.

The breadth of the palliative care approach is advantageous as an augmentation to the prison hospice model for a number of reasons. There are a number of barriers to the establishment of hospice broadly throughout the prison system. Implementing a full-scale hospice program in every prison is not practical. Some prison systems are very small and have less than 2000 beds (Harrison and Beck 2006). In the larger prison systems such as the Federal Bureau of Prisons, Texas, or California, by contrast, they approach 200,000 inmates. In these systems it makes more sense to develop palliative care. In California, for instance, there were 18,274 inmates who were 50 years or older at year-end 2005 distributed across the California Department of Corrections' 33 state prisons and 38 conservation camps (California Department of Corrections and Rehabilitation 2006).

In late 1998, the Grace Project was funded by the Robert Wood Johnson Foundation's Promoting Excellence in End-of-Life Care program. The acronym GRACE stands for Guiding Responsive Action in Corrections at End-of-life. The project took an in-depth look at four state and federal prisons from disparate regions in the United States: Coxsackie, New York; McCain, North Carolina; Salem, Oregon and Forth Worth, Texas. In addition to identifying key issues relevant to the delivery of hospice in prisons and core components of best practices in prison hospice programs, the Grace Project produced End-of-Life Care Standards of Practice, intended to assist existing programs in evaluating and improving their hospice care delivery and to offer guidance to prison hospice programs being designed and implemented (GRACE, 2000).

In reviewing the literature, and the hospice Standards of Care developed by the Grace Project, it is clear that correctional systems would have to designate specific facilities within their systems to be the locus of hospice care delivery. In states with many prisons distributed over a large geographic area (such as Texas, California, or Florida), a centralized hospice would separate inmates from their families during their dying. In states with fewer facilities, or a single prison that holds all inmates sentenced to terms of life imprisonment (such as Angola prison in Louisiana), or states that contract out-of-state for prison services, a single prison may be isolated, difficult to reach, situated without readily available services or accommodations for visitors from a distance, or may in fact be in an another state altogether.

Compassionate Release

Another way that jail and prison systems can assist terminally ill prisoners to die with dignity is to release them into the care of family members before their sentence has expired. Many prison systems have routinely made such compassionate releases available. Typically these releases have been granted when the inmate is so debilitated that they pose no threat to the public. In some cases judges who are responsible for evaluating the release are reluctant to release an inmate if the officials cannot guarantee that the prisoner will not re-offend (Mara, McKenna and Sims 2000). During an era when prisoners are seen in an unsympathetic light by the public, however, it is unlikely that many prison officials would support the compassionate release of a person convicted of a violent offense or a sexual crime. In the current climate correctional systems are most likely to err on the side of caution, placing public safety as the highest priority.

Anno and colleagues report that "compassionate releases were available in 43 (87.8%) of the 49 responding agencies. The average annual number of requests for compassionate release was 18, and the average number granted was 8"(2004:13). However averages don't tell the entire story. In some cases, the vetting process for requests is so rigorous that few requests get through the process to the approval or denial decision. Those that do may face nearly uniform approval, or denial, or some balance point in between. Further, some compassionate release processes are lengthy, and by the time patients are sufficiently incapacitated to protect the public safety, they are too ill to survive until the process has run its course. Requests can advance to decision-makers in as little as two weeks and as much as several months.

Anno and colleagues (2004) found that compassionate release procedures vary from state to state. As a result, there is no common definition for the compassionate release of dying inmates. In some instances prisoners or family members can initiate a request for compassionate release. More often, some member or team from inmate health services initiates the request. Likewise, the final authority to grant or deny the request may reside with a parole board, the governor, a judge or a senior member of the corrections department.

Aday observes that most states have provisions for compassionate release, but that "one obstacle to widening compassionate release is the lack of a suitable community placement. Many families, who also may be dealing with their own issues of aging, do not have the time or resources to adequately care for a released prisoner" (2003: 210).

Another factor affecting the availability of suitable community placement is that some inmates are estranged from their family and former community. This is often dependent on the original committal offense, the number of years an inmate has been incarcerated and the condition of the family support system both before and during their incarceration. There are inmates whose only "family" is their fellow inmates; the only community they are attached to is the prison community. For these inmates, an in-prison hospice or palliative care program may be significantly more compassionate than compassionate release.

When compassionate release is being considered, there is a heightened need for pre-release planning. Inmates are not entitled to benefits under Social Security, Medicare, Medicaid and many other assistance or support programs for housing, employment, medical care, food and other services. When an inmate's release is being precipitated by terminal illness, the need to access health care and funding for basic needs immediately upon release is crucial to the success of the inmate's transition from prison to the community. Working in partnership with a hospice program in the community is often the best way to facilitate continuity of care, including insuring that the patient's medical care and prescription medication needs are being met and that they are in a safe and appropriate living situation.

Conclusions

Imprisoning over two million offenders (including an estimated one-quarter million prisoners with sentences longer than 20 years), has created the problem of increased numbers of aging inmates, many of whom will die behind bars of terminal illness or at the end of a chronic disease process like diabetes. Some jurisdictions have responded with a particular form of compassion for these inmates and have introduced hospice, compassionate release and palliative medicine programs. Such programs make it easier for inmates, their families, and the correctional facility to cope with dying prisoners. Yet, only a fraction of the state Departments of Corrections have established such programs, and there is a long way to go before all prison inmates can be afforded the ability to die with dignity.

Some states permit prison hospices to obtain state licensure. Where this option is allowed and pursued, inmates are assured care comparable with the free community. Operating within the Standards of Practice laid out by the GRACE Project also provide some assurance of the quality of hospice programs, promote care comparable with the community and serve to ensure greater uniformity of care across programs and settings.

Even through there is little public or political support for compassionate release programs, they represent an opportunity to reduce prison overcrowding, and allow the prison system to focus its health care resources on other inmates. In the United States, inmates who die in prison hospices generally receive excellent care. Altogether, providing hospice care is one small step towards humanizing the deprivations of prison life, and ensuring that inmates can die with dignity.

References

Aday, Ronald H. 2003. *Aging Prisoners: Crisis in American Corrections*. Westport, CT:

Praeger.
------. 2006. "Aging Prisoners' Concerns Toward Dying in Prison." *OMEGA* 52: 199-216.
Anno, B. Jaye, Camelia Graham, James E. Lawrence, and Ronald Shansky. 2004. *Correctional Health Care: Assessing the Needs of Elderly, Chronically Ill, and Terminally Ill Inmates.* Longmont, CO: National Institute of Corrections.
Bauersmith, Joan and Ruth Gent. 2002. "The Broward Jails Hospice Program: Hospice in the Jail." *Journal of Palliative Medicine* 5:667-670.
Boyle, Barbara A. 2002. "The Maryland Division of Corrections Hospice Program." *Journal of Palliative Medicine* 5:671-675.
Byock, Ira. 1997. *Dying Well: Peace and Possibilities at the End of Life.* New York: The Berkley Publishing Group.
California Department of Corrections and Rehabilitation 2005. *California Prisoners and Parolees, 2004*. Sacramento, CA: California Department of Corrections and Rehabilitation.
Continuum Care Hospice. 2006. *Hospice History*. Retrieved April 17, 2007 (http://www.hospicenyc.org/).
Estelle v. Gamble, 429 U.S. 97. 1976.
Evans, Carol, Ronda Herzog and Tanya Tillman. 2002. "The Louisiana State Penitentiary: Angola Prison Hospice." *Journal of Palliative Medicine* 5:553-558
Freeborne, Nancy, Joanne Lynn, and Norman A. Desbiens. 2000. "Insight About Dying From The SUPPORT Project." *Journal of the American Geriatrics Society* 48:199-205.
Guiding Responsive Action for Corrections in End-of-life. 2000. End-of-Life Care Standards of Practice for Inmates in Correctional Settings. Retrieved May 25, 2006 (http://www2.edc.org/lastacts/archives/archivesMay00/standards.asp).
Harrison, Paige M. and Allen J. Beck. 2006. *Prisoners in 2005.* Washington, DC: Bureau of Justice Statistics.
Hightow-Weidman, Lisa and Justin Smith. 2007. *The Mythology of the Down Low: A Critical Exploration of Black Men Who Have Sex With Men and HIV Transmission. Infectious Diseases in Corrections Report* 9: 1, 3-4.
Hospice Association of America. 2006. *Hospice: A Historical Perspective.* Retrieved May 25, 2006 (http://www.hospice-america.org/history.html).
Jacob Arriola, Kimberly R., Braithwaite, Ronald L., and Cassandra Newkirk. 2006. "At the Intersection Between Poverty, Race, and HIV Infection: HIV-Related Services for Incarcerated Women." *Infectious Diseases in Corrections Report* 9:1-5.
Kuhlmann, Robynn and Rick Ruddell. 2005. "Elderly Jail Inmates: Problems, Prevalence, and Public Health. *Californian Journal of Health Promotion* 3:50-61
Linder, John, Sheila Enders, Elizabeth Craig, Joan Richardson, and Frederick J. Meyers. 2002. "Hospice Care for the Incarcerated in the Unites States: An Introduction." *Journal of Palliative Medicine* 5:549-552.
Linder, John, Keith Knauf, Sheila Enders, and Frederick Meyers. 2002. "Prison Hospice and Pastoral Care Services - California Medical Facility, Vacaville. *Journal of Palliative Medicine* 5:903-908.
Kay, Susan L. 1991. *The Constitutional Dimensions of an Inmate's Right to Health Care.* Chicago: National Commission on Correctional Health Care.
McGuire, M. Dyan. 2005. "The Impact of Prison Rape on Public Health." *Californian*

Journal of Health Promotion 3(2):72-83.

Mara, Cynthia M., Christopher K. McKenna, and Barbara Sims. 2000. Unintended Consequences of Sentencing policy: Key Issues in Developing Strategies to Address Long-term Care Needs of Prison Inmates. Retrieved April 17, 2007 (http://www.ncjrs.gov/pdffiles1/nij/grants/197030.pdf).

Maruschak, Laura M. 2005. *HIV in Prisons, 2003*. Washington, DC: Bureau of Justice Statistics.

Mumola Christopher. 2005. *Suicide and Homicide in State Prisons and Local Jails.* Washington, DC: Bureau of Justice Statistics.

------. 2007. *Medical Causes of Death in State Prisons, 2001-2004.* Washington, DC: Bureau of Justice Statistics.

Murphy, Daniel. 2005. "Healthcare in the Federal Bureau of Prisons: Fact or Fiction." *Californian Journal of Health Promotion* 3(2):23-37.

National Association of Social Workers. 2007. *Code of Ethics of the National Association of Social Workers*. Washington DC: Author.

National Hospice and Palliative Care Organization 2006. *NHPCO Facts and Figures.* Retrieved April 17, 2007 (http://www.nhpco.org).

Ratcliff, Margaret. 2000. "Dying Inside the Walls." *Journal of Palliative Medicine* 3:509-511.

St. Christopher's Hospice. 2006. *St. Christopher's Hospice*. Retrieved May 25, 2006 (http://www.stchristophers.org.uk/page.cfm/link=13)

Smyer, Tish, Marcia D. Gragert, and Sheena La Mere. 1997. "Stay Safe, Stay Healthy: Surviving Old Age in Prison. *Journal of Psychosocial Nursing and Mental Health Services* 35:10-17.

Snell, Tracy L. 2006. *Capital Punishment, 2005.* Washington, DC: Bureau of Justice Statistics.

Wellman v. Faulkner, 715 F.2d 269, 274 (7th Cir. 1983).

World Health Organization. 2000. *WHO Definition of Palliative Care.* Retrieved April 17, 2007 (http://www.who.int/cancer/palliative/definition/en/).

CHAPTER TWELVE

Doing Time Together: Correctional Officer Health

Amanda Mathias Humphrey

What is a chapter on correctional officers doing in a book about correctional health? While the preceding chapters have outlined some of the major challenges that inmates confront, correctional officers also "live" in the same conditions as the prisoners they supervise. If inmates are at high risk of contracting communicable diseases, so are correctional officers. Furthermore, they are at high-risk of violence. One of the challenges that correctional administrators realize is that when officers are healthier, they are less likely to be cynical, angry, and disgruntled, the all-to-typical outlook that many correctional officers share. As a result, this chapter addresses some of the health-related issues that correctional officers confront.

The major health issue for correctional officers is job-related stress. Stress has a negative impact on the physical and emotional health of correctional officers, and was defined by McCraty, Atkinson, Lipsenthal, and Arguelles as "negative perceptions, feelings, and emotions that are triggered by a perceived challenge or threat, whether real or imagined" (2003:3). Stress often is not a one-time experience for many people (Pearlin 1989). Correctional officers experience elevated levels of job stress on a daily basis. This stress is more severe than that experienced by employees in almost every other occupational group. The severity of correctional officer stress is in part a result of overcrowded correctional institutions, the austere environment they work within, and the risks of communicable diseases or violence that correctional officers and staff confront on a daily basis.

Correctional work has been described as fragmented, routinized, and menial. As a result, it is characterized by a lack of job satisfaction, professional recognition, and opportunities for achievement (Zupan 2002). Although job security, benefits and steady pay are assets of the correctional officer occupation, most officers receive lower pay and job prestige when compared to law enforcement officers. In fact, Richards writes about spending time in a Charleston jail in the 1980s, and reporting that, "turnkey guards who were paid minimum wages (they actually showed the prisoners their paycheck stubs), and appeared nearly as economically desperate as the prisoners" (2003:131). It is no surprise then that some research labels correctional officers as a "disaffected group" who suffer from, cynicism, alienation, and low job satisfaction. These issues along with a variety of emotional and physical health problems are often the long-term consequences of correctional careers.

This chapter outlines the issue of correctional officer health by identifying the sources of stress for correctional officers, and the short- and long-term consequences. In addition, the types of interventions and programs that are intended to reduce work-related stress and improve the physical and emotional health of correctional officers are examined. Such interventions include stress reduction programs operated or provided by correctional facilities, and are increasingly intended to help officer families as well. Finally, this chapter highlights several programs that focus on correctional officer wellness and health promotion.

Sources of Correctional Officer Stress

One important source of correctional officer stress is the work environment. Environmental stressors for correctional officers include: inmate assaults or critical incidents, interactions with prisoners, and conflicts with co-workers (Finn 2000). These work-related stressors are also classified as the social climate and physical environment stressors (Armstrong and Griffin 2004). The most important of these stressors is safety and security. Research has consistently identified that the unsafe or uncertain environment of correctional institution is the most important source of correctional officer stress (Cracy 2005; Lombardo 1989; Tripplett et al. 1996). The value of safety and security as a stressor is underscored by the fact that the workplace violence rate for correctional officers is higher than the rate for all other occupational classification except law enforcement (Duhart 2001).

Although Mumola (2005) outlines how rates of inmate murders in prisons and jails have decreased significantly, for correctional officers the risk of assaults is still high (Camp and Camp 2002; Duhart 2001). In the last ten years security and safety concerns among correctional officers have increased due to the overcrowded conditions in many facilities. The New

Jersey Department of Corrections notes how growing "inmate populations, more stringent sentencing laws, and restricting inmate releases" as increasing safety and security concerns within their institutions (see Hepner 2005). In addition to the direct risk of violence, correctional environments are often chaotic places, and this uncertainty also contributes to the stress that a correctional officer experiences during a shift. The greater these security and safety concerns the more likely correctional officers are to experience chronic job stress. Stress levels among correctional officers also rise after incidents of inmate violence against officers (Van Voorhis, Cullen, Link and Wolfe 1991).

Interacting with inmates is another stressor which stems from the correctional environment. The core task of correctional work is the supervision of inmates who Lipskey (1980) termed a "hostile group." It is the responsibility of correctional officers to deprive an inmate's liberty, thus creating an inherently conflict-ridden relationship between the officer and inmate. The correctional officer is the visual symbol of the correctional institution (Webb and Morris 2002). Therefore, as Zupan writes, inmates are not "respectful, appreciative or supportive" (2002) of the work of correctional officers. Correctional officers must then deal with the negative attitude, hostility, demands and manipulations directed at them by inmates (Childress et al. 1999; Lombardo 1989). These stressful interactions with inmates are what Webb and Morris (2002) identify as the "daily hassles" correctional officers experience when supervising inmates.

The third work-related stressor for correctional officers is conflict with co-workers. According to Finn (2000), disputes between fellow correctional officers can stem from negative attitudes, competition for desirable schedules and assignments, concern over a co-workers ability to perform their job duties, and coping with their co-worker's unethical conduct. Correctional officers often feel that they don't have the support of their managers. These feelings of isolation or lack of support have been identified as an important source of stress for correctional officers (Auerbach, Quizh and Pegg 2003; Triplett et al. 1996). In fact, Marston (1993) observed that many correctional officers viewed conflicts with co-workers as the second most important factor—behind security and safety—in contributing to officer stress.

Administration

The second source of correctional officer stress comes from the day-to-day operations of working within jails or prisons. Stressors resulting from administrative issues include: shift work, understaffing, overtime, supervisor demands, role conflict, and role ambiguity (Finn 2000). One cause of jail and prison officer stress is rotating shift work, which impacts an officer's family life along with their readiness to work (Childress et al. 1999). Shift work often leads to fatigue and irritability and also creates family frustration when officers are unable to attend important family events or spend holidays with their loved ones (Gerstein, Topp, and Correll 1987). In addition, officers have historically received relatively low wages, and rates of job turnover are high, and as a result, understaffing is a significant problem in many correctional facilities (Auerbach et al. 2003). Paoline, Lambert and Hogan (2006) found that the organizational characteristics of county jails were a better predictor of self-reported job satisfaction and stress than individual characteristics.

Officers working in under-staffed facilities are often unable to complete all of their assigned duties, which include head counts, searches, and paperwork (Finn 2000). In other cases, officers are required to work mandatory overtime on their days off, or stay after their assigned shift ends. Jail and prison officers also suffer from heightened security and safety concerns if there are not enough staff to effectively respond to incidents or disturbances (Childress et al. 1999). Correctional officers consistently report their supervisors as a source of stress because of the demand placed on them to complete work without being provided adequate resources or personnel to accomplish the duties (Wells 2003). As a result of understaffing, many correctional facilities require officers to work overtime and rarely allow officers to refuse these shifts (Finn 2000). Working these additional shifts adds to physical and psychological responses by exhausting the officer and further reducing time spent with family.

Other commonly cited stressors affecting correctional officers are role conflict and ambiguity (Auerbach et al. 2003; Lombardo 1989; Ray 2001). Role conflict is defined by Ivancevich and Matteson as a condition resulting when "compliance with one set of pressures makes compliance with another set difficulty, objectionable or impossible" (1980:11). Finn (2000) points outs that officers face ambiguity in their position because they must adhere to complex policies and regulations and rules, are expected to effectively and efficiently perform those duties, but are not given the resources to accomplish their mission. Role ambiguity is also increased as strictly following all rules and regulations is almost impossible, so officers have to establish priorities (Wells 2003). Adding to the stress is the fact that correctional officers are seldom provided with the resources or infrastructure necessary to accomplish the goals of treatment (Webb and Morris 2002).

Officers often want to exercise their discretion when dealing with inmates, but are sometimes prevented from utilizing their expertise by administrative demands to strictly follow facility rules and regulations (Armstrong and Griffith 2004). Officers are also expected to balance the opposing goals of security and rehabilitation and must determine how to best fulfill these goals (Webb and Morris 2002). As Schrag (1961), concludes, correctional officers have one-on-one contact with inmates thereby making them a unique source for determining "what works and what doesn't work" in dealing with the custody and treatment of inmates, yet they have almost no input in decision-making process regarding the rules and regulations for interacting with inmates. Webb and Morris (2002) echo this observation and suggest that officers often have a "better understanding of inmates than administrators." Altogether, some officers report that their interactions with administrators are more stressful than working with prisoners.

Consequences of Stress

The negative effects experienced as a result of exposure to stress cause a variety of physiological and psychological reactions. These reactions are referred to as the "stress response" (McCraty et al. 2003). The human body's response to stress, particularly to chronic stress, can also contribute to weight gain or loss, high blood pressure, cardiovascular disease, cancer, diabetes, and gastrointestinal disorders (Eysenck 1993; McCraty et al. 2003). Cheek (1984) revealed that the average life span for correctional officers was shorter than the national average life span, and the 1998 Metropolitan Life Statistics indicated that correctional officers now have an average life expectancy of only 58 years (Hepner 2005). In addition the suicide rate for corrections workers was thought to be much higher than other professions including peace officers (Stack and Tsoudis 1997). Unfortunately, there doesn't seem to be much conclusive data about suicide rates by profession, as no national-level organization collects these statistics.

Responses to stress can include psychological symptoms such as frustration, anger, worry, anxiety, fear, insecurity, depression, irritability, tension, and resentment, in addition to physiological responses (McCraty et al. 2003). These symptoms are often associated with marital problems and emotional disorders. Research indicates that some correctional officers have difficulty separating their roles as correctional officer from their role as spouse (and parent) causing them to respond to their loved ones as if they were inmates (Ray 2001; Wells 2003). This condition is referred to as the "spill over" effect (Hepner 2005). Research indicates that some correctional officers vent their frustration onto loved ones thereby damaging their relationships (Ray 2001; Wells 2003). This may also lead to an increased risk of domestic violence in families of correctional officers. Gambling, alcoholism, overeating and other addictive or self-medicating behaviors are also cited as emotional disorders that result from the stress of correctional work (Crary 2006; Ray 2001). One long-term condition relating to these types of psychological responses to stress is often labeled as burnout.

Malash and Jackson defined burnout as "a syndrome of emotional exhaustion and cynicism that occurs frequently among individuals who do 'people work' of some kind" (1981:99). Specifically, Maslach and Jackson (1981) identify three conditions that are characteristic of burnout. Those conditions include: feeling overextended and exhausted, depersonalization, and the absence of feelings of personal accomplishment from a job. Burnout has been identified as a common outcome of correctional work (Hays and Tompkins 1986; McShane and Williams 1993). High levels of burnout have a significant impact upon the administration's ability to efficiently and effectively operate a correctional facility (Cornelius, 1994).

Administrative Costs of Stress and Burnout

The effect of burnout is a major concern of correctional facility administrators because staff who are suffering from this condition negatively affect the operational ability of the facility. Problems associated with burnout include low morale, the unnecessary use of sick leave, excessive disability retirements, and turnover (Cornelius 1994; Slate, Vogel and Johnson 2001). Low morale is an important issue for correctional administrators because it reduces officer productivity and creates negative interactions between officers and inmates (Auerbach et al. 2003; Crary 2006).

The physical and emotional responses of long-term exposure to stress often leads to excessive use of sick leave. Absenteeism is often used by officers to cope with the stressful conditions in corrections (Crary 2006; McShane and Williams 1993). For example, Finn (2000) found that in one jurisdiction, approximately 20 percent of correctional officers utilized sick leave because they were suffering from the effects of burnout. This high use of sick leave has direct financial consequences on administration because other officers must be paid overtime to work the shifts left vacant (Wells 2003).

The financial effect of stress on correctional administrators is compounded by high rates of disability retirement among officers. Stress has been identified as a leading factor in disability retirements among correctional officers (McShane and Williams 1993; Wells 2003). These payments can be expensive to federal, state, and local governments. In addition to the direct financial costs, these retirements also add to the high turnover rates among correctional officers (Crary 2006; Wells 2003). Estimates of the annual turnover rate among correctional officers runs from 12 to 25 percent depending upon the organization (Finn 2000)—although there is some variance in these estimates and Petersilia (2006) reported that the California Department of Corrections and Rehabilitation had a turnover rate of just three percent, while Kentucky's rate was over 30 percent. This high rate of turnover increases costs, as agencies must continually spend money on recruiting, hiring, and training new officers (Lambert 2006; Wells 2003). Unfortunately, a high percentage of these officers may quit before the costs associated with hiring them can be recouped.

The presence of inexperienced officers also has safety implications for correctional facilities and staff. Due to elevated rates of turnover, experienced officers frequently are forced to work with inexperienced officers. Unfortunately, these officers are not always able to respond effectively to the demands of the job, particularly with handling conflict (Finn 2000). This inexperience may also lead to mistakes that jeopardize the safety and security of the facility. As a result of the high costs of managing stress and burnout, correctional administrators have a vested interested in reducing this problem. One response of jail and prison administrators to the problem of stress has been the creation of stress reduction programs.

Reducing Correctional Officer Stress

Finn (2000) provides an overview of some "best practices" in correctional stress reduction programs including the Multnomah County (Oregon) Peer Support Program, Massachusetts Stress Unit, South Carolina Post-Trauma Resources Program, and California Counseling Team Program. The Multnomah County Peer Support Program and the Massachusetts Stress Unit are both in-house programs that are staffed by correctional officers working as peer supporters. The following paragraphs briefly outline examples of programs from these three approaches.

The Massachusetts Stress Unit relies on the work of a part-time program coordinator and five correctional officers who volunteer as full-time peer supporters and provide assistance to the 4000 staff members within the state's correctional system (Finn 2000). The Multnomah County (Oregon) program, on the other hand, is operated in the county jail and provides services to approximately 500 correctional officers. The

Multnomah County program is also facilitated by a part-time coordinator who doubles as the department's chaplaincy coordinator (Finn 2000). This program maintains three peer support teams that address the problems of substance abuse, trauma, and debriefing (Finn 2000). Each of the team members includes correctional officers, deputies, and civilian employees who are directly supervised by a team coordinator (Finn 2000). Both of these programs provide peer support services, referrals to external professional counselors, and services to family members. However, only the Multnomah County program provides critical incident debriefing services for correctional officers and their families (Finn 2000).

In contrast to in-house stress programs, South Carolina's Post-Trauma Resources (PTR) and California's Counseling Team are examples of stress reduction programs that are privately operated. The PTR is a for-profit agency that provides critical incident debriefing services to the 4,850 officers employed by the South Carolina Department of Corrections, but does not provide assistance to family members (Finn 2000). In addition to its critical incident debriefing responsibility, PTR also provides short-term individual counseling to correctional officers when an officer is referred to PTR by the state's Department of Corrections (Finn 2000). Similar to the South Carolina approach, the Counseling Team located in San Bernardino California is a corporation that provides a broad range of stress reduction services to both sheriff's departments and correctional facilities in Southern California on a fee-for-service basis. The services provided by the Counseling Team include individual evaluation and counseling, critical incident debriefing, peer support training, and in-service training on topics such as burnout (Finn 2000). Unlike South Carolina's PTR, the Counseling Team provides services to the families of correctional officers.

There is some variation among stress reduction programs. Finn (2000) outlines several "distinguishing features" including whether or not the program offers professional counseling and/or peer support, and addresses chronic stress and critical incidents. Other features that differentiate these programs are whether or not the program conducts academy or in-service training and offers services to family members (Finn, 2000). The differences between stress reduction programs make it difficult to select an "ideal" program. Implementation of an approach is dependent on the nature of the organization (e.g., whether it is a jail or prison), its history, the relationships between officers and administrators, the availability of funding, and the strength of collective bargaining. Finn writes that "programmatic diversity means correctional administrators have the freedom to tailor the various components of their program to the particular needs of their facilities and employees and to the characteristics of their department's structure, history, size and resources" (2000:22).

Benefits of Stress Programs

There are three main benefits to correctional officer stress programs: 1) Better job performance, 2) Increased institutional safety, and, 3) cost-savings. The reduction of stress among correctional officers and their families can have a direct impact of the attitude of correctional officers while at work and how these officers perform their job. Correctional officer attitudes are improved because there is a sense among the officers that they are supported by their managers and that the administration is concerned about their needs. This translates into increased agency morale (NIC 1996). Similarly, officers whose stress levels are reduced are a "healthier work group" because they use fewer sick days and are less likely to be involved in conflicts with inmates and other staff members (Finn 2000; NIC 1996).

The presence of a "healthier work group" not only improves job performance but also increases the safety of the institution. This is because officers who are able to control their stress levels are less likely to lash out at an inmate or other staff (NIC 1996). The safety of the institution also rises because officers who are not distracted by stress will perform their job task more attentively than their stressed-out counterparts (Finn 2000). In addition, a decrease in the use of sick time and a reduction in turnover increase the overall experience levels of officers. Experienced officers tend to be more capable of handling inmate conflicts and diffusing potentially critical situations than "rookie" officers (Finn 2000; NIC 1996).

The reduction in sick leave, disability, and early resignations as outcomes of stress reduction services, not only increase the safety within correctional institutions but also lead to significant cost savings. A reduction in the number of officers on disability or who take early retirement automatically reduces the amount of money jurisdictions are forced to spend on disability and early retirement payouts (NIC 1996). Reduction in turnover also saves on human resource costs. For example, research indicates that when correctional officers resign their position approximately 71 percent of them do so in the first two years (Delprino 2002). Therefore, in order to keep up with turnover, jails and prisons must continually spend money for the recruitment, hiring, and training of new officers (NIC 1996). Despite the advantages of stress-reduction programs, there are several factors that must be considered before implementing these changes in jails or prisons.

Creating Effective Stress Reduction Programs

There are three main challenges that correctional administrators must consider while developing interventions to reduce officer stress (Finn 2000). The first consideration is program staffing, training and networking. The second factor is to ensure that staff members participate in these programs once developed. Last, the final category involves evaluation of the effectiveness of these interventions.

With regard to program staffing, training, and networking effective stress reduction programs have used different staffing models, including: professional staff, peer supporters, supervisor training, and developing a network of reliable referral resources (Finn 2000). The use of counselors with experience or training in the area of corrections is important because officers respect, trust, and respond to these counselors during the therapeutic process (NIC 1996). In addition to professional staff, utilizing peer supporters who are carefully selected and adequately trained is also an important component in these programs. Peer supporters are an essential part of a stress-reduction program because these officers have first-hand knowledge of the stressors of correctional work, allowing them to relate to and gain the respect of fellow officers (NIC 1996). And since peer supporters are located within the facility, they are often more available to correctional officers (Finn 2000).

The second key component for effective stress-reduction programs is to ensure participation in these interventions, and to reduce the organizational sources of stress (Finn 2000). In order for a stress program to be successful it is vital that all staff members support and utilize the intervention. Administrators and supervisors have an important role because they are responsible for providing the personnel and funding. Another way to encourage the participation of correctional officers in these programs is to collaborate with the union during their development. As Finn observes, "As the bargaining unit and officers' primary representation with management, the officers' union is in a unique position to stymie or promote a stress program" (2000:58). Union support is important because it also increases the respect and credibility of the program in the eyes of front-line officers (NIC 1996). This support may also facilitate correctional officer participation in a stress reduction program, but in order to encourage participation, outreach activities must also be directed toward line officers.

Combating sources of organizational stress is another important consideration for correctional administrators. Individuals providing stress reduction interventions are in a unique position to pinpoint sources of stress within a facility and provide suggestions to administrators and supervisors on how to reduce those stressors (Finn 2000). Another important organization source of stress is critical incidents - one of the unfortunate realities of correctional work is that officers will be exposed to suicides, unintentional injuries, and violence. Critical incident debriefing involves a comprehensive examination of these incidents in a supportive environment. The incorporation of critical incidents debriefings is a best practice because they can provide immediate emotional support to officers. Finn (2000) suggests that debriefings help officers deal with feelings of guilt, clear up inconsistencies in the events surrounding an incident, and serve as a sign of administrative support.

The final element for effective stress-reduction programs is evaluation. The evaluation of a stress program is critical in determining if the program is accomplishing its goals. Evaluations of stress-reduction programs should assess the implementation of the interventions (including the number of persons served, and the types of services delivered), their impact, and cost (Finn 2000). To determine the impact of a stress program an evaluation would include a determination regarding stress levels among officers and their family members before participating in the program and their stress levels after participating. According to Finn (2000), the impact evaluation should also include an analysis of changes in levels of absenteeism, substance use, emotional and physical health problems, resignation, disciplinary actions, and attitudinal changes. The determination of the costs and benefits of such programs is absolutely critical to ensure long-term funding.

Health Promotion

The future of correctional officer health programs resides with the development of services designed not only to reduce officer stress and combat those accompanying physical, emotional, and administrative consequences, but also to improve their physical and emotional wellness. The establishment of wellness or fitness programs designed to promote exercise, nutrition and emotional health of employees is increasing due to spiraling health care costs employers have to cover (DiNubile and Sherman 1999; Kielyl and Hodgson 1990). These expenditures are increasing because of rising health care costs in general, and poor employee health (DiNubile and Sherman 1999). As a result, employers are also responsible for the expense associated with sick leave, disability, and lower levels of productivity. As a result, more employers are concerned with managing those expenditures and focusing their efforts on prevention by encouraging employees to maintain a healthy lifestyle (DiNubile and Sherman 1999; Kielyl and Hodgson 1990). This effort is spilling over into corrections as more facilities are offering wellness and/or fitness programs.

Wellness or fitness programs in law enforcement had previously been limited to police agencies, but they are now being introduced by local and state correctional agencies as well. These wellness/fitness programs initially began as a way to combat correctional officer stress, as the psychological benefits of exercise are clearly established. However, administrators are now incorporating these wellness and fitness programs into their existing stress reduction programs in an effort to improve the overall health of their officers. Evidence of the benefits of wellness and fitness programs were reported in an analysis of a health risk reduction program (McCraty et al. 2003). These investigators evaluated the stress and health levels of correctional officers before and after participating in a three month health risk reduction program. The results of the analysis revealed significant decreases in cholesterol and glucose levels, heart rate, and blood pressure (McCraty et al. 2003). In addition, officers who participated reported significant decreases in feelings of anger, fatigue, hostility, and impatience (McCraty et al. 2003). The results of the study also showed an increase in officer productivity, attitude, and positive perceptions of administrative support (McCraty et al. 2003).

Some corrections departments are developing employee fitness centers within their facilities. The Pennsylvania State Correctional Institution at Houtzdale incorporated a fitness center into the design and construction of the facility. Standberg notes how the Assistant Superintendent at that facility reported that:

> Our fitness program helps keeps the staff healthy, active and in shape. I think it reduces sick leave and anyone more fit feels healthier and feels better about themselves. Its helps in the way they do their jobs. Stress reduction is also a key component (2006).

Recognizing the benefits of these programs, the New Jersey Department of Corrections (NJDC) and the Texas Department of Criminal Justice (TDCJ) are moving beyond stress reduction to healthy lifestyle promotion for officers and their families.

In 2001, for example, the NJDC was awarded funding from the National Institute of Justice to implement a test program that would be part of the federal Corrections and Law Enforcement Family Support Program (CLEFS). The New Jersey CLEFS program consists of four components: in-service training, supervisory training, wellness, and family services (Hepner 2005). Hepner notes how the in-service training component involves teaching "...correctional officers to identify the personal and organization causes and consequences of stress..." and designing "...stress management strategies in order to increase overall health and wellness" (2005). Similarly, the supervisory component involves training supervisors to identify the signs of stress and burnout in officers, teaching supervisors techniques for handling stress and how to communicate those to officers, and teaching supervisors how to refer officers to additional services.

Hepner observes that the goal of the wellness component is to "provide services designed to help employees identify specific risk such as high blood pressure, cholesterol, tobacco use, and to maintain and improve health by increasing physical exercise, improving nutrition and addressing stress" (2005). Finally, the family services component offers the families of officers with an "accurate understanding of corrections work and corrections-related stress, along with suggestions for coping with stress and sources for help" (2005). Altogether, such programs outline how health promotion programs can provide a "win-win" approach for correctional agencies and their staff.

One of the problems with the existing literature on correctional officer stress, burnout, and turnover, is that there is a significant gap when it comes to women working in jails and prisons. Over the past few decades Department of Corrections and local jails have made a considerable investment in recruiting women in officer positions. Griffin (2006) observes that these officers experience stress in much the same manner as males working in corrections. Yet, Lambert (2006), for found that female officers were more likely than their male counterparts to think about quitting. One important question that needs to be addressed is the extent to which individual, organizational, of family factors influence women working in corrections.

Conclusions

When correctional officers are less stressed-out, and more physically fit, they are better able to carry out the goals of the organization. Officers are also less likely to be cynical, angry, and hostile to the inmates. When officers are healthier, they are also more likely to provide better supervision, and this may reduce inmate-on-inmate violence, as well as other disruptive behaviors. As a result, the correctional health status of officers and inmates are inextricably intertwined.

A growing number of correctional agencies have recognized that developing stress reduction and health promotion programs for officers—and their families in some cases—is a sound investment for the agency.

Healthier officers may be less likely to quit, which increases the seniority on a shift, and reduces inmate misconduct. Less employee turnover is also cost effective, as agencies can divert more resources into rehabilitation, rather than constantly recruiting and training new officers. Moreover, higher levels of physical and psychological fitness may enhance the immune systems of these officers, and reduce the likelihood of contracting illness or disease.

Ultimately, a career correctional officer will spend over ten years behind bars—measured in eight or 12 hour shifts. Jails and prisons that provide supportive counseling, critical incident debriefing, stress reduction, and health promotion programs for their employees will benefit in cost savings, the officers will have a happier disposition, and the inmates will have one less challenge. Altogether, these programs are a "win-win" for all involved.

References

Armstrong, Gaylene and Marie L. Griffin. 2004. "Does the Job Matter? Comparing Correlates of Stress Among Treatment and Correctional Staff in Prison." *Journal of Criminal Justice* 32:577-592.

Auerbach, Stephen M., Ben G. Quick, and Philip O. Pegg. 2003. "General Job Stress and Job-Specific Stress in Juvenile Correctional Officers." *Journal of Criminal Justice* 31:25-36.

Camp, Camille G. and George M. Camp. 2002. T*he 2001 Corrections Yearbook: Adult Systems*. Middletown, CT: Criminal Justice Institute, Inc.

Cheek, Francis E. 1984. *Stress Management for Correctional Officers and their Families.* College Park, MD: American Correctional Association.

Cheek, Francis E. and Marie Di Stefano Miller. 1983. "The Experience of Stress for Correction Officers: A Double-Bind Theory of Correctional Stress." *Journal of Criminal Justice* 11:105–120.

Childress, Rebecca, Vincent Talucci, and Jennifer Wood. 1999. "Fighting the Enemy Within: Helping Officers Deal with Stress." *Corrections Today* December:70-72.

Cornelius, Gary F. 1994. *Stressed Out: Strategies for Living and Working with Stress in Corrections.* Laurel, MD: American Correctional Association

Crary, David. "High Stress, Low Glamour: Correctional Officers Struggle with Workplace Strains." Retrieved January 31, 2006 (http://www.policeone.com/pc_print.asp?vid=1000392).

Delprino, Robert P. 2002. *Work and Family Support Services for Correctional Officers and their Family Members: A National Survey.* Washington, DC: United States Department of Justice.

DiNubile, Nicholas, and Carl Sherman. 1999. "Promoting Physical and Fiscal Fitness in the Workplace: A Commentary." *The Physician and Sports Medicine* 27(2).

Duhart, Detis T. 2001. *Violence in the Workplace, 1993-1999.* Washington, DC: Bureau of Justice Statistics.

Eysenck, Hans J. 1993. "Prediction of Cancer and Coronary Heart Disease Mortality by Means of a Personality Inventory: Results of a 15-Year Follow-up Study." *Psychological Reports* 72:499-516.

Finn, Peter. 2000. *Addressing Correctional Officer Stress: Programs and Strategies.* Washington, DC: U. S. Department of Justice.

Gerstein, Lawrence, Charles Topp, and Gregory Correll. 1987. "The Role of the Environment and Person when Predicting Burnout Among Correctional Personnel." *Criminal Justice and Behavior* 14:352–369.

Griffin, Marie L. 2006. "Gender and Stress: A Comparative Assessment of Sources of Stress Among Correctional Officers." *Journal of Contemporary Criminal Justice* 22: 5-25.

Hepner, William. 2005. "Opening Remarks Commission on Safety and Abuse in American's Prisons." Presented at the Commission on Safety and Abuse in America's Prisons Public Hearing #3, November 1, St. Louis, MO.

Ivancevich, John and Michael Matteson. 1980. *Stress and Work: A Managerial Perspective.* Dallas, TX: Scott, Foresman and Company.

Jette, Maurice and Kenneth Sidney. 1991. "The Benefits and Challenges of a Fitness and Lifestyle Enhancement Program for Correctional Officers." *Canadian Journal of Public Health* 82:46-51.

Keinan, Giora, and Ayala Malach-Pines. 2007. "Stress and Burnout Among Prison Personnel: Sources, Outcomes, and Intervention Strategies." *Criminal Justice and Behavior* 34: 380-398.

Kielyl, Julia and George Hodgson. 1990. "Stress in the Prison Service: The Benefits of Exercise Programs." *Human Relations* 43:551-572.

Lambert, Eric G. 2006. "I Want to Leave: A Test of a Model of Turnover Intent Among Correctional Staff." *Applied Psychology in Criminal Justice* 2: 57-83.

Lindquist, Charles and John Whitehead. 1986. "Burnout, Job Stress and Job Satisfaction among Southern Correctional Officers: Perceptions and Causal Factors." *Journal of Offender Counseling, Services and Rehabilitation* 10:5-26.

Lipskey, Michael. 1980. *Street-level Bureaucracy*. New York: Russell Sage.

Lombardo, Luicen X. 1989. Guards Imprisoned: Correctional Officers at Work. New York: Elsevier.

Marston, J. L. 1993. "Stress and Stressors: Inmate and Staff Perceptions." *American Jails* 7(4):21-30.

Maslach, Christina and Susan E. Jackson. 1981. "The Measurement of Experienced Burnout." *Journal of Occupational Behavior* 2:99-113.

McCraty, Rollin, Mike Atkinson, Lee Lipsenthal, and Lourdes Arguelles. 2003. "Impact of the Power to Change Performance Program on Stress and Health Risks in Correctional Officers." Report No. 03-017. Boulder Creek, CA: HeartMath Research Center.

McShane, Marilyn D. and Frank P. Williams III. 1993. *The Management of Correctional Institutions.* Independence, KY: Garland.

National Institute of Corrections. 1996. *Managing Staff: Corrections Most Valuable Resource*. Washington, DC: U. S. Department of Justice.

Paoline, Eugene A., Eric G. Lambert and Nancy Lynne Hogan. 2006. "A Calm and Happy Keeper of the Keys: The Impact of ACA Views, Relations with Coworkers, and Policy Views on the Job Stress and Job Satisfaction of Correctional Staff." *The Prison Journal* 86: 182-205.

Pearlin, Leonard I. 1989. "The Sociological Study of Stress." *Journal of Health and Social Behavior* 30:241–256.
Petersilia, Joan. 2006. *Understanding California Corrections.* Berkeley, CA: California Policy Research Center.
Ray, Gayle. 2001. "The Hidden Emotions Behind a Badge." *Corrections Today* October:98-105.
Richards, Stephen C. 2003. "My Journal through the Federal Bureau of Prisons." Pp. 120-149 in *Convict Criminology,* edited by J. I. Ross and S.C. Richards. Belmont, CA: Thompson.
Schrag, Clarence. 1961. "Some Foundations for a Theory of Correction." Pp. 100-119 in *The Prison: Studies in Institutional Organization and Change,* edited by D. R. Cressey. New York: Holt, Rinehart and Winston.
Shamir, Boas and Amos Drory. 1982. "Some Correlates of Prison Guards' Beliefs." *Criminal Justice and Behavior* 8:233-249.
Slate, Risdon N., Ronald E. Vogel and W.Wesley Johnson. 2001. "To Quit or Not to Quit: Perceptions of Participation in Correction Decision Making and the Impact of Organizational Stress." *Corrections Management Quarterly* 5:68–78.
Stack, Steven J. and Olga Tsoudis. 1997. "Suicide Risk among Correctional Officers: A Logistic Regression Analysis." *Archives of Suicide Research* 3(3):183-186.
Strandberg, Keith. "Fitness for Corrections." Sports Art Fitness. Retrived January 31, 2006 (http://www.sportsartfitness.com/fitness_corrections.php).
Triplett, Ruth, Janet L. Mullings and Kathryn E. Scarborough. 1996. "Work Related Stress and Coping among Correctional Officers: Implications from Organizational Literature." *Journal of Criminal Justice* 24:291–308.
Van Voorhis, Patricia, Francis T. Cullen, Bruce G. Link and Nancy T. Wolfe. 1991. "The Impact of Race and Gender on Correctional Officers' Orientation to the Integrated Environment." *Journal of Research in Crime and Delinquency* 28:472–500.
Walters, Stephen. 1988. "Correctional Officers' Perceptions of Powerlessness." *Journal of Crime and Justice* 11:47–59.
Walters, Stephen. 1991. "Alienation and the Correctional Officer: A Multivariate Analysis." *American Journal of Criminal Justice* 16:50–62.
Webb, Gary, and David Morris. 2002. "Working as a Prison Guard." Pp. 69-83 in *Exploring Corrections,* edited by T. Gray. Massachusetts: Allyn & Bacon.
Wells, Doris. 2003. "Reducing Stress for Officers and their Families." *Corrections Today* April: 24-25.
Zupan, Linda. 2002. "The Persistent Problems Plaguing Modern Jails." Pp. 37-63 in *Exploring Corrections,* edited by T. Gray. Massachusetts: Allyn & Bacon.

CHAPTER THIRTEEN

Opportunities for Change in Correctional Health

Rick Ruddell and Mark Tomita

During the week of May 23, 2006, some 1,300 prisoners and 14 staff members in eleven California state prisons became sick from a pathogen known as campylobacter—a bacterium that is found in contaminated food or water. Correctional and public health officials responded to the outbreak, and within a week or so, the incident passed. No staff or inmates died. Public health officials attributed the cause of the illness to bacteria in the milk supply. Such outbreaks regularly occur; for example on one occasion in 1996, one hundred staff and inmates within a juvenile hall became sick after eating a Thanksgiving meal (Parikh et al. 1997) and the Pennsylvania prison system experienced an outbreak of tuberculosis that infected several hundred inmates (*Austin v. Pennsylvania Department of Corrections*).

The conditions within jails or prisons—close confinement of inmates who may have suppressed immune systems—are ideal for the transmission of disease. One might speculate that the public health officials in California took a deep breath of relief that the recent illness was not severe acute respiratory syndrome (SARS) or the H5N1 avian bird flu that have very high rates of mortality. A virulent strain of influenza could move through a prison system in a short period of time (Schwartz 2006). In the 1918 influenza pandemic, one of the early sites for the virus was the Portsmouth naval brig, and later at least 500 inmates at San Quentin contracted this illness (Stanley 1919). While jails and prisons have avoided such misfortune, reading through this volume has probably convinced the reader that many correctional facilities have often been just one step away from disaster. To date correctional stakeholders (including staff and inmates) have been fortunate that the prevalence of communicable diseases has been held at current rates, as things could be much worse. Such is a credit to the efforts of correctional medical care staff (including infection-control nurses who work within larger prison systems) who have worked with public heath officials to isolate and treat these diseases. Such actions underscore the importance of correctional medical care, not only for disasters, but to respond to the day-to-day health care needs of the inmates.

Correctional administrators have to overcome a number of challenges, and the authors in this volume have highlighted many of the barriers to providing health care in prisons. Goldstein (2005) in testimony to the Commission on Safety and Abuse in America's Prisons outlined seven factors responsible for a lack of appropriate medical care:

- Healthcare is not a Priority
- Lack of Medical Autonomy
- Lack of Appropriate Funding and Resources
- Lack of Qualified Staff
- Lack of Adequate Space
- Attitude of Medical Staff
- Overcrowding

The first issue shapes all the others. If correctional health care was a priority, the contributors wouldn't have had enough material to write this book. The reality, however, is that correctional heath care has become a birth to death enterprise, and correctional administrators struggle with the best way to respond to infants born in custody, or what action to take when an elderly inmate is dying—do correctional officials return them to the community on a compassionate release, confine them in a hospice, or let them die in a prison hospital unit?

When providing appropriate health care in juvenile facilities or adult jails and prisons becomes a priority, governments will provide suitable funding to correctional administrators, who in turn, will ensure that qualified staff are hired, medical facilities constructed, supplied and maintained to NCCHC standards, and inmates treated with care and compassion. For now, in many institutions, however, the opposite is true. Gibbons and Katzenbach notes "In California, where control of health care in state prisons has been ceded to a federal judge, one prisoner was dying needlessly from medical malpractice or neglect every six to seven days as recently as October 2005" (2006:38). If this statistic is an accurate reflection of the national landscape, many more prisoners will die this year from factors such as benign neglect, medical misadventure, and malpractice.

One of the barriers to providing appropriate care to prison inmates is the anger that people harbor towards offenders, which has made us consider them as non-deserving at best, and monstrous at worst. While acknowledging that some offenders have been involved in horrible crimes, we must also remember that approximately one-half of prison inmates today were sentenced for committing non-violent offenses. The political nature of punishment, however, has contributed to an atmosphere where being "tough on crime" means that few politicians will publicly advocate for livable, rehabilitative, or safe jail or prison conditions.

Ultimately, correctional administrators must balance a number of competing goals. The foremost is to ensure the safety of the community, and the facility: by making certain that inmates don't escape and are not engaged in any misconduct while incarcerated. To our knowledge, few correctional administrators have been promoted on the basis of providing top-notch medical services, but some have been fired after an inmate escapes or a riot occurs. As a result, the core goal of correctional administrators is security and control and they evaluate every issue based on an assessment of risk (the 'worst case scenario').

A second goal of correctional administrators is to operate their facilities effectively and efficiently: in other words, to come in under budget and maintain the public's confidence. Jails and prisons are one of the few enterprises that consider "no news to be good news." As a result, correctional officials tend to operate "below the radar" whenever possible (few actively 'court' the media) and place a priority on services that enhance the internal efficiency of the organization, especially as it relates to safety and security. Providing medical care is an afterthought in many facilities and health care staff become important only after there is an emergency. The previous chapters, however, have illustrated how correctional health has an impact upon community health.

While many are apathetic towards the plight of prisoners, we have to remember that correctional and community health are inextricably intertwined: what happens in corrections will soon have an effect on the community. Given this reality one important question is how to convince policy-makers to make a better investment in correctional care.

Barriers to Prevention, Screening, and Treatment

The NCCHC has outlined four barriers to providing appropriate correctional health care: a lack of leadership, logistical barriers, limited resources, and correctional policies (2002:xiv). How do we get correctional administrators to shift their priority from safety and security to rehabilitation? In our opinion, the foundation for positive change rests with the promotion of good physical and psychological health. Like anything else, this will require policy-makers to reward administrators for providing correctional programs that are more rehabilitative, including offering appropriate health care to the inmates. This will not be an easy transition, as these changes involve some risk and increased correctional costs. Recent studies, however, indicate that the public generally supports offender rehabilitation (Applegate and King Davis 2005). One important policy question is: If taxpayers are spending $60.8 billion dollars a year on corrections (Hughes 2006), should they expect a better return on this investment beyond simply warehousing offenders, and providing nothing more than "three hots and a cot"?[1]

Most juvenile hall superintendents, jail commanders, and prison wardens, focus their attention on the internal operations of their facilities. As a result, correctional administrators have sometimes failed to establish or nurture long-term collaborations with community health care organizations. This issue is particularly troubling given that the same governments often fund both agencies: hence, the county jail receives funding from local governments, as does the public health agency. If the respective heads of these agencies see their role as complimentary, it enables more effective collaboration: after all the same population is often served by both organizations.

Logistical barriers, on the other hand, refer to problems in the marriage of corrections and medical care. The security within a facility, for instance, sometimes acts as a barrier to providing appropriate care. Jails and prisons are environments where medications and medical equipment must be tightly controlled, and as outlined in Chapter 1, some inmates cannot have unrestricted access to assistive devices, or potentially life-saving medications (such as an epipen [preloaded injector for epinephrine], or inhalers). In addition, medical care staff members have to be vigilant that inmates aren't attempting to manipulate them. Cornelius reported how a prisoner serving a term of life imprisonment for the murder of his wife faked paralysis and was confined to a wheelchair for almost a decade:

> While on a transport for x-rays of a suspected broken ankle, he got out of his wheelchair for the first time in seven years, overpowered the officer and took his weapon....the prison superintendent said "We had never seen him walk" (2001:45).

In an environment where everything is scarce, inmates will sometimes attempt to manipulate medical or correctional staff in order to make their time in jail or prison more enjoyable.

The third obstruction to providing correctional medical care is limited resources. All correctional operations are limited by financial constraints. Most correctional spending is for security and control—approximately 70 to 80 percent of budget is typically earmarked for salaries—and historically less than five percent of correctional budgets have been spent on rehabilitation. Even when administrators are successful in getting funding for correctional health care, many facilities are hamstrung by their physical structure. Jails and prisons tend to have a long service life and Ruddell and Mays (2007) found that the average age of small jails was over 40 years, and that jails built in the early 1800s were still in operation two centuries later. Architects fifty years ago never foresaw the need for sinks in examination rooms, extensive drug formularies, the space required for medical testing equipment, classrooms for health promotion, employee wellness centers, mental health units or providing hospice care. Creating space for medical care was an afterthought, and today many operations are restricted by this limitation.

The last barrier to providing effective evaluation and care are the policies of the correctional facilities. The NCCHC outlines these practices as:

> failure to specify minimum levels of required care in contracts with private health care vendors, delays caused by the need to escort inmates to medical treatment, poor communication between public health agencies and prisons and jails, and lack of adequate clinical guidelines (2002:xiv).

Today's managers are apt to have much more in-depth knowledge of medical care issues, especially given that medical care is the number one source of inmate litigation (Schlanger 2003).

Health care staff who work within jails and prisons are often well-meaning professionals. Puerini and Shelton (2006) outlined how prison physicians are often required to spend much of their time screening inmates for various special diets, work assignments, or other comforts. The concern is that time spent approving applications for extra blankets, inserts for shoes or sunscreen is time taken away from inmates who are legitimately ill. In an under-funded environment physicians are forced to establish priorities, and they want to invest their time and energies on cases where they can make a difference.

In order to deter inmates from seeking unnecessary treatment, a number of jurisdictions have implemented "user fees" (co-payments), in order to discourage all but the most serious cases. On this, Sheriff Rick Walter from Scott County, Missouri observes "Once the inmates found out they had to pay, they quit complaining about being sick" (Freeze 2006). These user fees were first introduced about a decade ago, and wherever they are implemented, the number of sick calls decreases. Stana (2000) found that enacting these polices reduces physician visits by 16 to 50 percent.

Although the actual user fee might be low by some standards (the California state prison fee was $2.00 in 2005) this figure represents a considerable cost in the inmate economy where a prisoner might only earn a few dollars a week. As a result, anecdotal accounts from prisoners suggest that some have foregone treatment because of these fees; but we question whether this may create a greater long-term health care cost later in their sentence. Gibbons and Katzenbach reported that a CDC study of an MRSA outbreak found "co-payments were singled out as a significant contributor to the spread of these serious and aggressive skin infections because they discouraged prisoners from seeking care" (2006:48).

Deterring physician visits broaches the larger problem of "pay now or pay later." Jail and prison administrators sometimes rely on temporary and band aide style solutions to address serious medical problems, hoping that the inmate will be discharged before his or her health worsens. While the prison might not have an obligation to provide preventative health care, it may be in the system's best interest as a long-term cost-saving measure. Since taxpayers are going to be stuck with the burden in either case—because most prisoners are indigent—it makes good economic sense to tackle these medical problems while they are relatively minor, and while the inmate's residence is stable.

Correctional Staff

The primary goal of adult corrections is security and control. Given this reality, one must ask the following question: how does an agency recruit (and retain) professional medical staff and correctional officers who are committed to making a significant difference in the lives of offenders? While such characteristics are a cornerstone of the juvenile justice system, it is more difficult to work towards offender rehabilitation in adult corrections. Many staff members start out with the best of intentions and quickly become burned-out, cynical, and pessimistic. Durham (1994) describes how American corrections have been driven by crisis and reform. Officers become cynical when a reorganization or reform lasts only as long as the Commissioner of Corrections (or jail commander; juvenile hall superintendent), and a new philosophy, practice, or reform is promoted by the incoming management. It is no wonder that correctional officers often take a "wait and see" attitude towards reformers. As a result, many policy analysts suggest that officers undermine positive changes, and while this certainly occurs, managers have to convince their staff that reforms will be sustained.

One of the reasons a chapter on the health of correctional officers was included acknowledges the difficulties in surviving long-term correctional careers. Staff members are as confined as the inmates, and constantly confronting prisoner behaviors, over the long-term, can have a significant impact upon an individual's outlook. In some cases, correctional officers become so disgruntled that they engage in unethical (and sometimes illegal) behaviors that actively work against inmate interests. While the increasing professionalism of correctional officers has reduced this inappropriate conduct (in conjunction with better selection, training and the threat of litigation) it still exists.

As previously mentioned, Vaughn and Smith (1999) outlined how officers and medical care staff have engaged in the ill-treatment or torture of offenders—what they called "penal harm medicine." Using self-reported information from jail inmates they found that some staff used medical care to humiliate prisoners, withheld medical care, exposed prisoners to temperature extremes and sleep deprivation, used dental care as a method of ill-treatment and torture, and falsified prisoner's medical records. In organizations where such acts occur, there are significant lapses in agency oversight as well as the retention of problem employees. While prisoners might have a motive for exaggerating their mistreatment, such examples serve as strong warning signs that something is amiss.

In a response to Vaughn and Smith (1999), Ken Kerle and colleagues argue that correctional health care has come a long way in the past several decades, and outline a number of indicators of success, including; reductions in correctional suicides, and note that, "of the nearly 500 lawsuits regarding health care.....only six or seven involved jails accredited by the AMA/ACA/NCCHC. Only one verdict went against the jail" (1999 :905). Thus, correctional agencies that engage in voluntary accreditation might be sending a powerful signal to staff members about the importance of correctional health care (see Paoline, Lambert and Hogan 2006). Ultimately the indicators outlined through this book—decreasing inmate deaths due to AIDS, suicide, and violence—are all signs that conditions within American jails and prisons have improved.

In some cases, persons who are unqualified to practice medicine or nursing anywhere else are working in correctional facilities. Gibbons and Katzenbach reported that:

> some states allow doctors who have scars on their professional records to practice under a special license that restricts their work to prison and jails. All too often correctional health care is being provided by doctors, nurses, and others who could not find employment elsewhere due to restrictions on their licensees or for other reasons (2006: 41).

Such accounts reduce our faith in correctional medical care. But, correctional administrators have also alienated the qualified medical care professionals working for them. Warren outlined how the California Department of Corrections and Rehabilitation was chronically late in paying medical specialists and that, "Some of the doctors have not been paid in four years. Some of their contracts have lapsed. And some who deliver cardiology, radiology and a wide range of other services to prisoners are no longer responding when called" (2006:1).

According to Useem and Piehl (2006), positive changes in corrections must start at the top. In order to operate jails and prisons more effectively, these agencies are more selective in recruiting staff members, officers are better-trained and more professional, and often see corrections as a long-term career. In part, some of these changes are due to higher wages, and decreased risk. Safer institutions for inmates are safer for staff as well. In California, for example, between 1985 and 2007, one correctional officer was killed on the job as a result of an assault. While not trying to minimize the sacrifice of the officer, when one considers that there are some 34,500 California correctional officers, the odds of being killed on the job are slim indeed. There is the very real possibility, however, that officers will be injured on the job due to assaults, or contract a communicable disease in their career.

Moving Towards Health Promotion in Corrections

Some of the contributors to this volume have written about health promotion activities in correctional settings. Inmates are a captive audience, and health educators are ideally situated to develop interventions to enhance the inmate health. The Joint Committee on Health Education Terminology defines health promotion as the "aggregate of all purposeful activities, designed to improve personal and public health through a combination of strategies, including the competent implementation of behavioral change strategies, health education, and health protection measures" (1991: 101). From a health promotion perspective, juvenile halls, jails, and prisons, are nothing more than small communities that are structurally contained, and where services are provided by health- and medically-related practitioners to a group of community members with few positive ties to each other. Health promotion in correctional facilities, then, is a health service process encompassing all of the activities designed to prevent residents from dying or becoming diseased or disabled, or to limit the progression of disease or disability without the use of medical therapies.

Unfortunately, the task of developing health promotion activities usually is given to correctional administrators and local health officers who are usually not health promotion professionals. Instead, most health officers are physicians, and the development of health promotion policy is not a traditional role of that discipline. Rather, the health promotion professional in collaboration with an organizing committee should be responsible for the development of goals and intervention programs. Without such motivation, programs will neither be sustainable nor effective. Health promotion must rely upon the motivation within the community to act as a driving force for change, and the creation of an environment for the development and maintenance of healthy values, attitudes, and behaviors.

This motivation from the community is not usually a primary concern when delivering traditional, top-down medical services; thus, the culture of the facility will need to change. Professionals and other staff will need to be educated about the process of health promotion and how it differs with medicine. Final approval, of course, will have to come from the facility administrator and director of health services, but the content of the policies and procedures should be written by health promotion professionals in collaboration with stakeholders.

There are several other challenges that make health promotion in correctional facilities a difficult proposition. The first problem is the transient nature of the population. Some residents—especially jail inmates or residents of a juvenile hall—may live within the correctional community for only a day or two. According to the Corrections Standards Authority (2007), the average length of stay in California jails was about 20 days in 2006. This is a very short period to engage a new resident in health promotion programming, especially when we consider that the individual will need a certain length of time to adjust to the new environment and may not be receptive during this period to health promotion programming.

Some prison inmates, by contrast, may reside in their community for life without the possibility of returning to society. As a result, health promotion programs will have to be tailored for specific populations based on the length of stay, and health educators have to be realistic about what can be accomplished. This means that comprehensive programming will not take place with populations that might only be held for a day or two. Still, we have to acknowledge that detention in a juvenile facility or jail is a time when uncertainty and motivation to make changes is high. Consequently, some inmates may be very receptive to short-term interventions, although it may be difficult to sustain this motivation to change once the arrestee returns to the community.

A second limitation of the health education model is the prevalence of mental illness in correctional populations (Hanser 2007; James and Glaze 2006). Health promotion program models are typically designed for well populations without serious mental health problems. Programming for persons with mental illnesses would be easier in a specialized mental health unit than in the general population of the correctional facility because the population characteristics are known, and the staff and other professionals are specially trained to deal with these individuals. In correctional facilities, it is difficult to classify persons with mentally illness according to their learning styles, and other psychological and social characteristics that may improve success of a health promotion program.

The third problem is the challenge of developing and delivering programming for individuals who lack normative values, attitudes, and behaviors. That is the reason for their incarceration. Some inmates may develop an "oppositional culture" that actually promotes anti-social goals (Cornelius 2001), and gang members might actively try to undermine the rehabilitative program of an institution. Health promotion models are not designed for this population, so staff implementing these programs have to develop strategies that acknowledge the resistance within this high-risk population.

Another obstacle that has to be overcome in juvenile halls, jails, and prisons is that correctional officers might not support the implementation of these programs. Lin (2000) outlines how correctional officers have actively undermined or sabotaged reforms. As a result, these stakeholders have to be engaged from the beginning. It may be helpful for the advocate of health promotion to tie the health promotion efforts with the self-interests of the correctional officers (e.g., by providing strategies for the inmates to reduce the spread of HIV/AIDS, the risk is reduced to correctional officers as well).

Given these challenges, is it feasible to provide health promotion activities in correctional facilities? Throughout this volume, the contributors have outlined very clearly that change in corrections is often slow, and reforms are often forced by litigation rather than the best interests of the correctional population. Changing the culture of the correctional system to include health promotion will not be easy. Administrators, politicians, as well as health and medical professionals must be educated about the differences between health promotion and medical services, and they must be motivated to change the existing structure of health services. The current correctional approach to care in most facilities is based on the medical model without a complementary health promotion model.

In recent years, correctional administrators have introduced policies that will increase long-term inmate health and decrease costs. One of the most significant is the ban on tobacco in most jails and prisons. Kentucky recently banned tobacco use, and Alford notes how even a politician who "opposed anti-smoking initiatives...finds no fault with the prison's no-tobacco policy...as a tough-on-criminals initiative" (2006:4). These policies have made tobacco the top contraband item in many facilities, replacing narcotics (Porter 2005).

Correctional meals have always been high in fat and starch. In response to this nutritional challenge, several county jails have reduced the size of portions for inmate meals, and coffee has been eliminated in many jurisdictions (although in most places inmates have access to beverages and snacks at the commissary, if they have funds to purchase these goods). Some prison systems have introduced more nutritious meals, including providing inmates with a greater number of fruits and vegetables. Mandeville interviewed correctional officials in Utah and found that, "male inmates in Utah gain an average of 34 pounds within their first year of incarceration, while their female counterparts add on an average of 17 pounds" (2006:1). In some places, prisons have introduced more nutritionally sound diets and offer fitness programs (Baron 2006). The correctional administrators who develop these interventions are not doing so to be "soft on criminals." Instead, they realize that healthier inmates represent a long-term reduction in health care costs. These programs don't have to be costly as many prison systems grow their own fruits and vegetables.

A number of preventative interventions—such as the distribution of bleach and condoms, as well as needle exchange programs—were examined in Chapter 4. These programs tend to be controversial. Hence while they have been introduced in Australian, Canadian and European prisons, opposition to introducing such programs still exists in the United States. By distributing condoms, bleach (for cleaning needles), and syringes we are giving tacit approval to behavior that is undesirable or illegal. In addition, bleach and needles can be used as weapons. Yet, reports from other countries suggest that inmates don't misuse these items, and they are successful in reducing the transmission of communicable disease (MacDonald 2005).

We argue that health promotion is a necessary and complementary health service in correctional facilities. The process complements medicine and other clinical services, and helps to prevent or slow the progression of disease, disability, and death. The motivation to change an unhealthy to a healthy correctional population, however, must come from within the system and from the community. As a result, one of the most important parts of the health promotion process is to form organizing committees composed of key stakeholders, including; prisoners, staff, and community residents and leaders living in the neighborhoods outside of the correctional facility. These committees can serve as the driving force behind the program and will improve the likelihood of success. Ultimately, much can be gained through the implementation of a health promotion model, and the benefits of preventing disease and disability far outweigh the costs.

Evidenced-Based Corrections

Another theme that has been repeated throughout this book is the growing importance of evidence-based corrections. Despite the fact that we spend some $60.8 billion dollars funding local, state and federal corrections (Hughes 2006), we have very little idea of "what works" (what interventions are effective), and who is most likely to benefit from this treatment (MacKenzie 2006). Private businesses fully understand the bottom line and the fact that many jail and prison systems do not have a grasp of who is most likely to benefit from correctional interventions (both rehabilitative and medical) is a horrible indictment of these systems. As a result, we have to invest more resources on researching programmatic interventions that have been demonstrated to work with correctional populations, and evaluate whether they can be exported to other institutions.

Latessa, Cullen and Gendreau (2002) contend that much of what has been done in corrections in the past several decades is based on "quackery," and that rehabilitative, educational, and vocational programs have often been delivered on the basis of questionable theories of crime. Rehabilitation should start on a foundation of positive physical and psychological health and a review of the contributions to this book suggests that good health is the cornerstone of making other positive attitudinal or behavioral changes. When one is suffering from chronic pain, for example, it is difficult to concentrate on learning how to program a computer, focus on addictions education, or improve their social skills.

Latessa and colleagues are critical of the failure to use evidence from research in the development of rehabilitative interventions. The rationale is simple—interventions of any sort are expensive—and it makes little sense to continue implementing programs that are not effective or actually have a negative effect. In addition, if some treatments aren't successful with any population, then we are setting up inmates to fail. Chapters 7 and 9 outlined that in the areas of addictions and mental health, for instance, funding agencies are now demanding that program administrators demonstrate the effectiveness of their programs. Treatment staff, however, are often reluctant to let someone evaluate their programs, and this is a tragedy, because out there somewhere may be interventions that can be inexpensively implemented and are effective with a broad range of offenders.

There is increasing use of the term evidence-based in the medical literature as well. In the NCCHC report on the health status of jail and prison inmates they raise the issue of, "interventions for which there is strong, and in many cases overwhelming, scientific evidence of the therapeutic effectiveness" (2002: iii). By better understanding the efficacy of different interventions, we can also develop better cost-benefit analyses. The NCCHC (2002) found that universal screening for syphilis, gonorrhea and Chlamydia as well as hypertension and diabetes are cost-effective correctional interventions. It is important that we start considering correctional facilities as a key component in the delivery of community health care. Because the populations within these facilities are at high-risk for medical problems, early detection and intervention are strategies that make good economic sense.

A jail inmate or prisoner in a state or federal facility has very few options when it comes to medical care. In the preceding pages a number of challenges to providing appropriate health care were outlined, including the perception that medical services are a peripheral interest, levels of funding, as well as recruiting and retaining qualified medical care staff. Correctional medical care is good in some institutions, haphazard in others, and dangerous in some places. Given these realities, many inmates have taken it upon themselves to enhance their own physical and psychological health.

Guerilla Health Care

We can learn a lot about medical care from correctional health care staff, scholars, and correctional officers. But we can also learn from the experiences of prison inmates. There is a growing body of research and commentary about prison life. This work can improve our understanding of medical care as well. A number of prisoners who served their sentences, and finished a post-graduate education, have become academics and label themselves "convict criminologists." These scholars have shared some important insights into the inmate subculture.

In an influential statement, Murphy (2003:257-259), a former federal prisoner turned-academic, outlined what he calls "guerilla health care techniques" to survive prison. He argues that formal prison health care is rationed and is in scarce supply for the average inmate. In order to survive, health-conscious inmates have adopted four different approaches to maintaining well-being, and these include: the walker, the health nut, the weight lifter, and the maintenance man. The alternative to staying healthy is what Murphy calls the sessile state: forgetting about health, getting little or no exercise and adopting an apathetic attitude. The walker, health nut, weight lifter and maintenance man aim to physically and mentally survive prison, and the following paragraphs outline some of their characteristics.

As the name implies, the walker keeps physically active by walking as much as they can, up to several hours a day. The weight lifter, by contrast, is becoming an obsolete classification since weights have been removed from many jails and prisons. Since prisoners are resourceful, many still adhere to exercise regimens that increase their strength and conditioning without weights. Murphy observes how the health nut survives on "nutrition and vitamins for health maintenance. These inmates practically exist on fruits and vegetables purchased on the prison black market" (2003:257).

Last, Murphy (2003) describes the maintenance man, a prisoner who searches for physical and psychological self-improvement. Prison is an austere environment and maintenance men make the most of a bad situation. These inmates have adopted a holistic approach to health care—through a combination of exercise, finding whatever nutritious food that the prison can provide—and "working the system" so that they can access as many opportunities as they can. One example of a maintenance man is Michael Santos, a federal prisoner who was sentenced to a 45-year prison term for his involvement in the drug trade.

Santos (2003) has written four books about his journey from a naïve 22-year old non-violent first-time offender (a 'fish' in many prison systems) to a middle-aged prisoner awaiting release. These books enlighten the reader about what to expect from life within a federal prison, including the type of health care inmates receive. Santos observes that health care is not only rationed, but that minor complaints are overlooked, and serious illnesses are only acted upon after the physicians can no longer ignore the problem. Inmates who require an elective surgery may be on a waiting list for years, and living in discomfort the entire time.

Ultimately, we can learn much from these inmates, but the key lesson is once sentenced to a term of incarceration, a prisoner is often "on their own." To survive rationed health care, poor diets, cynical or abusive officers or staff, the ever-present threat of violence or communicable disease, and the discouragement of being locked up, an inmate has to summon all of their internal and external resources, and develop a plan for healthy living. To ignore self-reliance in prison is to surrender to the very real possibility of chronic disease.

Recent evidence suggests that some inmates are very successful in their pursuits of a healthy lifestyle. A federal study of deaths in state prisons found that rates of mortality for some age groups are less than their community counterparts (Mumola 2007). Moreover, Mumola also reported that the mortality rate for African Americans in prison was some 57 percent less than African Americans living in the community (2007: 3). Follow up studies might shed some additional light on whether this finding is also true of jails and federal prisons.

Conclusions

There are a number of challenges that correctional systems still need to confront. Clear and Cole have outlined five distinct issues that deserve some special attention, and these include: 1) Corrections lacks a clear mission, 2) Corrections requires methods that match the organizational goals, 3) Corrections cannot influence its own fate, 4) Corrections requires good personnel, and 5) Costs are increasing (2003:538-543). A review of this book reveals that all of these dilemmas have shaped correctional health care—but that the lack of a clear mission is the factor that drives all others. Up until the 1970s the stated purpose of American corrections was offender rehabilitation. While there is some dispute whether we actually delivered on this goal, the nature of imprisonment shifted to punishment, retribution, deterrence, and incapacitation.

If the guiding philosophy of a correctional system is punishment, then we might expect that few people will find correctional health to be an important issue. Instead, the talk will center on statements such as, "If you do the crime, you can do the time" a sentiment heard in many facilities, and from many inmates. Yet, there seems to be an increasing interest in correctional rehabilitation in recent years. With some 2.3 million Americans behind bars, and hundreds of thousands of prisoners serving terms of life imprisonment on the "installment plan" both the public and policymakers are increasingly questioning whether there is a better way to ensure public safety. Each re-admission to jail or prison is an indictment on the correctional system's ability to correct an offender.

One predicament is the number of stakeholders—from politicians, associations of correctional officers, families of offenders, litigious attorneys, rural counties that lobby prison systems to build facilities in their communities, and the firms that supply facilities with goods and services—involved in the delivery of American corrections, and each have an agenda. With the exception of the inmates and their families, most of these stakeholders don't really want much change. Decreasing correctional populations threatens the self-interests of these groups.

This brings us to another challenge: the fact that of the entire criminal justice system (law enforcement, courts, and corrections), corrections is the element that is least able to control its fate. The police and courts are more autonomous, and the police can modify their workloads by selective enforcement. Courts, on the other hand, can also regulate their workloads through delays and dismissals. In some jurisdictions these agencies can increase revenue (e.g., writing more tickets) or impose surcharges to help pay for their operations. A correctional facility, however, is entirely at the mercy of the activities of both the police and courts. A jail cannot turn away arrestees, and sometimes can't let out offenders in response to demand (although exceptions exist). Prisons also have to accept the next bus load of inmates even if they have no beds for them. Unlike the police or courts, corrections has fewer sources of funding, and has few ways of extracting additional funds from its clientele, who are mostly impoverished in the first place.[2]

Incarcerating people can be very expensive. Imposing a 25-year sentence on a "third-striker" represents a multi-million dollar investment in some states (counting inflation and increasing health care costs as a prisoner ages). These costs are leading many scholars and public policy analysts to question whether this is an appropriate way to sanction offenders, and whether prison is the most effective solution to the problem of crime. While some offenders need to be imprisoned to ensure public safety, we might not be gaining much of an economic benefit by imposing lengthy prison terms on drug or property offenders. In 2002, for instance, the average federal prison sentence for drug possession was

79 months, while the average term of imprisonment for a homicide offender was 109 months (Durose and Langan 2004). A sentence for a drug offender, in some jurisdictions, has become almost the same as a violent criminal.

A necessary first step in developing successful health care interventions (including health education or health promotion) is to identify the boundaries of the topic, and this volume has defined the problem, and the authors have highlighted some best practices that correctional health care providers have used to respond to the problems of addictions, mental health, communicable disease, special needs populations (such as women, juveniles and the elderly), suicide and violence reduction, and dental care. There are some issues that the contributors did not address, such as the ethical questions about corrections departments paying for sex-change medications or operations, providing medical services to death row inmates (they tend to receive less care than their counterparts in the general inmate population), or the question of giving organ transplants to prisoners who might never be released from prison. While such issues sometimes appear on the news, they tend to distract us from the most pressing issue in correctional medicine, the day-to-day care of inmates.

It is unlikely that correctional administrators will soon introduce comprehensive health promotion interventions, provide high levels of addictions treatment, respond to the large numbers of persons with mental illness, or address the special needs of inmates. Instead, most change in U.S. correctional medical care has come about because of lawsuits. Schlanger (2003) outlined how medical care was the number one source of correctional litigation in her survey of jails and prisons. Yet, litigation doesn't have to be the "end of the world" for correctional policy-makers. In fact, Schlanger (2003) found that some of the reforms that came from prisoner lawsuits were viewed as positive by the administrators who responded to her survey.

Providing correctional medical and health care is a challenge, but is also an opportunity for positive change. If we integrate the medical services in juvenile halls, jails, and prisons with those provided by community health agencies we can improve community health care. One important component is to form a bridge between corrections and the community. We have to start focusing on prisoner reentry and actually help inmates make a better transition into the community. When inmates fail (are re-arrested or violate the conditions of their release), everybody's safety has been jeopardized.

As a result, we challenge legislators and policy-makers to be smart on crime. Each year, federal and state officials discharge some 650,000 inmates from the prisons to our communities (Office of Justice Programs 2007), and providing basic health education, preventative health care, and correctional facilities that are as free of violence as possible is an important long-term investment in community health. Travis (2005) outlines how the "iron law of corrections" is that with the exception of the few inmates who actually die in prison, some 98 percent return to their communities. Subsequently, these prison inmates become our neighbors. Therefore it is in everybody's best interest when these individuals return to the community as healthy, sane, and well-adjusted citizens.

Endnotes

1. Few jails or prisons offer more than one hot meal per day, and in many cases, don't guarantee a cot. Inmates in overcrowded facilities are given a mattress and are expected to sleep on the floors of offices, gyms, and similar spaces.
2. Correctional agencies do however, extract money from their inmates by sharing in the profits of collect calls, selling commissary items to inmates, setting "user fees" on health services, and many jails are now charging inmates (at least the middle class ones) for the cost of housing.

References

Alford, Roger. 2006. "Prison Smokers Steaming: Total Ban on Tobacco Elevates Tension." *Kentucky Enquirer*. May 8, 2006.

Applegate, Brandon and Robin King Davis. 2005. "Examining Public Support for "Correcting" Offenders." *Corrections Today* 67:94,102.

Austin et a. v. Pennsylvania Department of Corrections, __ F. Suppl., ____ (E.D. PA., January 17, 1995), 1995 WL 65458.

Baron, Joan. 2006. "Women's Prison: Goodbye Macaroni, Hello Broccoli." *Casper Star Tribune*, January 17, 2006.

Clear, Todd R. and George F. Cole. 2003. *American Corrections.* Belmont CA: Wadsworth.

Cornelius, Gary. 2001. *The Art of the Con: Avoiding Offender Manipulation.* Alexandra VA: American Correctional Association.

Corrections Standards Authority. 2007. *Jail Profile Survey, 4th Quarter 2006*. Sacramento, CA: Author.

Durham, Alexis M. 1994. *Crisis and Reform: Current Issues in American Corrections.* Boston MA: Little, Brown and Company.

Durose, Matthew R. and Patrick A. Langan. 2004. *Felony Sentences in State Courts, 2002.* Washington DC: Bureau of Justice Statistics.

Freeze, Jennifer. 2006. "Scott County sees Decreased Inmate Medical Demand after Refusing to Pay." *Southeastern Missourian.* February 28, 2006.

Gibbons, John J. and Nicholas de B. Katzenbach. 2006. *Confronting Confinement: A*

Report of the Commission on Safety and Abuse in American Prisons. Retrieved June 9, 2006 (http://www.prisoncommission.org/report.asp).

Goldstein, Joe. 2005. *Health Care in Correctional Facilities Barriers to Humane and Adequate Care.* Testimony submitted to the Commission Safety and Abuse in America's Prisons, July 20, 2005.

Hanser, Robert D. 2007. *Special Needs Offenders in the Community.* Upper Saddle River, NJ: Pearson.

Hughes, Kristen A. 2006. *Justice Expenditure and Employment in the United States, 2003.* Washington, DC: Bureau of Justice Statistics.

In the News. 2006. "NYC Jails Stop Routine TB Skin Testing." *Correct Care* 20:10.

James, Doris J. and Lauren E. Glaze. 2006. *Mental Health Problems of Prison and Jail Inmates.* Washington, DC: Bureau of Justice Statistics.

Joint Committee on Health Education Terminology. 1991. "Report of the 1990 Joint Committee on Health Education Terminology." *Journal of Health Education* 22:97-108.

Kerle, Ken, Stan Stojkovic, Richard Kiekbusch and Joe Rowan.1999. "A Rejoinder to Vaughn and Smith's "Practicing Penal harm Medicine in the United States: Prisoner's Voices from Jail." *Justice Quarterly* 16:897-906.

Lamb, H. Richard, Linda E. Weinberger, and Walter J. DeCuir. 2002. "The Police and Mental Health." *Psychiatric Services* 53:1266-1271.

Latessa, Edward J., Francis T. Cullen, and Paul Gendreau. 2002. "Beyond Correctional Quackery - Professionalism and the Possibility of Effective Treatment." *Federal Probation* 66:43-59.

Lin, Ann Chih. 2000. Reform in the Making: The Implementation of Social Policy in Prison. Princeton, NJ: Princeton University Press.

MacDonald, Morag. 2005. A Study of the Health Care Provision, Existing Drug Services and Strategies Operating in Prisons in Ten Countries from Central and Eastern Europe. Helsinki, Finland: European Institute for Crime Prevention and Control.

MacKenzie, Doris L. 2006. *What Works in Corrections: Reducing the Criminal Activities of Offenders and Delinquents.* New York: Cambridge University Press.

Mumola, Christopher. 2007. *Medical Causes of Death in State Prisons, 2001-2003.* Washington, DC: Bureau of Justice Statistics.

Murphy, Daniel S. 2003. "Aspirin Ain't Gonna Help the Kind of Pain I'm In: Health Care in the Federal Bureau of Prisons." Pp. 247-266 in *Convict Criminology,* edited by J. I. Ross and S. C. Richards. Belmont CA: Wadsworth.

National Commission on Correctional Health Care. 2002. *Health Status Report on Soon-To-Be-Released Inmates.* Chicago, IL: Author.

Office of Justice Programs. (2007). *Reentry.* Retrieved April 19, 2007 from (http://www.ojp.usdoj.gov/reentry/learn.html).

Paoline, Eugene A., Eric G. Lambert and Nancy Lynne Hogan. 2006. "A Calm and Happy Keeper of the Keys: The Impact of ACA Views, Relations with Coworkers, and Policy Views on the Job Stress and Job Satisfaction of Correctional Staff." *The Prison Journal* 86: 182-205.

Parikh, Arit I., Michele T. Jay, Diamond Kassam, Terry Kociemba, Bobbe Dworkis, Pamela D. Bradley, and Kenneth Takata. 1997. "Clostridium Perfringens Outbreak at a Juvenile Detention Facility Linked to a Thanksgiving Holiday Meal." *Western Journal of Medicine* 166:417-419.

Porter, Janet. 2005. "Clearing the Air on Tobacco Use in Corrections." *Correct Care* 19:1, 22.

Puerini, Stephen and Michael Shelton. 2006. "When Requests for Comfort and Care Collide." *Correct Care* 20:1, 16.

Ruddell, Rick and G. Larry Mays. 2007. "Rural Jails: Problematic Inmates, Overcrowded Cells, and Cash-strapped Counties." *Journal of Criminal Justice* (35): 251-260.

Santos, Michael G. 2003. *About Prison.* Belmont, CA: Wadsworth.

Schlanger, Margo. 2003. "Inmate Litigation." *Harvard Law Review* 116:1555-1701.

Schwartz, Rachel D. 2006. "Pandemic Flu Preparedness and Response in Corrections Facilities." *Infectious Diseases in Corrections Report 9* (10): 1, 3-4.

Stana, Richard M. 2000. *Federal Prisons: Containing Health Care Costs for an Increasing Inmate Population.* Retrieved June 10, 2006 (http://www.gao.gov/archive/2000/gg00112t.pdf#search='Federal%20Prisons:%20Containing%20Health%20Care%20Costs%20stana').

Stanley, L.L. (1919). *Influenza at San Quentin Prison,* California. Retrieved May 8, 2007 (http://statelibrary.dcr.state.nc.us/iss/influenza/PDFfiles/USPHR050919.pdf).

Travis, Jeremy. 2005. "Prisoner Reentry: The Iron Law of Imprisonment." Pp. 64-71 in *Key Correctional Issues, edited by R. Muraskin.* Upper Saddle River, NJ: Pearson Prentice Hall.

Useem, Burt and Anne M. Piehl. 2006. "Prison Buildup and Disorder." *Punishment & Society* 8:87-115.

Vaughn, Michael S. and Linda G. Smith. 1999. "Practicing Penal Harm Medicine in the United States." *Justice Quarterly* 16:175-232.

Warren, Jennifer. 2006. "State Prisons Ordered to Pay Millions Owed to Doctors." *Los Angeles Times.* March 31, 2006

Cases Cited

Allen v. Hemingway
Austin v. PA Department of Corrections
Badea v. Moran
Bell v. Wolfish
Berry v. Lee
Board v. Farnham
Brad H. v. City of New York
Brownlee v. Conine
Chance v. Armstrong
Cooper v. Schriro
Creech v. Nguyen
Davis v. Norris
Dellier v. Williams
Estelle v. Gamble
Farmer v. Brennan
Farrow v. West
Foster v. Hori
Hallett v. Morgan,
Harris v. Hegmann
Helling v. McKinney
Hoptowit v. Ray
Hunt v. Dental Department
James v. O'Sullivan
Kinney v. Kalfus
Laube v. Campbell
Lopez v. Smith
Mallette v. Dunning
Minniecheske v. Gudmanson
Mitchell v. Duckworth
Mt. Healthy City School District Board of Education v. Doyle
Murphy v. Bray
Penrod v. Zavaras
Plata v. Schwarzenegger
Poirier v. Casperson
Rhodes v. Chapman
Shepherd v. Malan
Taylor v. Christain
Trop v. Dulles
Wagner v. United States
Wellman v. Faulkner
Wilkins v. Correctional Medical System
Wilson v. Wilkinson
Wynn v. Southward

Subject Index

Breinigsville, PA USA
08 January 2010
230415BV00004B/128/P

9 780979 645501